Health Program Planning, Implementation, *and* Evaluation

·

Creating Behavioral, Environmental, and Policy Change

Edited by

Lawrence W. Green · Andrea Carlson Gielen · Judith M. Ottoson
Darleen V. Peterson · Marshall W. Kreuter

Foreword by

Jonathan E. Fielding

JOHNS HOPKINS UNIVERSITY PRESS
Baltimore

Johns Hopkins University Press
2715 North Charles Street
Baltimore, Maryland 21218-4363
www.press.jhu.edu

Library of Congress Cataloging-in-Publication Data

Names: Green, Lawrence W., editor. | Gielen, A. C. (Andrea Carlson),
    editor. | Ottoson, Judith M., editor | Peterson, Darleen V., editor.
    | Kreuter, Marshall W., editor.
Title: Health program planning, implementation, and evaluation : creating
    behavioral, environmental, and policy change / edited by Lawrence W.
    Green, Andrea Carlson Gielen, Judith M. Ottoson, Darleen V. Peterson,
    Marshall W. Kreuter ; foreword by Jonathan E. Fielding.
Description: Baltimore : Johns Hopkins University Press, 2022. | Includes
    bibliographical references and index.
Identifiers: LCCN 2021017905 | ISBN 9781421442969 (paperback ; alk. paper)
    | ISBN 9781421442976 (ebook)
Subjects: MESH: Community Health Planning—organization & administration
    | Health Promotion—organization & administration | Models, Organizational
    | Program Evaluation | Health Policy
Classification: LCC RA427 | NLM WA 546.1 | DDC 362.12—dc23
LC record available at https://lccn.loc.gov/2021017905

*Special discounts are available for bulk purchases of this book. For more information,
please contact Special Sales at specialsales@jh.edu.*

This book is dedicated to the talented public health professionals who will plan, implement, and evaluate the programs and policies that protect and promote the health of everyone; and to the people in communities throughout the country and the world who will engage in and benefit from their good work. In that spirit, the authors dedicate this text also to those who, through up and down times, are so supportive of our work and give us hope for the future . . .

Beth, Doug, Madeleine, and Chloe; Jennifer, César, Gabriel, and Teresa (LWG and JMO)

Price; Ryan, Katy, Robin, and River; Matthew, Brittany, Huck, and Grey (ACG)

Joel (DVP)

Martha; Matthew, Charlene, and Cal, Will; Ellen, Nalin, Sam, and Oscar (MWK)

Contents

Part I. Hallmarks of the PRECEDE-PROCEED Model

Part II. PRECEDE-PROCEED Phases: Planning, Implementation, and Evaluation

Foreword

Health Promotion Planning, Implementation and Evaluation: Creating Behavioral, Environmental and Policy Change. While that title is precise, the authors have found a way to help practitioners, researchers, and policy makers alike address the subtle complexities inherent in effective planning, implementation, and evaluation to promote community and population health.

We live in an era of short social media texts as the preferred mode of interpersonal communications. Accordingly, this foreword is brief.

For more than 40 years, the PRECEDE-PROCEED model has been effectively applied throughout the world to address a broad range of health issues: risk factors like tobacco and lack of exercise; social determinants of health such as lack of access to transportation and safe housing; major disease challenges like heart disease and guinea worm disease; and holistic health outcomes as well. This volume aligns with the enormous and rapid changes in conceptions of the boundaries of disease prevention and health promotion. It also incorporates the range of available tools to facilitate progress in these domains.

Contributors to this volume have broadened the perspective from personal and proximal "risk factors" to "distal social health determinants." They expand the boundaries of health promotion planning by emphasizing ecologic assessments and multisectoral contributions to population health. The framework is practical and flexible, creates intervention approaches using the best evidence from research and practice, and incorporates rapid changes in availability and use of population data. It also emphasizes economic impact and provides a thoughtful integration of planning, implementation, and evaluation. This volume also recognizes new approaches to communication and fresh methods for reaching both communities and individuals.

Editors Larry Green and Marshall Kreuter, internationally acclaimed experts in public health improvement, wrote four previous volumes over the past four decades. Three new, talented coeditors and public health leaders, Andrea Carlson Gielen, Judith Ottoson and Darleen Peterson, add contemporary experience with the model and its applications in research, policy, practice, and evaluation (including accreditation of public health degree programs). They are joined in this new endeavor by 18 chapter coauthors, who bring both their academic expertise and experience in the field. The result is a rich set of perspectives, both domestic and global, on the broad and widely applied utility of the PRECEDE-PROCEED model for program planning, implementation, and evaluation of policies and programs.

This text will be widely used in MPH, advanced undergraduate, and other graduate courses as well as by governmental, not-for-profit, and private organizations. Experience with the model is documented in over 1,200 published articles. These citations and other supportive materials are found at http://www.lgreen.net.

Simply put, *Health Program Planning, Implementation and Evaluation: Creating Behavioral, Environmental and Policy Change* is an up-to-date powerhouse for global health promotion at all levels.

Jonathan E. Fielding, MD, MPH, MBA
Distinguished Professor of Health Policy and Management
Distinguished Professor of Pediatrics
UCLA Schools of Public Health and Medicine

Preface

Those entering the public health workforce face the challenges and opportunities posed by a complex array of contemporary health issues: global warming; infectious diseases such as COVID-19, Ebola, HIV, and the Zika virus; the continuing growth of opioid, vaping, and mass shooting epidemics; chronic diseases such as heart disease, diabetes, and cancer; and behavioral health conditions. The principles and practices of public health program planning, implementation, and evaluation to control these public health challenges (at the individual, community, state, national, and international levels) constitute the focus of this book.

This version of the PRECEDE-PROCEED model highlights the practical insights gained from more than four decades of applying the model, as it has been tailored to address numerous health problems endemic in a wide range of settings, populations, and circumstances. The more than 1,200 publications of field-tested PRECEDE-PROCEED applications around the world (see the searchable bibliography with links at http://www.lgreen.net) demonstrate both the utility and benefits of using the model to plan, implement, and evaluate public health policies and programs. The cross-cultural value of the model is reflected in the translations of previous versions of the book, in whole or in part, into Chinese, Japanese, Portuguese, French, and other languages.

To ensure that the content of this textbook addresses the global health challenges of the 21st century in a way that is accessible to students and faculty, Green and Kreuter recruited three talented and widely experienced colleagues to be coeditors:

- Andrea Carlson Gielen (professor of health, behavior and society and former director of the Johns Hopkins Center for Injury Research and Policy, Johns Hopkins Bloomberg School of Public Health)
- Judith M. Ottoson (retired, San Francisco State University and former associate professor, Andrew Young School of Policy Studies, Georgia State University and the University of British Columbia)
- Darleen V. Peterson (professor and the director of certificate, MPH, and DrPH programs at the School of Community and Global Health, Claremont Graduate University, where she is the associate dean for academic affairs)

These three distinguished scholars bring extensive public health practice, teaching, research, publishing, and consulting experience. In addition, as highlighted in the acknowledgments, 18 eminent public health scholars are chapter coauthors.

The hallmarks of the PRECEDE-PROCEED model (described in chapter 1) are its flexibility, evaluability, community participation, and its process for using and adapting evidence-based practices and practice-based evidence. The model's approach is consistent with calls for the future of public health to use multisectoral strategies (DeSalvo et al. 2017), build "a Culture of Health" (Chandra et al. 2016), and address the leading causes of disease and disability, including their underlying causes in health disparities and health equity. The Coronavirus Response Coordinator for the White House Coronavirus Task Force noted on March 31, 2020, that "there is no magic bullet, no magic vaccine or therapy. It's just behaviors."* As this book goes to press, efforts to address the COVID-19 pandemic have benefited from the kinds of planning approaches offered by the model. As effective treatments, behavioral strategies, and vaccines continue to emerge, the strategies outlined in this book will be needed to ensure that effective prevention and control strategies are adapted and implemented in all communities, especially communities of color and low-income neighborhoods. Allegrante, Auld, and Natarajan (2020) described how COVID-19 can best be addressed through the application of behavioral sciences and ecological thinking. The PRECEDE-PROCEED model is ideally suited to structure and guide such applications because it facilitates the development of multilevel interventions that are informed by theory, evidence, and community participation.

ORGANIZATION OF THE BOOK

The first chapter offers the core principles the PRECEDE-PROCEED model uses for program planning, implementation, and evaluation. Chapter 2 addresses participation and community engagement. Chapters 3–9 sequentially describe the model's core elements: **Social Assessment**, including quality of life; **Epidemiological Assessment**, including population health assessment and behavioral and environmental factors; **Educational and Ecological Assessment**, including identification of the most important and most changeable factors influencing change; and **Health Program and Policy Development**, including strategies for **intervention**, **implementation**, and **evaluation** that strategically build from the prior assessments.

Chapters 10–13 provide in-depth descriptions and evidence-based analyses of **Applications** of the PRECEDE-PROCEED model in different settings: **Community**, **Occupational**, **School**, and **Health Care Settings**. Chapter 14 addresses

---

*Deborah Birx. "There is no magic bullet, no magic vaccine or therapy. It is just behaviors." C-SPAN; 31 March 2020.

innovative approaches to applications of the model using new **Communication Technologies**.

To assist faculty and students, we have included an Appendix A, which provides a compilation of **Frequently Asked Questions** based on years of teaching the PRECEDE-PROCEED model. Brief answers are provided, along with where to find a more detailed discussion of the issue within the chapters. Faculty and students may find this a helpful resource as they learn about and apply the model. Additional teaching and learning resources will be found online at http://www .lgreen.net and on the Johns Hopkins University Press website.

The Council on Education for Public Health (CEPH)—the independent agency recognized by the US Department of Education to accredit schools of public health and public health programs—has revised its criteria to include a set of required foundational competencies for each level (bachelor's, master's, and doctoral). All graduates from accredited programs must demonstrate attainment of the new CEPH competencies. Thus, schools must indicate how their curricula address them and identify at least one specific, required assessment activity for each competency. This volume has been brought into conformity with these changes. Appendix B provides a table that outlines, by chapter, which **Public Health Competencies** are addressed and can be incorporated into readings, activities, assignments, and assessments for students as they progress in their respective health degrees.

In addition, because the National Board of Public Health Examiners (NBPHE) has been certifying graduates of CEPH-accredited programs since 2008, this volume addresses the 10 domain areas contained in the latest NBPHE 2017 content revision, which were also covered in the 2019 Certified Public Health (CPH) examination. This volume is included as a study guide resource in the Association of Schools and Programs in Public Health (ASPPH) study guide to prepare current students and graduates of CEPH-accredited programs for the new CPH examination. We believe these additions are particularly relevant given the ever-evolving landscape of public health professional preparation and credentialing.

The editors are most appreciative of the practitioners, researchers, teachers, and authors whose work has contributed to the development, evaluation, and evolution of the PRECEDE-PROCEED model. We are equally grateful to the thousands of students who have also contributed to advancing the model through their active participation in learning about it and sharing their insightful questions. The collective wisdom from all of these parties and experiences has provided the true foundation of this book.

References

Allegrante, J., Auld, M.E., & Natarajan, S. (2020). Preventing COVID-19 and its Sequela: "There's no magic bullet . . . It's just behaviors." *American Journal of Preventive Medicine, 59*(2), 288–92. https://doi.org/10.1016/j.amepre.2020.05.004

Chandra, A., Miller, C.E., Acosta, J.D., et al. (2016). Drivers of health as a shared value: Mindset, expectations, sense of community, and civic engagement. *Health Affairs, 35*(11), 1959–63. https://doi.org/10.1377/hlthaff.2016.0603

DeSalvo, K.B., Wang, Y.C., Harris, A., et al. (2017). A call to action of public health to meet the challenges of the 21st Century. *Preventing Chronic Disease, 14*, E78. http://dx.doi.org /10.5888/pcd14.170017

Acknowledgments

The model presented in this text is the product of four decades of the cumulative experience of the authors and our colleagues in practice, research, policy and program planning, implementation, and evaluation applied in both public health service and academic settings. At the outset, the PRECEDE portion of the model included key elements of:

- Ronald Andersen's Behavioral Model of Families' Use of Health Services;
- Albert Bandura's Social Learning Theory;
- Godfrey Hochbaum and Irwin Rosenstock's Health Belief Model;
- J. Mayone Stycos's decision model on couples' adoption of family planning methods;
- Kurt Lewin's force-field analysis; and
- methods and strategies in community-based participatory research.

The PROCEED portion of the model was further influenced by key aspects of:
- the Health Field Concept of Laframboise;
- the Lalonde Report for Health Canada;
- the Ottawa Charter of WHO; and
- the collective experiences of our global colleagues.

Our thoughts about implementation were also influenced by our experience in the US initiative in disease prevention and health promotion, particularly *Healthy People: Objectives for the Nation*. Our focus on implementation issues was greatly influenced by the work of a host of colleagues, both academic scholars and practitioners who have implemented the model in settings throughout the world. To date, the PRECEDE-PROCEED Model has been globally applied in more than 1,200 published applications.

After 40 years of applying this model globally, it has been our pleasure to create this volume in partnership with a team of outstanding scholars and practitioners who have brought the latest science and practical experience to their chapters. Accordingly, we gratefully acknowledge the insightful chapter contributions of Amelie Ramirez, Cam Escoffery, Chris Lovato, Gerjo Kok, Guy Parcel, Faten Ben Abdelaziz, Holly Hunt, Janey C. Peterson, John P. Allegrante, Lloyd J. Kolbe, María E. Fernández, Michelle Kegler, Nico Pronk, Patricia Chalela, Paul Terry, Robert S. Gold, Rodney Lyn, and Shelley Golden.

To all of these scholars and our other students, colleagues, and mentors whom we have recognized in the four previous volumes, we offer our appreciation and gratitude for their feedback on the model and its applications.

Finally, this volume has been made more readable and interpretable by the experienced editorial hand of Nicole Lezin and the talented graphics skills of Violet Anna Lieby in converting hand-drawn and dated software versions of many of the graphics and figures. We are also especially grateful for the graphic and administrative skills and good cheer of Jolanda Lisath and to Bree Hemingway, to Alice Rhoades for her reviews with a student's eye on proposed content and reference organization, and to Virginia Young for her help on the glossary. We appreciate the technical and administrative support of Keegan Edgar and Edith Jones from the Johns Hopkins Bloomberg School of Public Health. We offer our appreciation to Joel L.A. Peterson, managing partner of Pintoresco Advisors LLC, for project management consultation. Finally, we thank our families for their support, encouragement, and patience during the preparation of this volume.

Yes, it takes a village.

About the Editors

Andrea Carlson Gielen is professor of health, behavior and society and former director of the Johns Hopkins Center for Injury Research and Policy at the Johns Hopkins Bloomberg School of Public Health, where she taught program planning for health behavior change for three decades, teaching hundreds of graduate students across multiple platforms including in person, online, and in compressed formats. Dr. Gielen has led numerous federally funded studies and intervention trials. Her research focuses on developing, implementing, and evaluating theory-based health promotion programs and campaigns addressing a wide array of public health issues, such as HIV/AIDS, smoking in pregnancy, domestic violence, and the prevention of injuries caused by fires, burns, falls, poisoning, and motor vehicles. Intervention strategies that Dr. Gielen utilizes include community mobilization, computer-tailored and m-Health communication, social marketing, and the creation of innovative safety resource centers for deployment in hospital and community settings. Prior to joining the faculty at Johns Hopkins, Dr. Gielen served as a community health educator for the Maryland Department of Health, where she worked to create the state's first child passenger safety program. Dr. Gielen received her ScM and ScD degrees from the Johns Hopkins Bloomberg School of Public Health.

As professor emeritus of epidemiology and biostatistics at the University of California at San Francisco, **Lawrence W. Green** has capped a turnstile career in public health, rotating between previous positions in program development, policy, and evaluation, and full-time academic positions at the University of California School of Public Health at Berkeley (where he also received his three degrees), the Johns Hopkins Bloomberg School of Public Health, Harvard University School of Public Health and Center for Health Policy Research, and as founding director of the University of Texas Center for Health Promotion Research and Development at Houston. In the 1990s, he was at the University of British Columbia as professor and director of the Center for Health Promotion Research and the Division of Preventive Medicine and Health Promotion in the Department of Health Care and Epidemiology. His professional rotations between these academic appointments were in policy and program planning, management, and evaluation, with a Ford Foundation project in family planning in Bangladesh, later with the US Department of Health and Human Services as director of the federal Office of Health Information and Health Promotion in the Office of the Assistant Secretary of Health, in the late 1980s as vice-president of the Kaiser Family Foundation, and in the early 2000s as distinguished scientist and founding co-director of the CDC-WHO Collaborating Center of Global

Tobacco Control and as acting director of the CDC Office of Smoking and Health, then as director of the CDC Office of Science and Extramural Research.

Marshall W. Kreuter, a retired professor of public health at Georgia State University, has extensive experience in the engagement of communities in the planning, implementation, and evaluation of public health programs. Prior to that, he was a distinguished scientist at the Centers for Disease Control and Prevention (CDC) where, for two decades, he served in several key leadership roles: as the director of the Division of Health Education, as the first director of the Division of Chronic Disease Control and Community Intervention, and as director of the Prevention Research Centers program. While at the CDC, he and his co-workers refined the epidemiologic study of physical activity, initiated research and programs focused on the early detection of breast cancer, and added a greater emphasis on school health. He and his CDC colleagues used the PRECEDE-PROCEED model to create the Planned Approach to Community Health Program (PATCH) at the state and local level; they also used the model to develop an intervention strategy that has led to the near-eradication of Guinea worm disease in Africa. He received his academic training at California State University at Chico and the University of Utah. He did his postdoctoral fellowship at Johns Hopkins University and held full professorships at the University of Utah and Georgia State University.

Judith M. Ottoson retired as an associate professor from the Andrew Young School of Policy Studies, Georgia State University. Previous to retirement, she served also as an associate professor on the Faculty of Education, University of British Columbia; subsequent to her retirement, she served as adjunct faculty in the Department of Health Education, San Francisco State University. Her educational preparation includes a BSN from the University of Minnesota; an MPH specializing in public health education from the University of Hawaii; and an EdD from Harvard University with a concentration on administration, planning and social policy. Dr. Ottoson had over 20 years of diverse practical experience as an administrator, consultant, educator, and evaluator before pursuing an academic career that spanned more than two decades. Her practice-infused teaching, research, and publications used program evaluation to focus on whether and how programs and policy make a difference and the implementation factors that influence those outcomes. She has consulted with various academic institutions, governmental agencies, private organizations, foundations, and voluntary agencies on the design, implementation, and evaluation of programs. She has taught or consulted internationally, including in Africa, Brazil, China, and Europe. Dr. Ottoson reluctantly (and productively) came out of retirement to work with her colleagues on this volume to contribute to its theoretical and practical understandings of planning, implementation, and evaluation in health programs and policies.

Darleen V. Peterson is a professor of community and global health at Claremont Graduate University (CGU). She also serves as the school's associate dean for academic affairs and is the founding and current director of the master of public health (MPH) and doctor of public health (DrPH) programs. She also serves as co-director of the positive health psychology program in the School of Social Science, Policy and Evaluation. Prior to joining the faculty at CGU, she served as an assistant professor of clinical preventive medicine at the University of Southern California (USC), where she was the assistant director of the MPH program. She has taught graduate courses in health behavior theory and health communications and supervised field training in public health. Her research interests include health communication, specifically the evaluation of statewide tobacco control campaigns and the assessment of pro-tobacco marketing activities on youth smoking. She currently provides consultation on public health program accreditation to new and existing programs. She received an MA in communications management from USC's Annenberg School for Communication, an MPH in community health education from California State University, Northridge, and a PhD in preventive medicine (health behavior research) from the Keck School of Medicine of USC. She is a masters-level certified health education specialist (MCHES).

Contributors

Faten Ben Abdelaziz, PhD
Coordinator of Health Promotion,
  Department for the Prevention of
  Noncommunicable Diseases
World Health Organization
Geneva, Switzerland

John P. Allegrante, PhD
Professor, Department of Health and
  Behavior Studies
Teachers College, Columbia University
Adjunct Professor, Department of
  Sociomedical Sciences
Columbia University Mailman School
  of Public Health
New York, New York, USA

Patricia Chalela, DrPH
Associate Professor, Department of
  Epidemiology and Biostatistics
The Institute for Health Promotion
  Research
The University of Texas Health Science
  Center at San Antonio, School of
  Public Health
San Antonio, Texas, USA

Cam Escoffery, PhD, MPH, CHES
Associate Professor, Department of
  Behavioral Sciences and Health
  Education
Rollins School of Public Health at
  Emory University
Atlanta, Georgia, USA

María E. Fernández, PhD
Professor and Director, Center for Health
  Promotion and Prevention Research
University of Texas Health Science Center
  at Houston, School of Public Health
Houston, Texas, USA

Robert S. Gold, PhD DrPH
Professor, Department of Behavioral and
  Community Health and Medicine
Co-Director, University of Maryland
  College Park Center of Excellence for
  Health Information Technology
  Research
University of Maryland School of Public
  Health
College Park, Maryland, USA

Shelly Golden, PhD
Assistant Professor, Department of Health
  Behavior
University of North Carolina, Gillings
  School of Global Public Health
Chapel Hill, North Carolina, USA

Holly Hunt, MA
Chief, School Health Branch
National Center for Chronic Disease
  Prevention and Health Promotion
US Centers for Disease Control and
  Prevention
Atlanta, Georgia, USA

Vanya C. Jones, PhD, MPH
Associate Professor
Department of Health, Behavior and
  Society
Johns Hopkins Bloomberg School of
  Public Health
Baltimore, Maryland, USA

Michelle C. Kegler, DrPH, MPH
Professor, Department of Behavioral
  Sciences and Health Education
Rollins School of Public Health at Emory
  University
Atlanta, Georgia, USA

Gerjo Kok, PhD, MSc
Professor, Department of Work and Social
 Psychology
Maastricht University
Maastricht Area, Netherlands

Lloyd J. Kolbe, PhD
Emeritus Professor, Department of Applied
 Health Science
Indiana University School of Public
 Health–Bloomington
Bloomington, Indiana, USA

Chris Y. Lovato, PhD
Professor and Co-Director, Department of
 Health Care and Epidemiology
University of British Columbia, School of
 Population and Public Health
Vancouver, British Columbia, Canada

Rodney Lyn, PhD, MS
Associate Professor and Associate Dean
 for Academic Affairs
Interim Director, Division of Health
 Management and Policy
Georgia State University School of Public
 Health
Atlanta, Georgia, USA

Guy S. Parcel, PhD, MS
Professor and Dean Emeritus, Division
 of Health Promotion and Behavioral
 Science
The University of Texas Health Science
 Center at Houston School of Public
 Health
Houston, Texas, USA

Janey C. Peterson, EdD, MS, RN
Associate Professor, Department of
 Medicine
Weill Cornell Medicine
New York, New York, USA

Nico Pronk, PhD, MA, FACSM, FAWHP
Chief Science Officer, HealthPartners
 Institute for Medical Education
Bloomington, Minnesota
Adjunct Professor, Department of Social
 and Behavioral Sciences
Harvard T.H. Chan School of Public Health
Boston, Massachusetts, USA

Amelie G. Ramirez, DrPH
Professor and Chair ad interim, Department
 of Epidemiology and Biostatistics
Institute for Health Promotion Research
The University of Texas Health Science
 Center at San Antonio, School of Public
 Health
San Antonio, Texas, USA

Paul E. Terry, PhD
President and CEO, Health Enhancement
 Research Organization (HERO)
Editor in Chief, *American Journal of Health
 Promotion*
Edina, Minnesota, USA

PART I

Hallmarks of the PRECEDE-PROCEED Model

A Model for Population Health Planning, Implementation, and Evaluation

•

Lawrence W. Green, Andrea Carlson Gielen, Marshall W. Kreuter, Darleen V. Peterson, and Judith M. Ottoson

Learning Objectives

After completing the chapter, the reader will be able to:

- Explain three key perspectives on the PRECEDE-PROCEED model's application in research and practice.
- Describe the importance of combining evidence-based practice and practice-based evidence for health promotion program planning.
- Explain the hallmarks of the PRECEDE-PROCEED model's applications over the past five decades.

If you're depressed by the state of the world, let me toss out an idea: In the long arc of human history, 2019 has been the best year ever.

The bad things that you fret about are true. But it's also true that since modern humans emerged about 200,000 years ago, 2019 was probably the year in which children were least likely to die, adults were least likely to be illiterate and people were least likely to suffer excruciating and disfiguring diseases.

—Nicholas Kristof, opinion columnist, *The New York Times* (2019)

On the other hand, a Swedish youth challenged the true but optimistic reflection of these trends as she faced the future of global warming for her generation:

People are suffering, people are dying, entire ecosystems are collapsing. We are at the beginning of a mass extinction.

—Greta Thunberg, climate change activist (2019)

Kristof's reminder to acknowledge the progress we have made is an important one; so is Thunberg's reminder that we have not done enough. We should recognize progress, but we also need to understand the trajectory of that progress, and dips in it, such as COVID-19. What worked to address these needs? Why and how? Which actions should we take in the future to yield even more progress? Which policies should we devise or tweak? These are the questions that inspire—and sometimes vex—planners and practitioners of population health programs. They are also the questions at the heart of the PRECEDE-PROCEED model.

Actions and policies for population health have their justification in the felt needs of populations. These, in turn, are based on the accumulation of evidence-based practices derived from research and on practice-based evidence derived from evaluations in the field (Fielding and Teutsch 2013). Failing to identify and quantify those needs, or losing sight of the goals for meeting them, can lead programs into problems or failures that might have been avoided. By applying the steps in the PRECEDE-PROCEED model, planners and practitioners can benefit from the experience of thousands of their counterparts over the past five decades and avoid some common pitfalls.

We begin this chapter with a clarification of three perspectives that you will find emphasized throughout the book. Health programs (1) are *problem*-based and *population*-focused, (2) use an ecological and educational approach to maximize potential impact, and (3) respect the settings, cultures, and contexts of their audiences. This chapter concludes with an introductory walk through the steps of the PRECEDE-PROCEED process for health program **planning**, **implementation**, and **evaluation**,* along with a discussion of some of the hallmarks of the process and the product that emerges.

The application of PRECEDE (and later the PRECEDE-PROCEED model) has been used in more than 1,200 published works around the world. Of these, hundreds were rigorously evaluated field trials that used the model to plan, implement, and evaluate a range of programs in communities, schools, health care settings, or workplaces. (Some of those studies and programs are cited in the notes at the end of chapters[1] highlighted in the relevant chapters of this text, and found in a frequently updated and searchable bibliography at http://www.lgreen.net.)

These field trials and programs have gradually accumulated examples covering a range of health issues, populations, and community settings around the world, yielding a rich inventory of applications with practical, real-world impact. Two of these applications are the global eradication of smallpox (Fenner 1982) and of dracunculiasis (*Guinea Worm Disease* 2019). The latter, commonly known as Guinea worm disease, is caused when elongated worms invade human and

---

***Boldface** words are defined in the glossary.

other hosts. It was most dominant in poor areas of the world. No vaccine to prevent it or medicine to cure it was available. In the mid-1980s, it was estimated that 3.5 million people a year in 21 countries in Africa and Asia were afflicted with the disease. Today, thanks to the global collaborative work by the Carter Center and its partners, including the US Centers for Disease Control and Prevention (CDC), the Peace Corps, and the affected countries themselves, the **incidence** of Guinea worm is so low that the disease is considered near eradication. By the end of 2018, it had been reduced by 99% to 28 cases—that is, from millions of cases to a few dozen! The implementation of key components of the PRECEDE-PROCEED model served as the basis for tailored community-based programs, including health education strategies documented to have been a core component leading to the near-global eradication of that disease (box 1.1).

BOX 1.1

Case Example: The Impact of Health Education on Guinea Worm Disease

In the late 1980s, an estimated 3.5 million Guinea worm cases occurred annually in Africa and Asia. Most of the victims were poor and lacked access to safe water. Then and now, neither drugs to treat the disease nor a vaccine to prevent infection were available. It was a major health problem not only because of its global impact, but also because

- there was no way to treat the limited water sources people needed;
- adult victims were unable to work nor were they able to provide much-needed family support; and
- children in endemic areas missed 25% of the school year.

Given these realities, Drs. Don Hopkins and Ernesto Ruiz-Tiben, leaders of the World Health Organization (WHO) Collaborating Center for Research, Training and Eradication of Dracunculiasis at CDC, secured funding from the United Nations to develop health education and community development guidelines that could be applied across endemic communities in Africa and Asia.

The purpose of the guidelines was to promote community mobilization targeted to implement specific, measurable, health education strategies designed to prevent the onset of Guinea worm disease across all at-risk communities. A committee of 17 international health education and public health scientists and practitioners was convened in Atlanta to develop the guidelines, which can be found here: https://www.ncbi.nlm.nih.gov/pmc/articles/PMC6090361/.

The guidelines were grounded in the key elements of behavioral and community change theories, including the PRECEDE model, and were designed to give local practitioners and leaders practical and culturally appropriate action steps to:

(continued)

- Engage community leaders and residents in community participation;
- Help those leaders and residents plan and implement specific prevention actions (e.g., obtaining and using water filters properly, discarding damaged filters, protecting existing water supplies);
- Assess and measure the extent to which those actions were implemented and linked to a reduction in the incidence of Guinea worm disease.

As of 2018, based on the implementation of the health education strategies delineated in the guidelines, the countries of Pakistan, Senegal, India, and Yemen were free of Guinea worm disease. At that time, the disease had been reduced worldwide by *99%—from over 3.5 million cases to 28 human cases.* In 2019, 1,102 animal cases were reported. Of those cases, 1,069 were in dogs, 32 in cats and one in a baboon (Lancet 2019). Since the eradication of Guinea worm disease is hampered by having a reservoir of the disease in animals, the WHO has moved the eradication target date from 2020 to 2030 (Roberts 2019).

Evaluation studies assessing the impact of Guinea worm eradication efforts consistently provide ***practice-based evidence*** and conclude that planned health education strategies, tailored to the cultural needs and realities of specific communities, constitute a major factor in the reduction to the near-eradication of this disease. In reviewing the accomplishments of the Guinea worm eradication program detailed in box 1.1, Donald Hopkins, MD, MPH, director of the program, indicated: "One of the most important lessons has been the potential power of health education. Before, it was thought you could only have an effective eradication program by using a vaccine, as with smallpox and polio. Guinea worm eradication is proving that health education can be as valuable as vaccine for some diseases that cannot be prevented through medical intervention" (Hopkins, pers. comm., Sept. 2018).

The extensive applications of the PRECEDE-PROCEED model's planning, implementation and evaluation components, as in the Guinea worm example, have served as the primary means for refining the model. The applications also have helped us identify the characteristics of the model that have made it particularly useful. Building programs using the model produces ***practice-based evidence***. Practice-based evidence is a crucial complement of the ***evidence-based practices*** from research studies that are also key, but often limited in generalizability to settings, populations, and circumstances where new or adapted programs are often urgently needed.[2]

KEY CONCEPTS IN THE PRECEDE-PROCEED MODEL

A "Population Health" Perspective on Program Planning

The word *program* has several meanings. In the world of technology, a computer program is a language of codes that guide and enable a computer to interpret and organize fragments of information. At the theater, a program tells the audience about the sequence of events that will occur during the performance. The notions of guidance, organization, and direction are also evident when we define a **health program** as *a set of planned and organized activities carried out over time to accomplish specific health-related goals and objectives*. This simple definition of *program* serves as a compass that reminds us to keep our planning energies focused on a specific destination: health and quality-of-life improvement. Like some journeys, however, those we take in pursuit of population health will bring us complex challenges. The principles and strategies described in this book are designed to give planners the tools they need to (1) anticipate those challenges, and (2) prevent or resolve them successfully. When fully utilized, these tools maximize the likelihood of program success.

The *scope* of a program refers here to the full range of intervention components (i.e., planned activities) that need to be implemented to bring about the intended changes in health and social outcomes. These components often include changing broader community, school, worksite, and clinical programs and policies. *Population health* program planning seeks to improve the health and quality of life among groups identified by the places where they live, work, go to school, or seek health services. This **settings approach** is more than merely identifying people by venue so they can be reached more effectively. It recognizes that settings help determine the conditions for health-related behavior and support. If asked to portray our traditional view of health visually, a photographer or artist would likely provide a close-up of a patient being treated or diagnosed by a physician for a disease or symptom. To get a population and social perspective of health, that photographer would have to change the lens, step back, and take a wider shot. This broader perspective would take us beyond the clinical, one-on-one aspect of acute health care. It would enable us to view the connections that people have with specific aspects of both their physical and social **environments**. An emphasis on population health in no way disparages the importance of the health care of individuals, as illustrated in chapter 13 on health care settings. Programs addressing both individual care and population health are needed to achieve improvements in public health, and both need to be viewed as complementary and essential components of public health and health care systems.

An Ecological and Educational Approach to Program Planning

Ecology is typically defined as the study of the relationships among organisms and with their environments. The key to that simple definition is the phrase *study of relationships*. Health status and quality of life are most influenced by a combination of our genetic predispositions, the actions we take or do not take as individuals and groups, and numerous social-environmental factors often referred to as *social determinants* of health (Berkman and Kawachi 2000; Green et al. 2015; Green and Allegrante 2011; Kahan et al. 2014; Last and McGinnis 2003; Marmot 2000; Marmot and Wilkinson 1999; Wallerstein et al. 2018). Social determinants include history and culture, including structural racism and other forms of systematic oppression; the levels, quality, and distribution of employment, income, and education; housing quality and opportunity; the availability, quality, and cost of health insurance; and the safety of neighborhoods.

The ecological approach to health program planning (box 1.2) recognizes that any serious effort to improve a population's health status and quality of life must take into account the powerful role played by the surrounding ecosystem and its **subsystems** (such as family, friendships, organizations, community, culture, and physical environment) (Golden et al. 2015; Wold and Samdal 2012). The **health care system** and the **public health system**, for example, are subsystems within the broader **system** that influences health. The health system, in turn, is part of its own broader ecosystem consisting of other sectors, such as the sectors responsible for the social determinants mentioned above (e.g., the educational system). These aspects of community and society are highly relevant to health, even though they are not designed for, or directed primarily at, health. Today's practitioners, however, will see some forward-thinking municipalities assess potential health impacts when they consider changing their transportation, housing, and other systems. This trend offers new partnership opportunities for health program planners as they consider how to address the impact of larger social structures and systems on the health and well-being of their communities.

It is not surprising that community health and public health textbooks often make ecology one of the four or five scientific foundations on which they build the community or population approach to health analysis and planning (IOM 2003a; IOM 2003b). Ecological approaches, however, have proved difficult to evaluate because the units of analysis do not lend themselves to the random assignment, experimental control, and manipulation characteristic of preferred scientific approaches to establishing causation. The linear, isolatable, cause-effect model of scientific problem-solving remains the point of departure for the training of health professionals and practitioners. Today's health program planners cannot ignore the contextual reality that a population's health status is influenced by a complex ecological system.

BOX 1.2
A Historical Note on the Ecological Perspective

The **ecological perspective** in the context of health is not new. In 1848, Rudolf Virchow, the father of modern pathology, identified socioeconomic factors such as poverty as key elements affecting disease, disability, and premature death (Ackerknecht 1953; Green et al. 1996). Florence Nightingale, the mother of professional nursing during the same era, drew what would now be seen as epidemiological maps to associate patterns of patients' illnesses with their social conditions of living, and later in that century promoted home visiting by "health nurses" to complement the work of "sick nurses." From their earliest formulations and applications, the methods of public health and related disciplines embraced ecological concepts (IOM 2003a; 2003b). They were influenced by the 19th-century development of biological, especially Darwinian, concepts of the "web of life" and the role of the environment and adaptation in the origin and survival of species.

John Snow's basis for removing London's Broad Street pump handle in 1854 to prevent people from using cholera-contaminated water is heralded as the first classic epidemiological study. By mapping the sources of drinking water among those who died of cholera, Snow demonstrated that his ecological analysis of the problem gave him the insight he needed to develop an effective intervention 30 years before Koch isolated the cholera organism.

In developed countries, epidemiology remained almost exclusively preoccupied with the physical, chemical, and biological environments until the 1960s, when it became evident that non-communicable diseases and injuries were replacing communicable diseases as the leading causes of death, disability, and impaired quality of life. Studying the causes of non-communicable or chronic diseases revealed even more of the complex ecosystems in which our daily lives and health outcomes are embedded. Like the photographer stepping back for a wider angle, health ecosystems reveal more and more factors affecting health.

The ecological systems around us, like global warming, are constantly, usually imperceptibly, changing. To address those systems in our planning, we must first be able to *see* them. For some simple examples of how rather subtle changes in ecological systems trigger events that influence health and quality of life, see table 1.1.

By definition, ecological subsystems do not operate in isolation from one another; they overlap, connect with, and constantly influence each other. Therefore, the patterns illustrated in table 1.1 present only part of the picture. The other part is more complex. It pertains to how the ecological subsystems interact with each other to influence health. Suppose we constructed a list of all of the factors that could influence the health and quality of life for those living in a given community. Suppose we then positioned each of those factors on a piece of paper and drew arrows to show (1) how each was connected to the health issue of interest, and (2) how the various factors were related to one another. This exercise would yield a kind of ecological map or web—a systems model—enabling us to visualize the causal networks of relationships among the factors that can influence health status.

Just such a map is presented in figure 1.1. It depicts the conceptual model of interactions among the key components (subsystems) in a landmark 20-year Finnish community-based cardiovascular disease prevention program called the North Karelia Project (Puska 2000; Puska and Uutela 2000; Puska et al. 1998; Vartiainen et al. 1998). In chapter 6, we present a more detailed and specific ecological map based on a *post hoc* analysis and interpretation of what actually occurred as a result of the program's activities in that project. Since the North Karelia Project, ecological thinking has been expanded to advance systems science methodologies, such as agent-based modeling and network analyses, that allow researchers to model the dynamic and complex relationships of factors that affect a population's health and well-being (Burke et al. 2015; Farquhar and Green 2015; Li et al. 2016; Northridge and Metcalf 2016).

TABLE 1.1. How changes in ecological subsystems can influence health status

Ecological/ Social Change	Increases the probability of . . .	Can result in . . .	Leads to . . .	Can contribute to . . .
Higher cost of living	Both parents working, possibly longer hours or on multiple jobs	Less time to prepare healthful meals and an increased demand for fast foods	Increased consumption of fats and carbohydrates	Overweight and obesity
Suburban sprawl	Not being able to walk to work, school, or shopping	Increased use of motor vehicles and public transportation	Decreased levels of physical activity	Lower levels of cardiovascular fitness; higher rates of obesity
Introduction of walking trails and bike paths	People having access to multiple means of physical activity	Increases in the portion of the population that walks, jogs, or bikes	Increases in levels of physical activity	Increased cardio-respiratory fitness; improved mental health; lower levels of obesity
Higher rates of unemployment and poverty	Lack of access to health services, good nutrition, adequate and safe housing	Deficiencies in preventive services, poor or undernutrition	Multiple risk factors	Disproportionately high rates of chronic diseases, violence, mental illness, poor school performance
Public denouncement of second-hand smoke	Laws and regulations to protect air quality	Less exposure to tobacco smoke	Decrease in asthma triggers	Improved quality of life of children with asthma

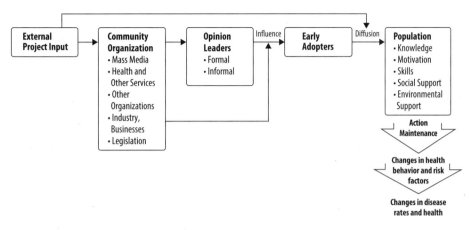

FIGURE 1.1. The North Karelia Project in Finland characterized its web of relationships as shown here, reflecting in part the relationships among organizations or sectors at the community level, in part the relationships among people whose behavior was affected by the program over a 25-year period, and in part the relationships among variables that needed to change to affect disease rates and health.

Sources: Puska, P., Nissinen, A., Tuomilehto, J., Salonen, J.T., Koskela, K., McAlister, A., Kottke, T.E., Maccoby, N. and Farquhar, J. (1985). The community-based strategy to prevent coronary heart disease: conclusions from the ten years of the North Karelia project. *Annual Review of Public Health*, *6*, 147–93. https://doi.org/10.1146/annurev.pu.06.050185.001051. Modified figure with permission from the *Annual Review of Public Health*, Volume 6 © 1985 by Annual Reviews. http://www.annualreviews.org. See also Farquhar, J. & Green, L.W. (2015). Community intervention trials in high-income countries. In Detels, R., Gulliford, M., Abdool Karim, Q., and Tan, C.C. (Eds.), *Oxford Textbook of Public Health* (6th ed., Vol. 2, pp. 516–27). Oxford University Press. https://doi.org/10.1093/med/9780199661756.003.0112

Education has multiple, layered meanings as we consider the strategies embedded in health education. Our commitment to an educational approach in population health planning is both empirical and philosophical. It is empirical to the extent that awareness, knowledge, and skills do influence the actions people take, which in turn shape the social and environmental capacity and systems in any community. It is philosophical to the extent that we and most health professionals remain committed to the principles of informed consent among those we serve, their active participation, and our cultural sensitivity and competence as we formulate programs for health improvement.

For this chapter's purposes—and for our approach to population health planning—we will highlight the following concepts relevant to health education: (1) individual and population-wide literacy, mathematics and science, and general knowledge; (2) population-wide programs and institutional approaches to impart skills, literacy, and knowledge; and (3) focused efforts to impart awareness and skills that assist in the population health interventions and assure greater equity in the distribution of benefits.

The general levels of a population's literacy, skills, and general knowledge have a direct impact on the effectiveness as well as the range of possible interventions for population health programs (Baker et al. 2011). A portion of this is the correlation between a population's socioeconomic level and its level of literacy, general skills, and knowledge. But there is also clear evidence that education in this sense is independently related to the range and effectiveness of possible population health interventions (Feinstein et al. 2006). Indeed, education might warrant a more central place in our definition of health, as some of those seeking to revisit the classic World Health Organization definition of health have suggested (Huber et al. 2011).

Populations and societies approach education in varying ways, with implications for equity and social justice. For example, they may offer free public education for all or limited access; offer gender-focused education (only for males or different content for males and females vs. the same for both sexes); or differ in terms of public support for higher education versus only for primary or secondary education. These choices have an impact on population health planning, programs, and interventions (Wu et al. 2004). In addition, the programmatic aspects and content of education institutions affect the range and efficacy of population health promotion and planning (Zimmerman and Woolf 2014). For example, if sex education is prohibited in public schools or the content of sex education is biased or limited, the range of policy and intervention options to prevent teenage pregnancies may be affected and intervention outcomes less effective than if sex education were more broadly and comprehensively taught as part of a public education program.

Educating stakeholders, participants, and policy makers on specific aspects or skills related to a population health intervention can have direct impacts on the intervention's outcomes. For example, educating a population on the mechanisms of pathogen transmission and the effectiveness of diligent hand-washing and wearing face coverings may improve the outcomes of interventions intended to reduce the transmission of communicable diseases (Zimmerman and Woolf 2014). Moreover, education and a commitment to the open exchange of ideas, values, biases, and assumptions help prevent planning from becoming a manipulative social engineering enterprise. Without **policy** supports for social change, however, educational efforts, shown to be effective on an individual basis, often prove to be too weak in mass media communications to yield a population-wide benefit.

Nancy Milio, an early advocate for more policy, organizational, economic, regulatory, and other environmental interventions to accomplish the goals of population health, conceded that we cannot justify abandoning health education as a critical channel for democratic, social, and behavioral change (1981). Planners who take an approach that is at once ecological and educational will understand the dynamic forces that influence health. They also will be more likely to commit to a policy of open, transparent, two-way communication with stakeholders.

Respecting People and Their Contexts in the Adaptation of Evidence-Based Practices

The notions of *best practices* and subsequently *evidence-based practice* were based on the view that the results of highly controlled research justified the choices of interventions in the planning and funding of programs by government agencies and foundations. Those notions have persisted, and deserve continued respect. But they also have been challenged because evidence from highly controlled, randomized trials of interventions, methods, and programs is limited in its generalizability or applicability to populations and settings in which they were not tested (Green 2008; Green and Glasgow 2006; Green and Kreuter 2000).

Population health programs unfold in places: in workplaces, health care facilities, schools, and communities. The ecological approach inherently recognizes the differences across those contexts. The educational approach recognizes that each place has its own history and traditions, enables people to perform their responsibilities in different ways, and reinforces its own way of doing things. A planner's sensitivity or insensitivity to these contextual characteristics can have a profound impact on a program's progress and effects. An example of planning programs that accommodate to context is shown in box 1.3.

BOX 1.3

Case Example: An Ecological Approach to Program Planning That Recognizes Context

Suppose a group of practitioners in Long Beach, California, is planning a tobacco control program for a segment of their community. They identify a promising combination of strategies documented in the CDC's publication *Best Practices for Comprehensive Tobacco Control Programs* as being effective in reducing tobacco sales and consumption in several states in the United States. Unlike the states where those strategies had been successfully applied, however, their community of interest consists primarily of first- and second-generation immigrants from Vietnam. In that Vietnamese population, 56% of men are smokers. Planners would need to take steps to adapt the CDC's proposed intervention strategies, taking into account the nuances of Vietnamese language and cultural traditions and beliefs. Such adaptation has at least two benefits: (1) it increases the probability that the population will see the intervention as relevant to their needs, and (2) the concern for cultural differences would be a manifestation of respect and a step toward building trust. Beyond these benefits, the practical value of linking program planning to cultural differences lies in assuring that the interventions selected or designed for the program will be culturally appropriate to the population, and therefore more likely to affect their behaviors and environments.

Not all contextual factors are obvious. For example, like most bureaucracies, the organizational infrastructure of state health departments or health ministries is typically divided into categorical units or divisions. Inevitably, several of these will share interests in the same health issues. If not coordinated, these common interests can result in territorial struggles and counterproductive competition. In such cases, leaders are disinclined to be cooperative, especially if limited resources are allotted to one division or unit at the expense of the others. Left unchecked, such circumstances can lead to a quiet downward spiral of mistrust, making subsequent collaboration almost impossible. Imagine yourself as a new employee, unaware of that context and being given the task of developing a cross-division collaborative effort. Sensitivity to the context is, in large part, a combination of one's understanding that places are unique and a belief (or attitude) that the characteristics that make them unique strongly influence what happens in that place.

Of course, the scenario just described can occur in reverse. The divisions involved may have a rich history of collaboration, linked by effective channels of communication. They may even have a flexible budgeting and accounting system that enables them to share and track resources and personnel. For a new employee, that context would constitute a substantial asset, but a new employee must proceed carefully to avoid appearing to devalue this finely honed collaborative structure. In the first phase of the PRECEDE-PROCEED planning and evaluation framework presented in this book, emphasis is placed on an assessment strategy that serves to sensitize the planner to cultural awareness through participatory approaches to planning.

THE PRECEDE-PROCEED MODEL

The PRECEDE-PROCEED model has demonstrated its widespread applicability and scalability; it has been applied effectively for five decades in hundreds of rigorously evaluated field trials that used it to plan, implement, and evaluate programs.[3] These efforts have addressed a wide range of health issues in communities, schools, health care settings and workplaces throughout the world. Some of those programs are highlighted in the subsequent chapters of this text, and a searchable bibliography of over 1,200 published applications is accessible to interested readers through the website http://www.lgreen.net/.

What are the phases of the PRECEDE-PROCEED approach to population health planning?

Besides the ecological and educational approach that simultaneously respects context and people, the salient features of this model are the phases and proce-dures that follow a logical sequence of steps aligned with a generic logic model or systems model of causes and effects. The primary purpose of implementing a population health program follows a straightforward and unambiguous for-mula: enhance a population's quality of life and health status by doing what is necessary to prevent illness and injury or mitigate their consequences. Popu-lation health programs may operate at one or a combination of three levels of prevention: primary (hygiene and health enhancement and health protection through environmental controls to prevent disease), secondary (early detection of disease and behavioral or environmental adaptations to support health main-tenance with chronic conditions), or tertiary (therapy to treat the disease or prevent sequelae or recurrence) (Reisig and Wildner 2008). All three of these prevention levels have been key to addressing the current COVID-19 pandemic, with experts prioritizing the need for each at different phases of the pandemic and for different sub-populations. For instance, primary prevention was recom-mended for all populations throughout the entire pandemic; tertiary prevention was critical early on and for older populations with co-morbidities; and the need for secondary prevention screening was called for by public health profession-als, but was often met with political resistance. As this textbook goes to press, all three levels continue to be critical in the United States and globally.

Regardless of the level that defines the scope of their work, planners will in-evitably be faced with myriad potential factors and conditions that are likely to have some degree of influence on health and quality of life. In most instances, many or even most of those factors and conditions will be amenable to change through planned programs and policy changes. Health programs must acknowl-edge that among the myriad factors are relatively intractable factors such as ge-netic predisposition, aging, or one's place of residence, which can have a strong influence on health and quality of life. Planners must also realize that such fac-tors are not "changeable" in a programmatic context in the same sense that pol-icies, services, environments, or behaviors are amenable to change.

To begin, let's start with a quick question. What does the phrase "faced with myriad potential factors and conditions" mean to you?

A. Complexity?

B. Confusion?

C. A lot of factors to juggle?

D. An overwhelming situation?

E. All of the above?

Complexity is the price one pays for embracing an ecological approach to health planning. If we accept the notion that everything influences everything else, however remotely, and carry that notion to its logical extreme, one might argue that average health practitioners would have good reason to shake their heads and circle "E" above. There is no getting around the reality that crafting an effective health program will almost always require you to sift and sort through many factors and set priorities. One of the key features of the PRECEDE-PROCEED planning process is that it provides planners with a simple but effective way to carry out that sifting and sorting process. It has a built-in mechanism that acts like a sieve, so that the factors with little or no relevance to your goal fall through the perforated openings. Those remaining will be those that (1) have the greatest influence on health and quality of life, and (2) are most amenable to change.

The framework has two components. The first set of phases consists of a series of planned assessments (or diagnoses) that generate information that will be used to guide subsequent decisions. This series of phases involves considerable sifting and sorting and is referred to as **PRECEDE** (for *p*redisposing, *r*einforcing, and *e*nabling *c*onstructs in *e*ducational/*e*cological **diagnosis**[4] and *e*valuation).

The second component is marked by the strategic implementation and evaluation of multiple actions based on what was learned from the assessments in the initial phases. This second component is named **PROCEED** for *p*olicy, *r*egulatory, and *o*rganizational *c*onstructs in *e*ducational and *e*nvironmental *d*evelopment. *Evaluation* is an integral part of both components and serves as the primary vehicle to assure the quality of the planning process. In PRECEDE, evaluation emerges immediately in the form of quantitative and qualitative information about quality of life and continues as information is gathered about population health status indicators and factors associated with those indicators, including social, economic, cultural, environmental, and behavioral factors. Each of the early phases of PRECEDE may be viewed as **formative evaluation**, in which diagnostic and assessment data serve to set program priorities, goals, objectives, and targets, and also as baseline measures for later **process** and **outcome evaluations**. In the PROCEED component, that prior information serves as the source of baseline data at the start of an intervention. It also supports the standardization of measures for monitoring progress toward or achievement of program goals and objectives, adjusting the objectives and course of action, and shifting resources accordingly.

PRECEDE and PROCEED work in tandem, providing a continuous series of steps or phases in planning, implementation, and evaluation. Identifying priorities generated in PRECEDE leads to quantitative objectives that become increasingly specific and quantified goals and targets in the implementation phase of PROCEED. These goals and targets become the standards of acceptability or criteria for success in the program's implementation and evaluation.

Operationalizing the PRECEDE-PROCEED Model

Applying PRECEDE and PROCEED is like solving a mystery. Using it requires a combination of inductive and deductive logic, starting with a shared vision of the desired ends and working backward to discover the forces that influence the attainment of that vision. Eight basic phases constitute the procedure (figure 1.2). The connecting lines and arrows represent not only the relationship among these phases and boxes, but also the dynamic process of implementation. (We refer the reader to chapter 8 on implementation for a deeper understanding). A final series of four levels of evaluation may be seen as phases during and following implementation. These levels of evaluation serve as monitoring and continuous quality improvement processes for ongoing programs or assessments for demonstration programs as they progress. (We refer the reader to chapter 9 on evaluation for more details.) As you review these individual phases, keep in mind that they are truly interdependent parts of an ecological planning system.

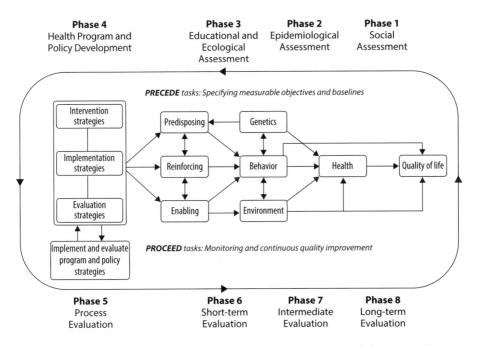

FIGURE 1.2. This generic representation of PRECEDE-PROCEED, with its phases of planning, implementation, and evaluation, also represents the underlying theoretical cause-and-effect relationships among the determinants of health and quality of life for populations.

Phase 1. Social Assessment. This initial phase signals a commitment to engaging the population of interest because it provides insights into the cultural and social circumstances unique to that population. An assessment of general hopes and problems of concern to the target population (patients, students, employees, residents, or consumers) is the starting point for obtaining indicators of quality of life. Specific methods designed to unveil quality-of-life indicators are described in detail in chapter 3. Some of the indicators of these subjectively defined problems and priorities will be described in chapter 3 as social indicators. Regardless of the methods employed, we urge planners to involve people in a self-study of their own needs and aspirations. The kinds of **social problems** a community experiences offer a practical and accurate barometer of its quality of life. They also can illuminate critical social and economic determinants and structural or systematic barriers to health and quality of life that need to be considered. In turn, these insights can lead to creative intervention strategies and community resources to support them.

Program success depends in part on a combination of organizational strengths and weaknesses and the degree to which those with a stake in the program's activities and its outcomes (sometimes called "stakeholders") are engaged. Furthermore, these factors tend to vary considerably across populations. The application of **situational analysis** tools (see chapter 3) during this phase will help planners detect the unique variations that require attention in the population they are serving.

Phase 2. Epidemiological Assessment. The initial task in Phase 2 is to identify the specific health goals or problems that may contribute to, or interact with, the social goals or problems noted in Phase 1. The use of available health data about the population enables the planner to rank several health problems or needs according to their importance and changeability. Vital indicators and other measures of population health are discussed in chapter 3, but we caution that death certificate data are not enough to characterize the leading causes of death in a population because the actual or underlying causes of death are often lifestyle factors that contribute large portions of attributable risk for death, such as with smoking and cancer (McGinnis and Foege 1993). Moreover, multiple sources of environmental, health behavior, morbidity and mortality comparative analyses give planners a rationale when they must decide which specific health issues or problem(s) are most deserving of scarce resources (Marmot and Wilkinson 2006).

A second task in the epidemiological assessment is the identification of factors or determinants of health in a population's genetics, behavioral patterns, and environment. Behavior, genetics, and social and physical environments are known to account for 90% of premature deaths (figure 1.3).

At this point, we need to pause for a reality check. Often, especially early

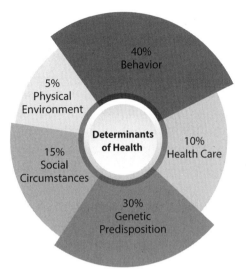

FIGURE 1.3. Compiled from multiple studies, the estimates of percentages of premature deaths attributable to the major determinants of health include 40% to behavioral patterns, 30% to genetic predisposition, and 30% to environmental factors. The last includes 5% to exposures in the physical environment, 10% to shortfalls in medical care, and 15% to social factors.

Sources: Data updated in Johnson, N.B., Hayes, L.D., Brown, K., Hoo, E.C., Ethier, K.A., & Centers for Disease Control and Prevention (CDC). (2014). CDC National Health Report: leading causes of morbidity and mortality and associated behavioral risk and protective factors—United States, 2005-2013. *MMWR Supplements, 63*(4), 3–27. https://www.cdc.gov/mmwr/preview/mmwrhtml/su6304a2.htm. From McGinnis, J.M., & Foege, W.H. (1993). Actual causes of death in the United States. *JAMA, 270*(18), 2207–12. https://doi.org/10.1001/jama.1993.03510180077038; and Mokdad, A.H., Marks, J.S., Stroup, D.F., & Gerberding, J.L. (2004). Actual causes of death in the United States, 2000. *JAMA, 291*(10), 1238–45. https://doi.org/10.1001/jama.291.10.1238. Erratum in: (2005), *JAMA, 293*(3), 293–4. https://doi.org/10.1001/jama.293.3.293

in their careers, health planners will be in situations where Phases 1 and 2 (or aspects of them) have already been undertaken. To varying degrees, local governmental and non-governmental health organizations will use information similar to that called for in Phases 1 and 2 as a part of their long-term planning. They may be focused on a specific range of health issues (e.g., a heart or cancer association) or behavioral issues (drug abuse, teen pregnancies). In those instances, health professionals are typically asked to develop a program aimed at a predetermined health issue or behavioral or environmental problem or **risk factor**, such as diabetes, specific injuries, smoking or vaping, physical activity, or drinking and driving. Thus, the user of the PRECEDE-PROCEED model would essentially be vaulted past the first phases of the framework into Phase 2 or even 3. For example, rather than starting with the social and epidemiologically defined problem of lung cancer, they might be directed to work on the behaviorally defined problem of smoking or vaping.

We strongly urge practitioners who find themselves in this situation to invest some time in reviewing the assumptions made in relation to the cause-effect linkages implied in the first two phases and who was involved or consulted in the process. This precautionary action ensures that the assumptions remain valid, or at least are explicit and understood by key stakeholders. For an example of the importance of taking the time for this step, see box 1.4; it will be time well spent for at least three practical reasons. First, it will lead to a better understanding of the assumptions upon which the priorities were based. Second, the practitioner will get a sense of who the stakeholders are and the extent to which they have been, or want to remain, engaged. Finally, the review may reveal some deficiencies or errors in Phases 1 or 2, or the need to update the data on which the conclusions are based. Left unattended, such problems can threaten the program's success.

A second part of Phase 2 is the assessment of the determinants of health, generally associated with the work of epidemiology. This phase focuses on the identification of those specific health-related genetic, behavioral, and environmental factors that could be linked to the health and social problems chosen as most deserving of attention. It has been well established that genetic, behavioral, and environmental factors combine to put people at greater or less health risk (Berkman and Kawachi 2000; Hernandez and Blazer 2006; Kawachi et al. 2002; Marmot and Wilkinson 2006; McGinnis et al. 2002).

The consideration of **genetic factors** is a relatively recent addition to the PRECEDE-PROCEED model, recognizing the gigantic leap in the available science and the rapid strides being made to isolate the genetic predispositions associated with various illnesses, risk factors, and biological conditions. Many

---

BOX 1.4

Conducting a Social Assessment When You Know the Health Problem

Suppose you are employed by a local health department and the director gives you the assignment of planning a community-wide breast and cervical cancer screening program aimed at populations known to be at high risk. For this planning endeavor, you are given some modest staff support and a budget for one year with continued funding contingent on progress made in that first year. You take the time to do your ex post facto review and find that the program is strongly supported by local health data. It is also apparent that members of the at-risk population and their constituencies have been actively involved in the process.

You also discover, however, that local physicians have not been involved and, consequently, are unaware of the proposed program. Trying to move a cancer prevention program forward without engaging the input and support of the local health care provider community could be problematic. On the other hand, their active support could have multiple benefits, including their endorsement of funding support to sustain the program in future years.

of these associations are complex interactions of genes with behavior and the environment (as reflected by the vertical arrows in figure 1.2), so they will seldom be treated as independent effects on health. Exceptions include a few genetic diseases such as phenylketonuria (PKU), sickle cell anemia, cystic fibrosis, and Tay-Sachs disease. For most of the gene-gene, gene-environment, and gene-behavior interactions, the science is not yet developed sufficiently for widespread application, but is developing quickly. Most controls on the gene-environment interactions depend on the behavior of individuals and populations in their exposure to environmental risks, so we place behavior between genetics and the environment in the model.

Behavioral factors refer to the patterns of behavior (and together with environmental circumstances that create **lifestyles**) of individuals and groups that protect them from or put them at risk for a given health or social problem. They also include the behaviors and actions of others. For example, the behavior of health care workers, parents, friends, or coworkers may influence the health status of a target population either in the aggregate, as through social norms, or individually, as in the exercise of social power over the behavior of individuals. Another example is the collective social action or behavior of individuals and groups (e.g., campaigning for votes) for or against relevant health policies.

Environmental factors are those determinants of health external to the person that can be modified to support behavior, health, and quality of life. Being cognizant of such forces will enable planners to be more realistic about the limitations of programs consisting only of health education directed at personal health behavior. It also offers additional intervention opportunities directed toward influencing powerful social forces: for example, through organizational and community mobilizing and advocacy strategies that can shape policies at the local, provincial, state, or national level.

In some instances, planners may strategically decide to intervene directly on a social or quality-of-life factor as an indirect means to influence health. In such a **strategy**, the outer arrows connecting behavior and environment to the quality-of-life box become the focus of this phase (see figure 1.2). The process of setting priorities on the basis of causal importance, prevalence, and changeability is important at each phase. It is especially important in the early phases because factors selected in early phases considerably magnify the factors that surface in the subsequent phases.

Phase 3. Educational and Ecological Assessment. On the basis of cumulative research on health and social behavior and on ecological relationships between environment and behavior, literally hundreds of factors could be identified that have the potential to influence a given health behavior, environment, or the interaction of genes with behavior and environment. In the PRECEDE component, these factors are grouped into three manageable categories: predisposing factors, reinforcing factors, and enabling factors. These categories are based on the theoretical mechanism through which they shape behavior, as well as the educational and ecological approaches needed to influence them through the program. The health program and policy strategies that can be used to influence these three factors are shown in figure 1.4, and are illustrated in the original research that led to the formulation and validation of the PRECEDE model (Green et al. 1979; Green et al. 1974; Hatcher et al. 1986).

Predisposing factors include a person's or population's knowledge, attitudes, beliefs, **values**, and perceptions that facilitate or hinder motivation for change. Figure 1.4 also shows how predisposing factors interact with genetic predisposition. Predisposing factors also include the early childhood experiences that created the attitudes, values, and perceptions in the first place. While such experiences may not be modifiable by the program being planned (e.g., Adverse Childhood Experiences or ACEs), understanding their long-term influences can foster intervention strategies that accommodate special needs of specific audiences (e.g., trauma-informed systems and programming).

Reinforcing factors are the rewards or satisfactions received and the feedback an individual receives from influential significant others following the adoption

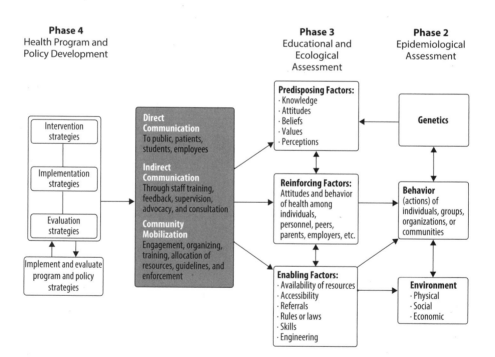

FIGURE 1.4. Phases 3 and 4 of PRECEDE address the strategies and resources required to influence the predisposing, enabling, and reinforcing factors, which, in turn, influence or support behavioral and environmental changes. Changes in these targets become the explanations for program success or failure.

of a behavior. These factors may encourage or discourage continuation of the behavior. Reinforcing behavior produces lifestyles (enduring patterns of behavior), which in turn influence the environment through social norms, political advocacy, consumer demand, or cumulative actions.

Enabling factors are those skills, resources, or barriers that can help or hinder the desired behavioral and environmental changes needed to achieve the desired health outcome. One can view them as vehicles or barriers, created mainly by societal forces or systems. Facilities and personal or community resources may be ample or inadequate, as might income or health insurance, and laws and statutes may be supportive or restrictive. The skills required for a desired behavior to occur also qualify as enabling factors. For example, providing sphygmomanometers for a hypertension self-care program would have minimal value if the participants lacked the skill or capacity to use the device to take their blood pressure readings. We have found it helpful to think of enabling factors as those things that *make change possible* when people want that change in a behavior or the environment (Green and Ottoson 1999; Green and Raeburn 1990).

In summary, the primary tasks of the third phase involve sorting, categorizing, and selecting the predisposing, enabling, and reinforcing factors that seem to have the greatest impact on the behavioral and environmental targets generated in previous stages, and which are the most changeable. Successful completion of these tasks will reveal which of the factors, or which combinations of them, deserve highest priority as the focus of intervention (Cantor et al. 1985; Kreuter and Green 1978; Levine et al. 1987; Morisky et al. 1982).

Phase 4. Administrative and Policy Assessment. Now, equipped with the information generated in the first three phases, the planner is poised for the final assessments of the PRECEDE component and the first phase of PROCEED. On the diagram, this corresponds to Phase 4: administrative and policy assessment. This is where the planner must match the prioritized predisposing, reinforcing, and enabling factors with the communication and mobilization methods and policies necessary for change. How will the plan be set in motion with intervention and implementation strategies and policies, anticipating resource requirements and policy restrictions or other constraints? In practical terms, these assessments are designed to answer the questions:

- What program components and interventions are needed to affect the desired changes specified in previous phases? (Intervention strategies)

- Does this program have the policy, organizational, and administrative capabilities and resources to make this program a reality? (Implementation strategies)

- On which criteria and by which methodology will program or policy success be decided? (Evaluation strategies, continued with Phases 5–8)

Most organizations will have limited readiness or capacity to design fully and implement a program that attempts to intervene on the wide range of forces influencing the social and structural determinants of health. Some of these limitations can be offset by cooperative arrangements with other local agencies or larger organizations at state, provincial, or national levels, or through the development of coalitions and political alliances at the local level.

Phase 4 is the turning point in the model where the diagnostic assessments of PRECEDE turn into the implementation and evaluation actions of PROCEED. The continuous outer circle around the model, in figure 1.2, intends to show the movement and turning points in the model. In the earliest stages of development, experienced planners will have an eye on Phase 4 as they rely on their experience with the range of possible interventions and their sensitivity to their organization's mission, policies, capacity, and readiness. Potential interventions and sensitivity to the sponsors' policies, capacity, and readiness will serve as important parameters to consider as they scale their programs in the earlier planning phases. But the policies, capacity, and readiness of one's own institution need not be the only factors. Information derived from their situational analysis in Phase 1 may yield insights into the probability of obtaining support from other organizations within their locality or resources from outside the community. Identifying and accessing these types of opportunities for support and partnerships can influence a program's success, sometimes to an even greater extent than the internal resources available in a single organization.

The planning and launching considerations specific to each of the major settings for health programs—communities, work sites, schools, health care settings, and the Internet or handheld devices—are discussed and illustrated in chapters 10 through 14. Pivoting from PRECEDE to PROCEED provides a focal point for describing principles and methods of program management and evaluation. As the planning process continues through the subsequent phases, the PRECEDE-PROCEED framework yields continuous feedback to adjust program components to fit the objectives, changing circumstances, and needs of various population segments.

PRECEDE was first developed as an evaluation model to aid practitioners in their efforts to document the cost-benefit effects of demonstration programs.[5] With the addition of PROCEED, it has evolved into the comprehensive planning, implementation, and evaluation framework presented in this book. Throughout this volume, we emphasize that in the context of health program planning, implementation, and evaluation, integral and continuous parts of planning are inseparably tied to measurable objectives generated from the beginning of the first steps of the process. For example, the results of the social and epidemiological assessments emphasize the importance of stating program objectives early on and routinely throughout the planning process. The primary evaluation task is one of *documenting* (through measurable objectives and other data and information deemed relevant) baseline indicators. As one turns the corner from PRECEDE to PROCEED in Phase 5 and moves from planning into implementation and evaluation, the principal evaluation task is one of *using* the information gained from monitoring those indicators to make program adjustments and to inform stakeholders of program progress. For those practitioners and researchers faced with the task of carrying out a demonstration program or research project to test the effects of a given intervention or strategy, PRECEDE-PROCEED provides a globally tested, generic planning framework and logic model.

HALLMARKS

The long history of PRECEDE-PROCEED applications and studies has helped us identify those characteristics of the model which, over time, are consistently associated with success. Collectively, these enduring characteristics represent the "hallmarks" of the model: (1) its flexibility and scalability, (2) its evidence-based process and evaluability, (3) its commitment to the principle of participation, and (4) its provision of a process for appropriate adaptation of evidence-based best practices to specific populations and circumstances. Each is briefly described below.

Hallmark: Flexibility

Whether one is involved in planning a large-scale, multinational health program, an integrated school health program, a vaccination program for a specific population, or a patient education program for a small target population, the principles and guidelines of the PRECEDE-PROCEED model apply. Considerable documentation is available about the application of the PRECEDE-PROCEED planning process across a wide range of populations, settings, disease prevention and **health promotion** issues, and specific disease management. The model has even been applied to planning and **evaluation** situations in which health outcomes were not an immediate issue, such as continuing education and staff development issues. Health departments have used the model as a guide to developing programs subsequently adopted by other jurisdictions and adapted into guidelines by national organizations. PRECEDE-PROCEED has been used by health care and public health professionals as an organizational framework for curriculum development, continuing education, research, and its translation and dissemination. (See the applications in chapters 10–14 for examples of the populations and settings to which the model has been applied.) For other specific examples and a searchable bibliography of published applications, extensions, descriptions, and reviews of the model as they relate to hundreds of varied populations, health issues, and contexts, visit our website at http://www.lgreen.net.[5]

Hallmark: Evidenced-Based and Evaluable

The PRECEDE-PROCEED process requires planners to begin with a clear picture of the desired final outcome (see box 1.5). The first question asked is: What is the ultimate concern or aspiration here, and what do we want to accomplish in relation to it? The desired goal of the program is articulated first as a vision or mission statement. Then, as the planning process continues, the goal is spelled out in the form of a measurable **objective** that includes quantitative estimates of the magnitude of the desired effect and the estimated time required to achieve that effect. Once the broad goal or vision has been agreed upon, planners turn to a series of assessment tasks designed to uncover the salient factors and conditions that, independently or in combination, influence the desired outcome. Questions relevant here include: Who will achieve how much of what benefit, and by when? Answers to these four questions, for each "who" or "what," constitute the identification of an objective. These objectives are often ranked or stratified in order of their causal importance, their prevalence in the population, and the evidence supporting interventions to affect them. Once those critical factors and conditions are identified, again in *measurable terms*, planners will be in a stronger position to ask and answer the next question: What actions are most likely to yield a desired outcome?

The complex ecological nature of population health challenges means that from the outset of planning a program through its implementation, changes are likely to occur that require adjustments or modifications. Because of the commitment to using measurable objectives throughout the planning process, the PRECEDE-PROCEED model acts as a kind of learning system with a built-in evaluation mechanism. This evaluation capacity provides an ongoing

---

BOX 1.5
PRECEDE-PROCEED Planning, Implementation, and Evaluation Questions

What is the *ultimate concern or aspiration* here and what do we want to accomplish in relation to it?

    Who will achieve *how much* of *what* benefit, by *when*?

    What *actions* are most likely to yield a desired outcome?

    How will we know the actions were *implemented* and the desired *outcomes* were achieved?

source of feedback that alerts planners to events or changes that might otherwise go undetected. In less rigorous planning efforts, these undetected (and sometimes unintended) events often surface as problems after the program has been implemented—hence the term "unanticipated consequences." But in the PRECEDE-PROCEED model, these unanticipated events represent opportunities to refine and strengthen the planning process, at a point when changes can still be useful and improve results.

Hallmark: Participation

In the context of a population health program, **stakeholders** are those people or groups with a vested interest in that program or aspects of it. Those who participate in or receive program services are stakeholders. Those who participate in the planning and implementation of the program and are leaders in the organizations they represent are also stakeholders. If health programs were a business, the former would be thought of as customers and the latter as the retail workforce or representatives of the company who interface with the customers. In the PRECEDE-PROCEED planning process, participation is central to both of these categories of stakeholders, as is at least a well-maintained line of communication with the agency's leadership. Participation is more than a philosophical principle. Evidence from decades of research and experience on the value of participation in learning and behavior change indicates that people will be more committed to initiating and upholding changes they helped design or adapted to their own purposes and circumstances (Bjãrås et al. 1991; Minkler and Wallerstein 2003; Schiller et al. 1987; Wandersman and Florin 2000).

Consider those for whom a program is designed. Population health programs seek to redress a wide range of health issues, from noncommunicable diseases, HIV/AIDS, and injuries to bioterrorism, environmental pollution, malaria, and new viruses such as COVID-19. These health concerns, and their behavioral and environmental precursors, are value-laden and, to varying degrees, culturally defined. Intervention strategies—including policy dictates from a distant central government, especially in pluralistic, democratic societies—will have little chance of being effective without the participation and understanding of those who will be affected by the policy and those who implement it, as seen in chapter 2. Many issues that affect health outcomes (such as sexual behavior, obesity, and domestic violence) are not amenable to traditional surveillance and regulation. The constitutional and civil rights of citizens protect most individual behaviors, including bearing arms in the United States, sexual practices among consenting adults, advertising unhealthful products, or even producing pornography. Governments such as those of Australia, Canada, and the United States limit the powers of the central government in favor of state or provincial rights in many health matters. Most of these powers are ceded to local governments with the expectation of dissemination of successful programs (Green et al. 1999; Green and Ottoson 2004).

The most appropriate *center of gravity for population health programs* usually will prove to be the community. This does not exclude state and national levels of support needed by communities, or institutional and family levels of support to individuals (Roussos and Fawcett 2000; Sanchez 2000). State and national governments can formulate policies, provide leadership, allocate funding, and generate data for health promotion. At the other extreme, individuals can govern their own behavior and control the determinants of their own health, up to a point, and should be allowed and encouraged to do so. But the decisions on priorities and strategies for *social* change affecting the more complicated lifestyle issues can best be made collectively, as close to the homes and workplaces of those affected as possible. This principle assures the greatest relevance and appropriateness of the programs to the people affected and offers the best opportunity for people to be actively engaged in the planning process themselves. It also augurs well for sustaining successful programs into the future. A 2012 Institute of Medicine (now renamed the National Academy of Medicine) committee report entitled *Improving Health in the Community* recognized limitations in a community-based approach to health improvement insofar as many factors affecting health in a community will originate elsewhere and may not be modifiable by efforts within the community. This caution also applies well to today's recognized need for social and racial justice changes in structures and policies that shape community life inequitably for many. The COVID-19 pandemic underscored the fluid circumstances of vaccines being tested, adapting to new variants, reaching communities, and the priorities and uneven reach and scheduling of vaccines in geographic and racial or ethnic segments of the population.

Participation by health program planners from multiple disciplines is also critical given the complex nature of the challenges they face. After nearly five decades of evolution and application, the PRECEDE-PROCEED model bears the imprints of many professional disciplines. These include epidemiology, **health education** and **health promotion**, anthropology, sociology, psychology, social psychology, political science, economics, health administration, health communication, and management sciences. Philosophers have often reminded us of what we know intuitively: that there are different ways of knowing and different interpretations of reality (Wilber 1998). Participatory research in public health has taught us that an epidemiologist, an anthropologist, a health educator, and a layperson are likely to view a given problem through different lenses (Minkler and Wallerstein 2003). Because each is quite likely to detect a glimpse of reality that the others may miss, it is in the planner's best interest to actively support multidisciplinary input into the process. The PRECEDE-PROCEED approach to planning ideally would tap into the representation of disciplines or the literature of health practitioners, epidemiologists, social, behavioral, communications, economic, and political scientists, and certainly those the program would seek to serve; they are expected to jointly explore how their various views of reality can be combined to generate a sound and effective program. Furthermore, planning cannot be limited to tidy boundaries of health institutions, for much of what relates to the health of human populations happens in other sectors, such as schools, industry, social services, and welfare. Participation will be productive to the extent that (1) it occurs at the outset of the planning process, (2) time is dedicated to allow such discourse to occur, and (3) those discussions are carried out in an atmosphere of mutual *respect and trust.*

Hallmark: A Platform for Evidence-Based Practice and Practice-Based Evidence

Within the health field, the term *best practices* generally has been applied to specific medical interventions that had been shown in randomized, controlled research trials to be effective across the human species. That is, other than adjustments of dosage by age and sex, a "best practice" should be effective regardless of culture, socioeconomic condition, or historical precedent in social customs, laws, and policies. Experimental studies that yield *bona fide* "best practices" must rely heavily on the ability to control factors in the environment that may in any way confound the results.

Immunization is often held up as the ultimate "best practice" in public health. Consider how vaccines are developed. The process begins with laboratory experiments, followed by carefully controlled animal studies, and eventually moves on to randomized controlled clinical trials among humans. The only difference between the experimental and control samples of the population being studied is that members of the experimental group receive the actual vaccine while members of the control group receive a placebo. Only after the evidence shows that virtually every administration of the vaccine will prevent the adverse effects of the microbe in question, with minimal or no danger of side effects, do scientists and regulatory agencies declare the vaccine to be safe and effective for distribution to the public. It is precisely this kind of scientific rigor that has armed both medicine and public health to achieve the prevention and control of many infectious and communicable diseases.

Setting aside the current COVID-19 pandemic, bringing communicable diseases under control in the recent past contributed to a shift often referred to as the **epidemiological transition**. It is a process of substitution wherein infectious diseases as primary cause of death—especially premature deaths—were replaced by a predominance of chronic and degenerative diseases that afflicted many, as they live longer but with more suffering (Sepúlveda 1998). This transition also has led to related shifts associated with epidemiological methods (Carolina and Gustavo 2003; Hackam and Anand 2003).

In our discussion of the ecological approach, this chapter has emphasized that the underlying causes of health priorities are embedded in the social, economic, and cultural circumstances that surround people where they live and work. Because these conditions vary considerably from place to place, a program shown to be effective in redressing a health problem in one community, or in one study, may not fit the circumstances of another community experiencing the same health problem (Green 2001; 2006; 2007; 2008; Green and Kreuter 2000; Green and Ottoson 2004; Green et al. 1999). In short, the creation of consistently effective, generalizable population health interventions that apply everywhere (like a one-size-fits-all or fits-most vaccine) is not attainable. However, the process of customizing planning to a community's unique situation, while complex, pays off in terms of improved health outcomes and community engagement in addressing them. In the context of population health planning, this book contends that the notion of "best practice" should be viewed not as a static intervention, but as a process of careful, evidence-based planning that enables planners to *tailor* strategies and methods, using unique practice-based evidence, to any given place, population, or circumstances.

We recognize that generalizability or external validity is clearly one of the criteria of good science, but the scientific products of such research usually must be qualified as to its generalizability to other populations, settings, health issues, and circumstances. Accordingly, research into population health programming can promise to produce reasonably reliable guidelines for *good* practices. More importantly, population-based research will produce findings that can guide a generalizable *process for planning for a population*, not a generalizable *plan for all populations*. The products of such research should be generalizable in suggesting ways of engaging the community, ways of assessing the needs and circumstances of the community or population, ways of assessing resources, ways of planning programs, and ways of matching needs, resources, and circumstances with appropriate interventions. The PRECEDE-PROCEED model provides a platform for such a process.

SUMMARY

This chapter introduces the key features of a model of health program planning that has been applied globally and reflected in the Association of Schools and Programs of Public Health's (ASPPH) recommended public health competencies, as shown in appendix B. Those features emphasize a blending of ecological and educational approaches into a collaborative and participatory, evidence-based, community-diagnostic, capacity-building strategy for population health programs. It argues for an approach to using evidence-based best practices that are sensitive to the contexts or settings where they are to be applied (which are usually different from those where the controlled experimental research that established the efficacy of these best practices was conducted). It also makes the case that a population health program must consider the many ecological levels and relationships between environmental and behavioral determinants of health. Accordingly, planners then develop intervention strategies that are "tailored" to the needs of populations in their respective settings.

An overview of the PRECEDE-PROCEED model summarizes eight phases: (1) social assessment, (2) epidemiological assessment, (3) educational and ecological assessment of the highest-priority health problems and determinants identified in Phase 2, and (4) administrative and policy assessment to identify intervention, implementation, and evaluation strategies for the highest-priority predisposing, enabling, and reinforcing factors identified in Phase 3. Phases 5–8 are the evaluation of process, short-term, intermediate, and long-term objectives. Evaluation is built into each of the first four phases, including formative evaluation of the priorities, determinants, and potential interventions; establishing baseline measures and quantitative targets as part of the setting of objectives in each phase; and, in Phase 5, evaluating the program process, as well as the match or fit of potential interventions with the priority changes they are required to affect. Phases 6–8, during and after the implementation of the program, provide for ongoing monitoring and continuous quality improvement and for evaluation of the short-term, intermediate, and long-term effects of the program.

The hallmarks of PRECEDE-PROCEED include its flexibility and scalability, evidence-based process and evaluability, commitment to the principle of participation, and process for appropriate adaptation of evidence-based best practices to the practice-based evidence for specific populations and circumstances in which these are to be applied.

EXERCISES

1. What trends have you noticed in recent years, in your community or among your friends, in health behaviors, conditions of living, and health concerns? Can you find any objective data to support your observations? If not, how would you go about verifying your personal view of these trends?

2. Identify at least three national or international health campaigns or programs spanning several years. How do you account for the public concern about these different health problems at different times? What were the

major features of these programs? Why have different problems at different times required different health program methods?

3. Identify and describe the demographic characteristics (geographic location, size, age and sex distribution, etc.) of a population (students, patients, workers, or residents) whose quality of life you would like to improve. Follow the population you choose through most of the remaining exercises in this book. Look ahead at the upcoming exercises and make sure the population you choose is appropriate for the assessment and planning steps that will be required. If not, adjust accordingly and retrace your steps. (After all, adaptation and flexibility are encouraged in applying the PRECEDE-PROCEED model!)

Notes

1. Early research trials and reviews that helped validate and shape the representation of the PRECEDE-PROCEED model (sometimes referred to as its earlier version, the PRECEDE model) included applications by numerous faculty, postdoctoral fellows, and doctoral students at Johns Hopkins University. Some of the more recent trials and other tests and applications of the model can be found in other chapters of this volume. For the full searchable online bibliography of over 1,200 published applications and adaptations of the model for various purposes, go to http://www.lgreen.net/bibliographies.

2. The phrase "If we want more evidence-based practice, we need more practice-based evidence" was originally coined by Green during his tenure as director of the Office of Science and Extramural Research at the CDC from 2000 to 2005. Since that time, PRECEDE-PROCEED has been a recognized resource for developing practice-based evidence to complement evidence-based practice, which comes primarily from highly controlled research that neglects external validity for the sake of greater internal validity. See also the arguments and evidence supporting the call for more practice-based evidence to justify or adapt "evidence-based practices": Alderman et al. (1980); Green (1998; 2001; 2006; 2007; 2008); Green and Ottoson (2004); Truswell et al. (2012); Kokko et al. (2014); Wold and Samdal (2012).

3. A brief history of the PRECEDE-PROCEED model: It originated as a cost-benefit evaluation framework (Green 1974) from converging streams of research and experience in public health (Rogers 1962), medical care (Andersen 1968), family planning (Green 1970a), psychological (Green 1970b) and social factors in health behavior (Green 1970b), diffusion and adoption theory (Green 1970a; 1975), and other models of change (Green 1976), and the demands of that period on health programs to demonstrate their effectiveness through evaluation in cost-effectiveness and cost-benefit metrics. The model was applied systematically in a series of clinical and field trials by faculty, doctoral students, and postdoctoral fellows at Johns Hopkins University and collaborators in other populations and institutions. These confirmed the model's utility and predictive validity as a planning tool as well as an organizing framework for the variety of social, behavioral, epidemiological, and administrative sciences bearing on the planning and evaluation of programs (see note 1 above). The first edition of this book appeared in 1980 with the coinage of the acronym PRECEDE (Green et al. 1980), with the further history of the model being traced in the successive editions (Green and Kreuter 1991; 1999) and in the evolution of the PROCEED components of the model (Green and Kreuter 2005).

4. Referring to the PRECEDE-PROCEED phases as "diagnoses" or as "assessments": In the first and second editions of this text, we used *diagnosis* to describe each stage of the PRECEDE planning process (e.g., social diagnosis and epidemiological diagnosis). In the third edition, we replaced diagnosis with *assessment,* mainly in response to users who felt uncomfortable with the term *diagnosis.* Though we still consider *diagnosis* to be an appropriate denotation for the processes described in each phase, its connotation tends to associate the model, uncomfortably for some, with clinical procedures. For some, it also tends to imply that all the assessments must start with or find a problem. Positive approaches to health and assets-based approaches to community assessment call for at least part of the planning process to be concentrated on aspirations, assets, and strengths, not just on needs, weaknesses, deficits, problems, and barriers. We will use the terms interchangeably in this edition, with "diagnosis" when a problem focus is intended and "assessment" when a more assets-based assessment, or combined assets-and-problems assessment, is intended.

5. The website at http://www.lgreen.net contains a searchable online bibliography of over 1,200 published applications and adaptations of the model for various purposes and with multiple audiences. For instance, searching by using the key words "child" or "children" yielded 72 titles; samples of the more recent work include Lam et al. (2016); Loureiro et al. (2009); Manios et al. (2012); and Mizumoto et al. (2013). Many of the references are also hyperlinked on this website to their abstracts or online full text. Many other hyperlinks are found on the website that are not listed in this book to minimize the problem of broken links (URLs that change) and the need for the reader to type in complicated URLs.

References

Ackerknecht, E. (1953). *Rudolf Virchow: Doctor, Statesman, Anthropologist.* University of Wisconsin Press. https://doi.org/10.1001/jama.1953.02940320082034

Alderman, M., Green, W., & Flynn, B.S. (1980). Hypertension control programs in occupational settings. *Public Health Reports, 95*(2), 158–63. Reprinted in Parkinson, R. (Ed.). (1982). *Managing Health Promotion in the Worksite.* Mayfield Publishing Co.

Andersen, R. (1968). *A Behavioral Model of Families' Use of Health Services* (Research Series No. 25). Center for Health Administration Studies, University of Chicago.

Baker, D.P., Leon, J., Smith Greenaway, E.G., Collins, J., & Movit, M. (2011). The education effect on population health: A reassessment. *Population and Development Review, 37*(2), 307–32. https://doi.org/10.1111/j.1728-4457.2011.00412.x

Berkman, L.F., & Kawachi, I. (2000). *Social Epidemiology.* Oxford University Press.

Bjãrås, G., Haglund, B., & Rifkin, S. (1991). A new approach to community participation assessment. *Health Promotion International, 6*(3), 199–206. https://doi.org/10.1093/heapro/6.3.199

Burke, J.G., Lich, K.H., Neal, J.W., Meissner, H.I., Yonas, M., & Mabry, P.L. (2015). Enhancing dissemination and implementation research using systems science methods. *International Journal of Behavioral Medicine, 22*(3), 283–91. https://doi.org/10.1007/s12529-014-9417-3

Cantor, J., Morisky, D.E., Green, L.W., Levine, D.M., & Salkever, D. (1985). Cost-effectiveness of educational interventions to improve patient outcomes in blood pressure control. *Preventive Medicine, 14*(6), 782–800. http://doi.org/10.1016/0091-7435(85)90071-4

Carolina, M.S., & Gustavo, L.F. (2003). Epidemiological transition: Model or illusion? A look at the problem of health in Mexico. *Social Science and Medicine, 57*(3), 539–50. https://doi.org/10.1016/S0277-9536(02)00379-9

Dubos, R. (1987/1959). *Mirage of Health: Utopias, Progress, and Biological Health.* Rutgers University.

Farquhar, J. & Green, L.W. (2015). Community intervention trials in high-income countries. In Detels, R., Gulliford, M., Abdool Karim, Q., and Tan, C.C. (Eds.), *Oxford Textbook of Public Health* (6th ed., Vol. 2, pp. 516–27). Oxford University Press. https://doi.org/10.1093/med/9780199661756.003.0112

Feinstein, L., Sabates, R., Anderson, T.M., Sorhaindo, A., & Hammond, C. (2006). *What are the effects of education on health?* Proceedings of the Copenhagen Symposium, Organisation for Economic Co-operation and Development.

Fenner, F. (1982). Global Eradication of Smallpox. *Reviews of Infectious Diseases, 4*(5), 916–30. Retrieved May 20, 2021, from https://www.jstor.org/stable/4452859

Fielding, J.E., & Teutsch, S.M. (2013). *Public Health Practice: What Works.* Oxford University Press. https://doi.org/10.1093/acprof:oso/9780199892761.001.0001

Golden, S., McLeroy, K., Green, L.W., Earp, J.A., & Lieberman, L.D. (2015). Upending the social ecological model to guide health promotion efforts toward policy and environmental change. *Health Education and Behavior, 42*(Suppl. 1), 8S–14S. https://doi.org/10.1177/1090198115575098

Green, L.W. (1970a) Identifying and overcoming barriers to the diffusion of knowledge about family planning. *Advances in Fertility Control, 5,* 21–9. Reprinted in *Journal of the Institute of Health Education, 9,* 2–10. https://doi.org/10.1080/03073289.1971.10805995

Green, L.W. (1970b). Should health education abandon attitude change strategies: Perspectives from recent research. *Health Education Monographs, 1*(30), 24–48. Reprinted in Simonds, S.K. (ed.), *The SOPHE Heritage Collection of Health Education Monographs* (Vol. 1, pp. 215–39). Third Party Publishing Co.

Green, L.W. (1974). Toward cost-benefit evaluations of health education: Some concepts, methods and examples. *Health Education Monographs, 2*(Suppl. 2), 34–64. Reprinted in *Supplement to the Report of the President's Committee on Health Education.* (1974). National Health Council. Reprinted in *U.S. Congress: Disease Control and Health Education and Promotion* (pp. 939–65). (1975). Reprinted in *The SOPHE Heritage Collection of Health Education Monographs* (Vol. 3, pp. 129–54). (1982). Third Party Publishing Co.

Green, L.W. (1976). Change-process models in health education. *Public Health Reviews, 5*(1), 5–33.

Green, L.W. (1998). Prevention and health education in clinical, school, and community settings. In Maxcy, K.F., Rosenau, M.J., Last, J.M., & Wallace, R.B. (Eds.), *Maxcy-Rosenau-Last Public Health and Preventive Medicine* (14th ed., pp. 889–904). Appleton & Lange.

Green, L.W. (2001). Foreword. In Sussman, S. (Ed.), *Handbook of Program Development for Health Behavior Research and Practice* (pp. iii–iv). SAGE Publishing. http://dx.doi.org/10.4135/9781412991445

Green, L.W. (2006). Public health asks of systems science: To advance our evidence-based practice, can you help us get more practice-based evidence? *American Journal of Public Health, 96*(3), 406–9. https://doi.org/10.2105/AJPH.2005.066035

Green, L.W. (2007). The Prevention Research Centers as models of practice-based evidence two decades on. *American Journal of Preventive Medicine, 33*(Suppl. 1), S6–S8. https://doi.org/10.1016/j.amepre.2007.03.012

Green, L.W. (2008). Making research relevant: if it is an evidence-based practice, where's the practice-based evidence? *Family Practice, 25*(Suppl. 1), i20–4. https://doi.org/10.1093/fampra/cmn055

Green, L.W., & Allegrante, J.P. (2011). Healthy people 1980–2020: raising the ante decennially or just the name from public health education to health promotion to social determinants? *Health Education & Behavior, 38*(6), 558–62. https://doi.org/10.1177/1090198111429153

Green, L.W., & Glasgow, R. (2006). Evaluating the relevance, generalization, and applicability of research: Issues in external validation and translation methodology. *Evaluation & the Health Professions, 29*(1), 126–53. https://doi.org/10.1177/0163278705284445

Green, L.W., Hiatt, R.A., & Hoeft, K.S. (2015). Behavioural determinants of health and disease. In Detels, R., Gulliford, M., Karim, Q.A., & Tan, C.C. (Eds.), *Oxford Textbook of Public Health*

(6th ed., pp. 218–33). Oxford University Press. https://doi.org/10.1093/med/9780199661756
.001.0001

Green, L.W., & Kreuter, M.W. (1991). *Health Promotion Planning: An Educational and Environmental Approach.* Mayfield Publishing Co.

Green, L.W., & Kreuter, M.W. (1999). *Health Promotion Planning: An Educational and Ecological
Approach* (3rd ed.). Mayfield Publishing Co.

Green, L.W., & Kreuter, M.W. (2000). Commentary on the emerging Guide to Community
Preventive Services from a health promotion perspective. *American Journal of Preventive
Medicine, 18*(Supp. 1), 7–9. https://doi.org/10.1016/s0749-3797(99)00131-2

Green, L.W., & Kreuter, M.W. (2005). *Health Program Planning: An Educational and Ecological
Approach* (4th ed.). McGraw-Hill Publishing Co.

Green, L.W., Kreuter, M.W., Deeds, S.G., & Partridge, K.B. (1980). *Health Education Planning:
A Diagnostic Approach.* Mayfield Publishing Co.

Green, L.W., Levine, D.M., Wolle, J., & Deeds, S. (1979). Development of randomized patient
education experiments with urban poor hypertensives. *Patient Counselling and Health
Education, 1*(3), 106–11. https://doi.org/10.1016/s0738-3991(79)80027-0

Green, L.W., & Ottoson, J.M. (1999). *Community and Population Health* (8th ed.). WCB/
McGraw-Hill.

Green, L.W., & Ottoson J.M. (2004). From efficacy to effectiveness to community and back:
Evidence-based practice vs practice-based evidence. In Green, L., Hiss, R., & Glasgow, R.
(Eds.), *Proceedings from Conference: From Clinical Trials to Community: The Science of
Translating Diabetes and Obesity Research* (pp. 15–18). National Institutes of Health.

Green, L.W., Ottoson, J.M., Garcia, C., & Hiatt, R.A. (1999). Diffusion theory and knowledge
dissemination, utilization and integration in public health. *Annual Review of Public
Health*, 30, 151–74. https://doi.org/10.1146/annurev.publhealth.031308.100049

Green, L.W., & Raeburn, J. (1990). Contemporary developments in health promotion:
Definitions and challenges. In Bracht, N. (Ed.), *Health Promotion at the Community Level*
(pp. 29–44). SAGE Publishing.

Green, L.W., Richard, L., & Potvin, L. (1996). Ecological foundations of health promotion.
American Journal of Health Promotion, 10(4), 270–81. https://doi.org/10.4278/0890-1171
-10.4.270

Green, L.W., Wang, V.L., & Ephross, P.H. (1974). A 3-year, longitudinal study of the impact of
nutrition aides on the knowledge, attitudes, and practices of rural poor homemakers.
American Journal of Public Health, 64(7), 722–24. https://doi.org/10.2105/AJPH.64.7.722

Guinea Worm Disease Eradication: A Moving Target. (2019). *The Lancet, 393*(10178), 1261.
https://doi.org/10.1016/S0140-6736(19)30738-X

Hackam, D.G., & Anand, S.S. (2003). Commentary: cardiovascular implications of the
epidemiological transition for the developing world: Thailand as a case in point.
International Journal of Epidemiology, 32(3), 468–9. https://doi.org/10.1093/ije/dyg167

Hatcher, M.E., Green, L.W., Levine, D.M., & Flagle, C.E. (1986). Validation of a decision model
for triaging hypertensive patients to alternate health education interventions. *Social
Science and Medicine, 22*(8), 813–9. https://doi.org/10.1016/0277-9536(86)90235-2

Hernandez, L.M., & Blazer, D.G. (Eds.) (2006). *Genes, Behavior, and the Social Environment
Moving Beyond the Nature/Nurture Debate.* The National Academies Press. https://doi.
org/10.17226/11693

Huber, M., Knottnerus, J.A., Green, L., van der Horst, H., Jadad, A.R., Kromhout, D., Leonard,
B., Lorig, K., Loureiro, M.I., van der Meer, J.W.M., Schnabel, P., Smith, R., van Weel, C., &
Smid, J. (2011). How should we define health? *The BMJ, 343*(d4163). https://doi.org/10.1136
/bmj.d4163

Institute of Medicine. (2003a). *The Future of the Public's Health in the 21st Century.* The
National Academies Press. https://doi.org/10.17226/10548

Institute of Medicine. (2003b). *Who Will Keep the Public Healthy?: Educating Public Health*

Professionals for the 21st Century. The National Academies Press. https://doi.org/10.17226/10542

Institute of Medicine. (2012). *An integrated framework for assessing the value of community-based prevention.* National Academies Press. https://doi.org/10.17226/13487

Johnson, N.B., Hayes, L.D., Brown, K., Hoo, E.C., & Ethier, K.A. (2014). Centers for Disease Control and Prevention (CDC). CDC National Health Report: leading causes of morbidity and mortality and associated behavioral risk and protective factors—United States, 2005–2013. *Morbidity and Mortality Weekly Report, Suppl. 63*(4), 3–27. Retrieved May 20, 2021, from https://www.cdc.gov/mmwr/preview/mmwrhtml/su6304a2.htm

Kahan, S., Gielen, A., Fagan, P., & Green, L.W. (Eds.) (2014). *Health Behavior Change in Populations.* Johns Hopkins University Press.

Kawachi, I., Subramanian, S.V., & Almeida-Filho N. (2002). A glossary for health inequalities. *Journal of Epidemiology and Community Health, 56,* 647–52. http://dx.doi.org/10.1136/jech.56.9.647

Kokko, S., Green L.W., & Kannas, L. (2014). A review of settings-based health promotion with applications to sports clubs. *Health Promotion International, 29*(3), 494–509. https://doi.org/10.1093/heapro/dat046

Kreuter, M.W., & Green, L.W. (1978). Evaluation of school health education: Identifying purpose, keeping perspective. *Journal of School Health, 48*(4), 228–35. https://doi.org/10.1111/j.1746-1561.1978.tb03798.x

Kristof, N. (2019, December 28). "This Has Been the Best Year Ever." *The New York Times.* Retrieved May 20, 2021, from https://www.nytimes.com/2019/12/28/opinion/sunday/2019-best-year-poverty.html

Lam, W., Dawson, A., & Fowler, C. (2016). Approaches to better engage parent-child in health home-visiting programmes: A content analysis. *Journal of Child Health Care, 21*(1), 94–102. https://doi.org/10.1177/1367493516653260

Last, J., & McGinnis, J.M. (2003). The determinants of health. In Scutchfield, F.D. & Keck C.W. (Eds.), *Principles of Public Health Practice* (2nd ed., pp. 45–58). Delmar Learning.

Levine, D.M., Green, L.W., & Morisky, D. (1987). Effect of a structured health education program on reducing morbidity and mortality from high blood pressure. *Bibliotheca Cardiologica, 42,* 8–16.

Li, Y., Lawley, M.A., Siscovick, D.S., Zhang, D., & Pagán, J.A. (2016). Agent-Based Modeling of Chronic Diseases: A Narrative Review and Future Research Directions. *Preventing Chronic Disease, 13.* http://dx.doi.org/10.5888/pcd13.150561

Loureiro, M.I., Goes, A.R., Maia, T., Paim da Câmara, G., & Saboga Nunes, L. (2009). Mental health promotion during pregnancy and early childhood: an action-research project in primary health care. *Revista Portuguesa De Saúde Pública, Número Especial 25 Anos,* 79–89. Retrieved May 20, 2021, from http://hdl.handle.net/10362/4415

Manios, Y., Grammatikaki, E., Androutsos, O., Chinapaw, M.J.M., Gibson, E.L., Buijs, G., Iotova, V., Socha, P., Annemans, L., Wildgruber, A., Mouratidou, T., Yngve, A., Duvinage, K., de Bourdeaudhuij, I., & ToyBox-study group. (2012). A systematic approach for the development of a kindergarten-based intervention for the prevention of obesity in preschool age children: the ToyBox-study. *Obesity Reviews, 13*(Suppl. 1), 3–12. https://doi.org/10.1111/j.1467-789X.2011.00974.x

Marmot, M., & Wilkinson, R. (Eds.) (1999). *Social Determinants of Health* (1st ed.). Oxford University Press.

Marmot, M., & Wilkinson, R. (Eds.) (2006). *Social Determinants of Health* (2nd ed.). Oxford University Press.

Marmot, M. (2000). Social determinants of health: From observation to policy. *Medical Journal of Australia, 172*(8), 379–82. https://doi.org/10.5694/j.1326-5377.2000.tb124011.x

McGinnis, J. M., & Foege, W.H. (1993). Actual causes of death in the United States. *JAMA, 270*(18), 2207–12. https://doi.org/10.1001/jama.1993.03510180077038

McGinnis, J.M., Williams-Russo, P., & Knickman. J.R. (2002). The case for more active policy attention to health promotion. *Health Affairs, 21*(2), 78–93. https://doi.org/10.1377/hlthaff.21.2.78

Milio, N. (1981). *Promoting health through public policy.* F. A. Davis. Reprinted by the Canadian Public Health Association. (1987).

Minkler, M., & Wallerstein, N. (2003). *Community-Based Participatory Research for Health.* Jossey-Bass.

Mizumoto, K., Takahashi, T., Kinoshita Y., Higuchi, M., Bachroen, C., & Da Silva, V. (2013). A Qualitative Study of Risk Factors Related to Child Malnutrition in Aileu District, Timor-Leste. *Asia-Pacific Journal of Public Health, 27*(2), 1398–408. https://doi.org/10.1177/1010539513486175

Mokdad, A.H., Marks, J.S., Stroup, D.F., & Gerberding, J.L. (2004). Actual causes of death in the United States, 2000. *JAMA, 291*(10), 1238–45. https://doi.org/10.1001/jama.291.10.1238. Review. Erratum in: (2005), *JAMA, 293*(3), 293–4. https://doi.org/10.1001/jama.293.3.293

Morisky, D.E., Levine, D.M., Green, L.W., & Smith, C. (1982). Health education program effects on the management of hypertension in the elderly. *JAMA Internal Medicine, 142*(10), 1835–8. https://doi.org/10.1001/archinte.1982.00340230077014

Northridge, M.E., & Metcalf, S.S. (2016). Enhancing implementation science by applying best principles of systems science. *Health Research Policy and Systems, 14*(74), 1–8. https://doi.org/10.1186/s12961-016-0146-8

Puska, P., & Uutela, A. (2000). Community intervention in cardiovascular health promotion: North Karelia, 1972-1999. In Schneiderman, N., Speers, M.A., Silva, J.M., Tomes, H., & Gentry, J.H. (Eds.), *Integrating Behavioral and Social Sciences with Public Health* (pp. 73–96). American Psychological Association United Book Press, Inc.

Puska, P. (2000). Do we learn our lessons from the population-based interventions? *Journal of Epidemiology and Community Health, 54*(8), 562–3. https://doi.org/10.1136/jech.54.8.562

Puska, P., Vartiainen, E., Tuomilehto, J., Salomaa, V., & Nissinen A. (1998). Changes in premature deaths in Finland: successful long-term prevention of cardiovascular diseases. *Bulletin of the World Health Organization, 76*(4), 416–25.

Reisig, V., & Wildner, M. (2008). Prevention, Primary. In Kirch, W. (Ed.), *Encyclopedia of Public Health.* Springer, Dordrecht. https://doi.org/10.1007/978-1-4020-5614-7_2759

Roberts, L. (2019). Exclusive: Battle to wipe out debilitating guinea worm parasite hits 10-year delay. *Nature, 574,* 157–8. https://doi.org/10.1038/d41586-019-02921-w

Rogers, E.M. (1962). *Diffusion of innovations* (1st ed.). Free Press of Glencoe.

Roussos, S., & Fawcett, S.B. (2000). A review of collaborative partnerships as a strategy for improving community health. *Annual Review of Public Health, 21,* 369–402. https://doi.org/10.1146/annurev.publhealth.21.1.369

Sanchez, V. (2000). Reflections on community coalition staff: Research directions from practice. *Health Promotion Practice, 1*(4), 320–2. https://doi.org/10.1177/152483990000100407

Schiller, P., Steckler, A., Dawson, L., & Patton, F. (1987). *Participatory Planning in Community Health Education: A Guide Based on the McDowell County, West Virginia Experience.* Third Party Publishing.

Sepúlveda, J., & Gómez, D.H. (1998). Origin, direction and destination of the health transition in Mexico and Latin America. In Sánchez, D.M., Bazzani, R., & Gómez, S. (Eds.), *Priorities in collective health research in Latin America.* GEOPS.

Thunberg, G. (2019, September 23). *Transcript: Greta Thunberg's Speech at the U.N. Climate Action Summit.* Retrieved May 20, 2021, from https://www.npr.org/2019/09/23/763452863/transcript-greta-thunbergs-speech-at-the-u-n-climate-action-summit

Truswell, A.S., Hiddink, G.J., Green, L.W., Roberts, R., & van Weel, C. (2012). Practice-based evidence for weight management: alliance between primary care and public health. *Family Practice, 29*(Suppl. 1), i6–i9. https://doi.org/10.1093/fampra/cmr058

Vartiainen, E., Paavola, M., McAlister, A., & Puska, P. (1998). Fifteen-year follow-up of smoking prevention effects in the North Karelia Youth Project. *American Journal of Public Health, 88*(1),81–5. https://doi.org/10.2105/ajph.88.1.81

Wallerstein, N., Duran, B., Oetzel, J.G., & Minkler, M. (Eds.). (2018). *Community-Based Participatory Research for Health: Advancing Social and Health Equity* (3rd ed.). Jossey-Bass.

Wandersman, A., & Florin, P. (2000). Citizen participation and community organizations. In Rappaport, J., & Seidman, E. (Eds.), *Handbook of Community Psychology* (pp. 247–72). Springer Science & Business Media. https://doi.org/10.1007/978-1-4615-4193-6

Wilber, Ken. (1998). *The Marriage of Sense and Soul: Integrating Science and Religion*. Random House.

Wold, B., & Samdal, O. (Eds.) (2012.) *An Ecological Perspective on Health Promotion: Systems, Settings and Social Processes*. Bentham Publishing. https://doi.org/10.2174/9781608053414 1120101

Wu, J., Liu, Y., Rao, K., Sun, Q., Qian, J., & Li, Z. (2004). Education-related gender differences in health in rural China. *American Journal of Public Health, 94*(10), 1713–6. https://doi.org/10.2105/ajph.94.10.1713

Zimmerman, E., & Woolf, S.H. (2014). *Understanding the relationship between education and health*. National Academies Press. https://doi.org/10.31478/201406a

CHAPTER 2

Participation and Community Engagement in Planning

•

Lawrence W. Green, Andrea Carlson Gielen,
and Marshall W. Kreuter

The fight for equity can be won only if vulnerable and oppressed communities can be fully engaged as partners in taking action to address the health and social problems about which they—not "outside experts"—know most deeply.

—Nina Wallerstein, Bonnie Duran, John G. Oetzel
and Meredith Minkler, 2018

Learning Objectives

After completing the chapter, the reader will be ready to:

- Describe why effective community program planning requires the active engagement of residents, community leaders and public and private partners at the most local level.
- Choose planning strategies that accommodate the diversity of values and needs within the specific population of interest.
- Explain why community members are more likely to participate in community public health efforts when they understand what you (and your collaborators) can and cannot do.

In chapter 1, we called out participation as a hallmark of the PRECEDE-PROCEED model. Participation sets the stage for the first step in program planning: deciding what kind of program or problem needs to be addressed. Planning any public health program—especially health promotion programs—should begin with engagement of the people who are most directly affected as potential subjects of public health surveillance or the objects of communications and programs or policy changes. That involvement should start with consideration of their overall quality of life, even before health assessments. Ideally, participation by local community members in formative, community-based research produces better planning, better plans, better programs and policies, and (most importantly) better outcomes.

ECOLOGICAL CONTEXT AND PROBLEMS AS THE FIRST CONCERN OF COMMUNITIES

Health programs do not spring from a social vacuum, nor should they be transplanted directly from a cookie-cutter manual of central-office health plans dictated or formulated great distances away from the people they are to serve. A population's needs typically emerge in community or organizational **settings**, and so should the programs to address these needs. Understanding these needs and programs demands both lay citizens' and professionals' knowledge of the people affected by the problems. The *ecological* perspective tells us that the policies and other factors influencing a population's health status and perceptions are shaped, modified, and maintained by people's interaction with the **community** environments and social structures in which they live their lives, as seen in figure 2.1 (Frankish et al. 2015). Population health programs can address the needs of different types of communities depending on their mandates and scope. Communities can be defined by geographic areas such as counties or states; organizations or settings such as workplaces, schools, places of worship, or health care delivery settings; or social groupings such as sororities, professional societies, or civic action committees.

The *educational* perspective tells us that people (1) learn continuously from their environmental surroundings and social structures, and (2) can develop, individually or collectively, the knowledge and skills to modify them. These two perspectives point us to the central themes of this book and the PRECEDE-PROCEED model: that people and their environments interact continuously, with reciprocal effects on each other. That is, people influence their social and physical environments through their attitudes and behavior (individually and collectively), and they learn and are influenced *by* their **environments** and their behavior, as shown in box 2.1. An essential starting point, then, is the engagement of people in defining their social conditions and quality of life concerns so that we can know what is important to them, beyond our relatively narrow health perspective.

Understanding the social context of communities from the perspective of those who live, work, study, worship or receive health care there is both a pragmatic and a moral imperative. It is pragmatic because the actions necessary to resolve contemporary health problems or to pursue equitable and just health goals require joint participation from multiple community institutions and

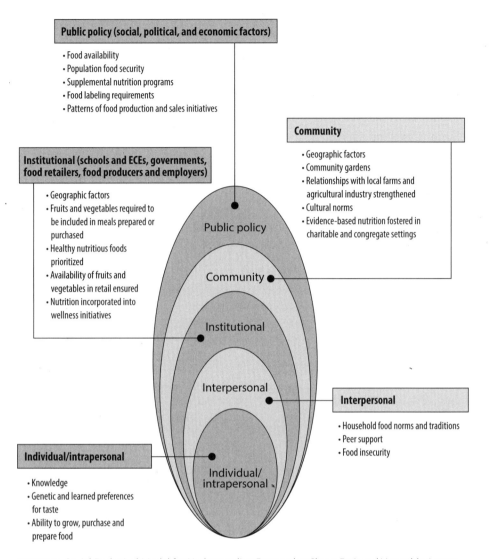

FIGURE 2.1. Social Ecological Model for Understanding Factors that Shape Fruit and Vegetable Access and Intake. *Sources:* Adapted from Rimer, B., & Glanz, K. (2005). *Theory at a Glance: A Guide for Health Promotion Practice.* US Department of Health and Human Services, National Institute of Health, and National Cancer Institute. Available from https://cancercontrol.cancer.gov/brp/research/theories_project/theory.pdf. See also: Institute of Medicine. (2003). *Who Will Keep the Public Healthy?: Educating Public Health Professionals for the 21st Century.* National Academies Press. For more information, see https://www.healthypeople.gov/2020/law-and-health-policy.

individuals. It is also pragmatic because people living day-to-day with the issues to be addressed will have experience, knowledge, and insights that professionals might not have. Without some mutual belief that the issue at hand is worthy of attention, time, and effort, joint participation is unlikely. The imperative also is moral, based on the principles of informed consent and respect. People should be informed and their views acknowledged, and whenever possible honored, in program and policy decisions. Failure to attend to this imperative would be both undemocratic and disrespectful, denying people personally or via their representatives the opportunity to register their concerns on matters that affect their health and quality of life.

Grounded in these two imperatives, **social assessment** is a first step in health program or policy planning, but aspects of it are repeated throughout the entire planning process, especially in health promotion planning. We define social assessment as *the application, through broad participation, of multiple sources of information, both objective and subjective, designed to expand the mutual understanding of people regarding social problems and quality of life issues that might relate to their aspirations for the common good.*

For this first phase of planning, the measurement of these sources of information is generally based on (1) social and economic indicators for the population, and (2) quality of life indicators for individuals. One purpose of the social assessment is to help planners expand their view by taking note of those community aspirations and social goals that could benefit from improved health, as well as those that might compete with health for resources and attention. Health planning must seek ways to link health to those potentially competing social

---

BOX 2.1

Case Example: Layers of Community Involvement in a Worksite Program

A highly trained team of Minnesota professionals and University of Minnesota investigators carried out a systematic application of PRECEDE-PROCEED to reduce wood dust exposure in woodworking shops. They formed a planning committee consisting of small woodworking shop owners, government officials, technical college instructors, health and safety professionals, and trade association representatives. They acknowledged that a "limitation of this study was the lack of involvement of employees in our planning activities other than as participants in a small focus group." Results of the study showed significant increases in worker awareness, increases in stage of readiness to change, and actual behavioral changes consistent with dust control. But the change in dust concentration fell short of statistical significance with a 10.4% reduction. The authors attribute the shortfall to problems of measurement and the resistance of employers to using expensive environmental controls or equipment. Would a more significant engagement of employees possibly also have produced more substantial commitment and change among both employees and employers? Would more attention to the financial and related concerns of employers have produced greater effort on theirr part to obtain and use equipment for dust control?

Source: Brosseau, L.M., Parker, D.L., Lazovich, D., Milton, T., & Dugan, S. (2002). Designing intervention effectiveness studies for occupational health and safety: The Minnesota wood dust study. *American Journal of Industrial Medicine, 41*(1), 54–61. https://doi.org/10.1002/ajim.10029

and quality of life goals and show how health improvements can contribute to them, or harmonize health goals with them so that health and social or quality of life benefits are seen as complementary. This chapter's phase of PRECEDE-PROCEED planning is concerned particularly with this understanding. The situation analysis that flows from a mutual understanding builds a shared sense of what is important and what resources are available to guide the health program planning, implementation, and evaluation processes that follow.

SOCIAL AND HEALTH CONDITIONS: A RECIPROCAL RELATIONSHIP

Diagrammatic representations of the PRECEDE-PROCEED model usually present it as a linear, cause-and-effect process where *inputs* (implementation of **health education**, policy and other interventions) cause certain changes that will eventually lead to *outcomes* (health and improved quality of life). Of course, some of these linkages, especially the relationships between health and the social or personal quality of life, are not actually one-way streets. A more realistic view is suggested in figure 2.2, representing the relationships between health problems and quality of life at the individual and community levels. The arrows indicate that health influences quality of life (QOL) at the same time that QOL and the social factors (including structural) associated with it affect health.

Social determinants of health include the cumulative effects of past and current **conditions of living** that combine to enhance or compromise optimum health, many of which are beyond any individual's control. These include history and culture, including structural racism and other forms of systematic oppression; levels, quality, and distribution of employment, income, and education; housing quality and opportunity; the availability, quality, and cost of health insurance; and the safety of neighborhoods (Berkman et al. 2014; Fielding and

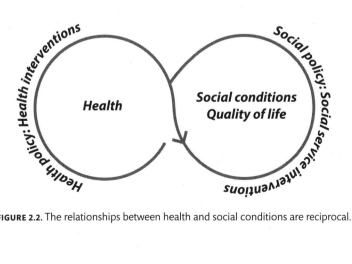

FIGURE 2.2. The relationships between health and social conditions are reciprocal.

Teutsch 2012; Green and Allegrante 2011; Green and Gielen 2015; Kahan et al. 2014; Marmot 2000; Marmot and Wilkinson 2006; Wallerstein et al. 2018). These determinants also lie beyond the purview of the health fields as conventionally defined, but they cannot be relegated entirely to other fields outside the health sector. Even within the health professions, greater attention to these social determinants and quality of life outcomes is needed from professionals whose scope is limited solely to medical care settings and health outcomes (Bunker 2001).

The arrow in figure 2.2 implies that social conditions and quality of life can lead to health problems or the capacity and will to cope with health problems. Health workers can effectively address this aspect of the reciprocal relationship mainly in cooperation with social workers, educators, housing and recreation professionals, law enforcement, community activists, and those in other sectors who shape social policy and social service programs.

Recognition that structures supportive of health need to be in place beyond the walls of our health care delivery system in order to improve the public's health has led to the promotion of *population* health and the preeminence of policy solutions for addressing today's public health problems, as also seen in chapter 1. It remains true, however, that community engagement is central to effective development and implementation of policy solutions. This reality has stimulated a growing emphasis on community coalitions to facilitate the collaboration and shared resources needed across sectors and organizations. It also has stimulated support and **advocacy** for changing social structures for improved **health equity**, even including environmental reforms to control global warming. Attention to issues of health equity is a practical response to addressing the cumulative, adverse effects of structures and systems that perpetuate inequities, as well as a moral imperative, as noted by Adler and Rehkopf: "Health disparities result from both biological differences and social disparities. We focus on the latter not just because the effect is greater, but also because they are avoidable and inherently unjust." (2008)

This collaborative and capacity building emphasis in community health has led in turn to a growing emphasis on **social capital** in the health literature, with its notions of interorganizational trust and cooperation to bond and bridge the complementary rather than competing capabilities of different sectors and organizations (Hawe and Shiell 2000; Kreuter and Lezin 2002).

The arrow in figure 2.2 also indicates that social conditions and quality of life are themselves influenced by health problems or concerns amenable to modification by policies and other interventions for health improvement or maintenance. PRECEDE-PROCEED, at this stage, emphasizes this aspect of the reciprocal exchange. At later stages of the planning process, we will address the organizational, policy, and regulatory ways in which health programs can alter social determinants of health. Meanwhile, recognizing at this stage the feedback loop in figure 2.2 from quality of life produced by health can make the health professional's job easier. That is because people will appreciate and support health innovations and policies (including regulations) if they can see clearly how such efforts address not only their health, but also their social and economic concerns and quality of life (see also Centers for Disease Control and Prevention 2000; Raeburn and Rootman 1998).

HEALTH AS AN INSTRUMENTAL RATHER THAN TERMINAL VALUE

The social assessment phase of the PRECEDE-PROCEED model is more than a step in a planning and evaluation framework; it is also a way of thinking. This becomes evident when we ask, "Among the many things in life we value, where does health fit?" Health is certainly a desirable state. Music, art, work, and play are also highly valued to different degrees, as are parenting or friendship, as well as daily pleasures such as eating. We value many good things in life—things that compete with each other for our investment of time, interest, energy, and resources. In day-to-day affairs, it is rare for people to engage in a given health-related behavior primarily because they believe the behavior is going to make them live longer lives. More likely, actions we deem to be healthful can be explained in terms of more immediate benefits as to how those actions make us feel, function, or look. In some cultures, health behaviors are tied to religious and spiritual tenets. Generally, health seems to be cherished because it serves other ends.[1]

The 1986 Ottawa Charter for Health Promotion put it this way: "Health is seen as a resource for everyday life, not the objective of living" (First International Conference on Health Promotion 1986; Kreuter et al. 2003). Last's *Dictionary of Epidemiology* added that "it is a positive concept, emphasizing social and personal resources as well as physical capabilities" (Last 2000; Last 2002, 520). The sociologist Talcott Parsons defined health as "the ability to perform important social roles" (McDowell 2002; Parsons 1964, 433). These functional views of health see it as a means to other ends and define health in terms of a person's ability to adapt to social and environmental circumstances. This puts health squarely into an educational and ecological perspective.

Planners who acknowledge that health is an instrumental value use that insight quite practically, at both the population and individual levels. When seeking collaboration with non-health organizations, health planners first identify the priority values of those organizations and then show how strategic health improvements can enhance those values. For example, corporate decision-makers are more likely to support health initiatives for their employees, or even for their communities, if they can see how those initiatives relate to their corporate missions. They respond most readily to those health programs that might affect their priorities such as performance, absenteeism, or excessive medical claims (as seen in chapter 11). Similarly, school officials are more likely to support integrated school health programs when they are presented with evidence that such programs reinforce their educational mission by affecting attendance and academic performance (as seen in chapter 12).

At the individual level, the application of tailored communications using technology has given health professionals the opportunity to apply our understanding of ultimate and instrumental values while taking a population approach to personal health, as shown in box 2.2 (Gold and Atkinson 2005, and also chapter 14 in this edition). In tailored health communications, an algorithm generates specific, personalized messages based on an assessment of an individual's characteristics, sometimes including those things they value and enjoy (Gielen et al. 2015; Gielen et al. 2018).

BOX 2.2

Case Example: Linking Health Behavior Communications to Instrumental and Ultimate Values

Suppose a large work site wants to implement a **health promotion** program, a part of which includes a tailored communication component designed to increase the level of physical activity across the entire workforce. Brief questionnaires are given to 450 employees. Communication messages are created for various combinations of responses to the questions. The responses of one of those employees, a 32-year-old woman named Ellie Watson, reveal that she has a keen interest in classical music and a passion for gardening. Among the hundreds of messages designed for the subsequent communication back to the 450 employees, Watson will receive a personally addressed message framed within the context of her self-declared interests: listening to classical music while exercising and earning physical activity points through gardening. In contrast to messages encouraging Watson to increase her level of physical activity because science says it will give her cardiovascular benefits over time, tailoring constitutes a planned effort to connect the **ultimate values** associated with music and gardening with the **instrumental value** of physical activity and health.

ELICITING SUBJECTIVE ASSESSMENTS OF COMMUNITY CONCERNS

Assessments that elicit information from community members about their subjective quality of life concerns provide the foundation for health planning; this is important for every type of community a planner is trying to serve—counties, schools, health clinics, and so on. Surveys, structured interviews, or focus groups are frequently used to gain insight on such concerns (see, for example, Buta et al. 2011; Frattaroli et al. 2006; Frattaroli et al. 2012; Johnson et al. 2012; McDonnell et al. 2011). The subjective assessment of quality of life through participatory research methods offers a view of a particular situation through the eyes of the community members themselves,[2] who share what matters to them and show where health lies in the context of their lives. Health promotion seeks to promote healthful conditions that improve quality of life as seen through the eyes of those whose lives are affected. Although health might have *instrumental value* in reducing risks for morbidity and mortality, its day-to-day value lies in its contribution to their terminal values of quality of life.

For example, Kaiser Family Foundation staff and members of the state governor's office conducted a social reconnaissance with the state of Mississippi. Prior to making health promotion grants in that state, they conducted structured interviews in local communities. The interviews revealed that the main concerns of the population centered on the quality of housing and economic development, which they related in part to the quality of schooling. These became central themes in the subsequent analysis of health problems and led to the coordination of planning with the state housing and economic development offices and with the local school boards (Butler et al. 1996; Geiger 2002). In the United States, health care delivery systems such as hospitals and health departments have completed community health assessments (CHAs) and community health improvement plans (CHIPs) as part of national accreditation processes. Such accreditation requirements are designed to highlight the importance of obtaining input from community residents and cross-sector partners to reach stronger consensus on the needs to be addressed.

RELEVANCE OF AN ECOLOGICAL AND ENVIRONMENTAL APPROACH

An ecological approach to planning stimulates our search for relevant connections among the broad factors that affect health and anticipates the potential impact of those connections. For example, health care and agency administrators who are unaware of the rationale for focusing on the association between health and quality of life may resist contributing their organizational support to broader social programs because they believe that finite health resources will be spent on non-health objectives, which they may perceive as a bottomless pit. However, there is growing support among those in health care and public health for transforming health systems in ways that increase their contribution to prevention and population health, particularly as they relate to reducing disease burden through improvements in the social determinants of health.

Achieving population health goals will require what the National Institutes of Health (NIH) calls a "macro" integration of biomedical, behavioral, and population-level sciences as part of an ecological worldview (Mabry et al. 2008). If preventive health programs are unable to attract the interest of the community or gain the trust and cooperation of non-health organizations, they stand a diminished chance of success in today's world. The application of PRECEDE-PROCEED planning is designed to help planners employ a sound educational effort, one that increases health care and agency directors' understanding that preventive health programs addressing the increasingly complex social and behavioral determinants of health will depend on the cooperation of other sectors. Unless the health sector can buy into the broader social goals addressing the primary concerns to the community, planners may find their organizations on the sidelines of the mainstream of community action and energy, isolated from community resources.

The social assessment phase of PRECEDE-PROCEED (see also chapter 3) is designed to help planners with two tasks:

- to identify and interpret the social conditions and perceptions shared among the community members, and
- to make the connection between those conditions and perceptions and the diversity of health program strategies that will be needed to accommodate the diversity of values and needs.

THE PRINCIPLE AND PROCESS OF PARTICIPATION

The social assessment is an important step that precedes the analysis of relevant epidemiological data in a given target population. It applies the principle of participation to ensure the active involvement of those intended to benefit from a proposed program or policy change. The importance of this principle, echoed for decades in various applied social sciences, has been confirmed in community experience in several fields. Notable among these for our application is the general literature on technical assistance, including public health (especially health education), health care services, family planning, and agricultural extension.[3] This literature has been most extensively reflected in community and rural economic development and participatory research from around the world, because the gaps between the technical assistance and research agencies and the communities they seek to help seem greatest in underserved rural and inner city areas and in developing countries (Green et al. 1995; Wallerstein et al. 2018). Another body of literature concerns community involvement through *concientación*, a process largely of Latin-American origin in the 1960s and early 1970s. It refers in our context to a consciousness-raising process whereby persons with limited means become conscious of the political realities and root causes of their situation and take collective action to address them (Shor and Freire 1987).

One rationale for participation based on the differing but complementary perspectives scientists and lay people have concerning health is presented in figure 2.3. Scientists tend to have a sharper focus on the objective indicators of health, whereas lay people tend to have a more diffuse perception of health, with greater emphasis on subjective indicators. Their view is textured by aspects of their lives other than the strictly biological, such as social, emotional, and metaphysical or spiritual dimensions of health. "Objective" should not be equated with "actual," any more than "subjective" indicators should be discarded as meaningless. The objective data may be less biased by personal perceptions of those taking the measures, but they are only as accurate a reflection of reality as the investigators' aptitude in knowing what to ask or what to look for. Health professionals who work more intensively with their community members can help bridge these sometimes divergent worldviews.

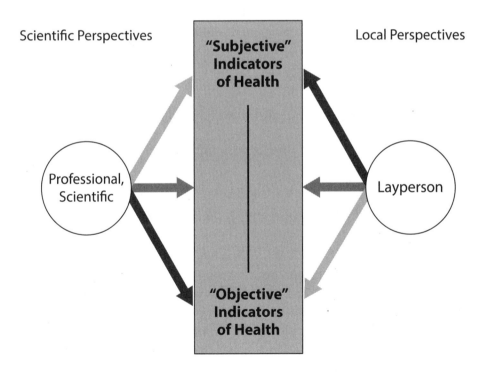

FIGURE 2.3. Professionals view health through a different set of lenses than do people viewing their own health or that of their community. The professional lenses have a greater acuity (represented by darker arrows) at the "objective" end of the spectrum of health and a less clear view of the "subjective" end of the spectrum (represented by lighter arrows). The public lenses are the opposite, with greater acuity at the "subjective" aspects of health and less clarity at the "objective" end of the health spectrum.

FORMS OF PARTICIPATION

Paulo Freire contrasted the extreme forms of participation as two theoretical approaches to community change. He characterized the first as "cultural invasion" and the second as "cultural synthesis." In cultural *invasion*, the actors from outside draw the thematic content of their action from their own values and ideology; their starting point is their own world, from which they enter the world they invade. In cultural *synthesis*, those who come from "another world" do not come as invaders. They come not to teach or transmit or give anything, but rather to learn about this new world along with the people in it.[4] Freire contended that those who are "invaded," irrespective of their level in society, rarely go beyond or expand on the models or innovations given to them, implying that there is little internalizing, little growth, and seldom much adoption, adaptation, and incorporation into their social fabric. In the synthesis approach, there are no imposed priorities: leaders and people work together to develop priorities and guidelines for action.

According to Freire, resolution of the inevitable contradictions between the views of leaders or outsiders and the views of the local people is only possible where the spirit of cultural synthesis predominates. "Cultural synthesis does not deny differences between the two views; indeed it is based on these differences. It does deny invasion of one by the other, but affirms the undeniable support each gives to the other." (Freire 1970, 183)[5]

The differences across cultures will vary depending on who the partners are. For example, health professionals of two or more organizations within the community may experience fewer cultural differences than between university researchers and local agency representatives, or between patients and clinicians. But cultural differences should always be considered and valued in the planning process (Huff et al. 2015).

Imagine a partnership project that involves the local fire department and injury researchers, who shared the goal of increasing the number of smoke alarms installed throughout their community (Frattaroli et al. 2012). Although the goal was the same, the approach between the two groups could be quite different, with the fire service leadership ready to instruct firefighters to make home visits immediately while the researchers wanted time to build teams that would confidently embrace new educational messaging, and data collection to facilitate follow-up and evaluation research. The clash between a culture of urgency and top-down decision-making versus one of emphasizing generalizability and team-building needed to be recognized so that a feasible and mutually agreeable approach to achieving the shared goal could be realized.

When members of a target audience are included in the planning process, as they should be, there are additional cultural considerations. Differences in sociocultural backgrounds, ethnicity, and education (among others) need to be respected and valued, and most importantly listened to in nonjudgmental ways. In the smoke alarm example, working within a predominantly Hispanic community required the planning team to appreciate not just language differences, but also community resident concerns about how their immigration status might be affected and how some residents could be worried by the presence of uniformed firefighters, perhaps even confusing them with police officers. Those who would deliver the smoke alarms would need to feel comfortable working with families from different backgrounds; building their skills and confidence in doing so is part of the program planning activities that will be discussed in later phases of the model (Frattaroli et al. 2012).

PARTICIPATION IN SETTING PRIORITIES

Because resources for health are finite, planners must set priorities to avoid the debilitating bind of trying to do too much with too little. The need to engender community participation and the need to set program priorities constitute mutually reinforcing reasons for putting the social assessment step at the beginning of the PRECEDE-PROCEED process. As you will discover in the next chapters, the careful analysis of epidemiological data on mortality and morbidity plays an important part in determining how resources will be allocated for health improvement efforts at the national, regional, provincial, state, or local levels. Political experience demonstrates, however, that priorities will not be based solely on statistical analyses indicating the pervasiveness of the problems, or even on their human burden and economic costs.

If planners set priorities based on objective health data without involving the community in the process, some of the priorities, judged to be of lower importance based on statistical criteria, will come back to haunt them on the grounds that the public's perceptions of what constitutes a priority was ignored. It would have been folly, for example, to ignore the anthrax concerns of the American public in 2001, even though only a handful of people had been exposed or suffered any health effects. The relatively enormous numbers dying of heart disease, cancer, diabetes, motor vehicle injuries, and other leading causes of death notwithstanding, the public's concern had to take priority for at least that brief period of time. The same is true of the late 2019/early 2020 emergence of the coronavirus (COVID-19) epidemic and growing public concerns about a pandemic, even in the early stages when cases and mortality remained relatively low.

The community will not often ask, "Why are you doing A or C?" They *will* ask, "Why aren't you doing F?" (as seen in figure 2.4). We are not calling for the abrogation of scientific evidence and professional judgment in favor of incorrect public understanding. Nor are we advocating for political decisions based on public polls. We *are* advocating for a sincere synthesis and search for common understanding as the basis for sound, effective program planning and implementation.[6]

PUBLIC PERCEPTIONS AND PROFESSIONAL DIAGNOSIS: COMMON GROUND

The need to discover common ground (area A) by bringing together the three key perceptions or assessments that influence planning is illustrated by figure 2.4: the public's perceived needs and priorities, health professionals' perceived "actual" or documented needs as indicated by scientific data, and policy makers' perceptions of resources, feasibilities, and policy. It is in area A where action is most likely, because it is here that policy makers and others who allocate resources see the greatest convergence of public sentiment and scientific data. The task of social assessment and the subsequent steps in health program planning is to bring the three spheres of perception into closer alignment, as shown in figure 2.5.

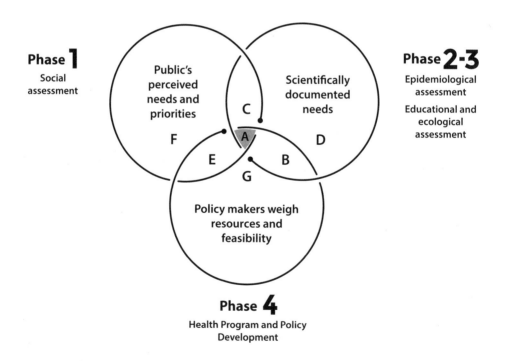

FIGURE 2.4. Finding common ground among the public's perception of needs, the health sector's measurements of needs, and policy makers' perception of resources and feasibility of meeting needs.

Usually, the public perceives its needs in ways that only partially overlap with what epidemiologists and other health scientists and professionals might view as "actual" or documented needs (figure 2.4, area C). Yet the view through lay lenses often carries as much weight (area E) with policy makers (elected legislators, appointed officials) as, if not more than, the scientific data brought to the table as "actual needs" by health professionals (area B). Priorities expressed by the public, who comprise political constituencies, will influence politicians in bringing resources to bear on issues of *common* concern and requiring organizational, policy, or regulatory action (area A). This is why public health education and media advocacy efforts to create an informed electorate are so important, especially when the actions to be taken involve not just individual health behavior, but policy and regulatory actions by politicians (Biglan et al. 2000; Chapman and Lupton 1995; Green et al. 2002; McLoughlin and Fennell 2000; Mindell 2001; Stead et al. 2002; Stillman et al. 2001).

The arrows in figure 2.5 indicate the directions in which each of the strategies in health program planning and development can pull or push the three spheres into greater alignment for common action. *Public health education* helps move the public's perception (area F) in the direction of what data and science have deemed to be the "actual needs" (area D), resulting in an increase for common

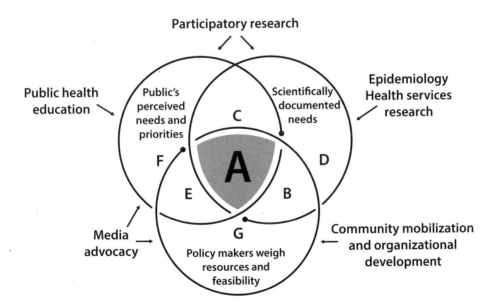

FIGURE 2.5. Bringing the three world views into closer alignment through public health education, participatory research, media advocacy, epidemiology, health services research, and community mobilization of resources enlarges the potential area for common action (A).

action (area A). *Media advocacy*, a more politicized form of health education directed at policy makers (area G) and to a lesser degree to the public (area F), seeks to pull the public's views and the policy makers' views into greater alignment, to further enlarge the area of action (area A). *Participatory research* engages the professional and scientific community (area D) in greater dialogue with the public (area F) on general community concerns or specific issues, thus enlarging common action in areas C and A. Finally, various strategies of **community organization**, mobilization of resources, grant-writing, organizational development, and strategic planning draw on documented needs from health services research (area D) to influence policy and resource allocation (area G) to further enlarge common action (area A).

One might assume that the principle of participation, so critical at the local level, is of lesser or even no importance at the national or state levels (Shoveller and Green 2002). Not so. When policies and priorities set at one level depend on implementation or compliance by people or institutions at another, planners must make every effort to solicit active participation, input, and even endorsement from that second level. Without such collaboration vertically, as well as horizontally within levels, the support and cooperation needed from the higher level will be developed more reluctantly and cautiously, if not defiantly.

Inattention to this simple principle, even at the highest levels, is at once a foolish and serious oversight. It is foolish because participation requires mostly simple acts of courtesy and respect, along with the time needed to foster dialogue and, ultimately, trust. It is serious because it often produces a threat to the proposed program. Continued failure to consult and reconcile differences fosters mistrust and undermines collaboration. Such mistrust explains much of the tension frequently observed between agencies at the national and state or state and local levels, and the cynicism of "street-level bureaucrats" employed by central levels to work at local levels (Lipskey 1980). It is also what marks a weakened democracy and fails to produce an informed electorate. As Rose described the function of open debate:

> "... more public information and debate on health issues is good, not just because it may lead to healthier choices by individuals but also because it earns a higher place for health issues on the political agenda. In the long run, this is probably the most important achievement of health education ... [that] in a democracy the ultimate responsibility for decisions on health policy should lie with the public." (Rose 1992, 123–240)

THE CAPACITY-BUILDING AND SUSTAINABILITY
CASE FOR PARTICIPATION

To this point, arguments for participation have emphasized the notions of cultural synthesis, cooperation, and facilitating a democratic process of planning. Another set of arguments centers on the pragmatic goal of transferring not only power of expertise and resources to local groups and organizations, but also the capacity to carry on after the external grants have expired—the **sustainability** case for participation (Green 1989).

An admittedly idealized characterization of health program planning in developing countries is presented in figure 2.6, based on World Health Organization (WHO) experience with anchor institutions or official agencies; see box 2.3. Although idealized, it is meant to provide a graphic vision of what health planners are trying to achieve through participatory planning. The twelve planning steps fall into two broad categories of actions separated by the vertical divider: community functions on the left and official agency functions on the right. In this instance, we view *community functions* as those closest to where the people whose needs are in question live or work. This could be a work team in a factory, a department or a floor of workers in an office building, an industrial plant, a classroom, a school, a neighborhood, a town, a county, or a district. *Official agency functions* refer to those taken by organizations operating under the auspices of government policies or public mandates at either the local, state or provincial, or national levels. Most often, this will be an official health agency or department, but it may also include a foundation or the headquarters of a private or voluntary health organization. Ideally, the needs and interests expressed at the local or subunit level would trigger the entire sequence. But because of the concentration of resources at higher levels of government or more central offices of other organizations, the process often starts as a top-down process.

EXAMINING THE STEPS OF ASSESSMENT

Functional Planning Steps. In figure 2.6, under "community functions," the three steps to the left at each level are those ideally initiated, implemented, and controlled by local people, or the people closest to the felt needs. These community functions are graphically drawn horizontally, side by side with official agency functions, rather than at the bottom of a vertical structure. This depiction seeks to avoid the perception of a necessarily hierarchical relationship characteristic of bureaucracies and levels of administration. The relationship between the communities and official agencies, regardless of their "level," need not (and ideally

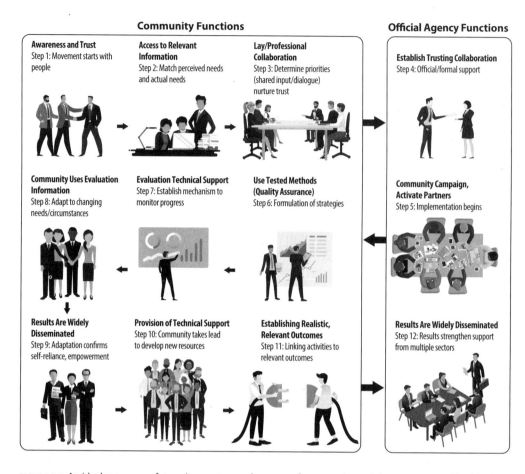

Community Functions

Awareness and Trust
Step 1: Movement starts with people

Access to Relevant Information
Step 2: Match perceived needs and actual needs

Lay/Professional Collaboration
Step 3: Determine priorities (shared input/dialogue) nurture trust

Official Agency Functions

Establish Trusting Collaboration
Step 4: Official/formal support

Community Uses Evaluation Information
Step 8: Adapt to changing needs/circumstances

Evaluation Technical Support
Step 7: Establish mechanism to monitor progress

Use Tested Methods (Quality Assurance)
Step 6: Formulation of strategies

Community Campaign, Activate Partners
Step 5: Implementation begins

Results Are Widely Disseminated
Step 9: Adaptation confirms self-reliance, empowerment

Provision of Technical Support
Step 10: Community takes lead to develop new resources

Establishing Realistic, Relevant Outcomes
Step 11: Linking activities to relevant outcomes

Results Are Widely Disseminated
Step 12: Results strengthen support from multiple sectors

FIGURE 2.6. An ideal sequence of steps in a system and process of community social assessment and health planning, leading to official agency or centralized support, intersectoral cooperation, a cycle of continuous capacity building in the community (Steps 7–10), and ultimately greater self-reliance. *Source:* Adapted from Green, L.W. (1983). New Policies in Education for Health. *World Health, xiii*(6), 13–17.

would not) be viewed or approached as bureaucratic. Bureaucratic structure implies a top-down command structure and bottom-up reporting structure. In planning for health programs, the ideal is for the initiative and the control to be vested at the most local level and for official agencies or legislatures to seek common elements of local needs and priorities that would benefit from their broader policy, regulatory, organizational, financial, or technical support, as with the supply of vaccine or face masks in a local COVID-19 epidemic.

Technical Support. All this talk about local initiative, autonomy, participation, and empowerment would seem to imply that the necessary skills and technical knowledge to carry out a systematic social diagnosis and planning process are extant in the local group or community. Clearly, communities do possess many of the skills and resources (although often untapped) needed to plan and implement an effective community-based health program.[7] At the same time, however, gaps

BOX 2.3
Anchor Institutions

In the United States, the term "anchor institutions" describes organizations that are anchored or securely tied to a particular place by a combination of "mission, invested capital, or relationships to customers, employees, residents, and vendors." Hospitals and universities are common examples of anchor institutions that have operated in one place for decades and are likely to be there for many more.

A growing number of anchor institutions have recognized that the communities in which they are embedded have economic and health profiles starkly at odds with the assets and relative prosperity of the institutions themselves. To address these disparities, some have adopted an "anchor mission" approach, including a commitment to deploy their considerable economic power in ways that benefit both the institutions and the communities surrounding them.

Source: Martin N. et al. (2017). *Advancing the Anchor Mission of Healthcare* (p. 10). The Democracy Collaborative.

usually do exist in local capacities and skills (Foster-Fishman et al. 2001; Hawe et al. 1997; Kreuter and Lezin 2002). With sufficient searching and encouragement, one can find indigenous skills and resources in the community, but they may remain dormant without concerted efforts to identify and bring those resources into play. When health planners nurture community participation, they:

- predispose the community by arousing indigenous community awareness, concern, and initiative;

- enable the community by providing technical assistance to those who wish to take initiative; and

- reinforce the community by connecting them with the sources of moral and tangible support needed from other levels of organization and generating systems of data that provide feedback on progress and accomplishments.

These are implicit, roughly in this order, in the three levels depicted by the three rows of the chart in figure 2.6. In other words, the community moves gradually from steps that predispose them to action to steps that enable them to take action, and then steps that reinforce their action.

Tasks Common Across PRECEDE Phases. In figure 2.6, the community functions are expressed in twelve steps. Cutting across all twelve are three essential elements that are applied, with some variation, in the first three phases of PRECEDE (this and the next four chapters)—the social assessment, the epidemiological assessment (including the health, behavioral, and environmental assessments), and the educational and ecological assessment. Those three steps are:

1. Self-study by the community (with or without technical assistance) of its needs, aspirations, and resources or assets (column 1);

2. Documentation of the presumed (and eventually measured, if possible) causes of the needs, or determinants of the desired goals (column 2);

3. Decision on the priorities to be assigned among the problems, needs, or goals, based on perceived importance and presumed changeability, and formulation of quantified goals, objectives, and strategies (column 3).

More technical skills are required for these three tasks in the epidemiological and the educational-ecological assessments, as shown in chapters 4, 5, and 6 of this volume. For example, a professional planning staff must use some epidemiology and some social-behavioral research in reviewing the scientific literature to document the causes or determinants of health. They need to incorporate principles because they provide the critical scientific evidence to reinforce the local insight reflected in the social and quality of life diagnosis. Step 3 in figure 2.6 will reveal a good deal about the level of collaboration between professionals and lay participants. Hawe notes that planners can take two routes to change (Blankertz and Hazem 2002; Hawe 1996). They can either base a proposed change on the needs of the community or consumer, or they can focus primarily on the needs of the managers or organization(s) they serve. This distinction made Hawe (1996) warn those engaged in community-based planning of the political temptation to seek community "endorsement" to support the planner's agenda: "They should recognize the danger in sublimating community interests in an orchestrated process of consensus building and priority setting, which has a high risk of having its deliberations ignored." PRECEDE-PROCEED suggests that a better option is to check assumptions and create situations that make it possible for the different perspectives to inform each other, ideally finding common ground and purpose.

Equipped with factual data on a community's problems and trends, professionals will come face-to-face with the felt needs of community members and their natural desire to acknowledge the strengths, not just the problems, of their community. Often the felt needs will rank low, if at all, on routine data listings of leading causes of mortality or morbidity. Reconciling these differences is central to the educational approach to health program planning featured by this book and the PRECEDE-PROCEED model.

Official Functions. In Step 4, an official health organization formalizes the plans or proposals submitted by one or more local community groups and generates a strategic plan for allocating its resources. Official agency resources include funding, material support, transfers of necessary authority, and technical assistance. Step 5 suggests the need for centralized agencies to coordinate their assistance with communities or subcommunities so that a harmonized flow of resources reaches the community proportionate to the distribution of the needs to be met by programs. Too often, the state and national organizations seeking to carry out their separate missions at the local level compete unwittingly for the time and effort of precious talent and energy in underserved communities. Accordingly, intersectoral and interagency coordination at the central levels will help reduce the confusing and often redundant signals communities receive.

Implementation and Evaluation. Steps 6 through 8 require central agencies to return selected implementation and evaluation functions to the community. Information and technical assistance number among the resources communities need to be able to carry out these functions. We are going beyond the social assessment phase here, but it should serve you at this stage to have a broad picture that anticipates how the whole process of community organization and development for health might play out.

The Capacity-Building, Self-Reliance, and Sustainability Cycle. Steps 7 through 10 engage the community in a progressively greater degree of responsibility for managing and evaluating their own progress. By Step 10, the "competent community"[8] will have unearthed or developed its own indigenous resources to maintain the program[9] or to move on to solve other problems on its priority list.[10] Rather than turning back to central agencies for more support at that point (Step 10), the community is "empowered" with its own "collective efficacy" and returns to Step 7, continuing the self-reliance and sustainability cycle outlined in figure 2.6 (Bandura 2004; Fetterman 2000; Green 2004; Minkler et al. 2002; Wandersman and Florin 2000; Zimmerman et al. 2004).

Evaluation, Demonstration, and Diffusion. Often, the payoff of central support to local community projects, from the point of view of the official or central agencies, is not only solving a local problem, but also demonstrating the problem-solving process by a typical community. The hope of most grant-making organizations is that their grants will inspire other communities or groups to emulate the example demonstrated by the grantee community. To maximize this potential, the evaluation of project impact and outcomes (Step 11) becomes a central priority. Evaluation results can not only inspire other communities as practice-based evidence, but can also help the funding organizations by providing documented examples of how they can improve their coordination with other central organizations (Step 12) and their technical assistance and support to other communities. Such demonstration, evaluation, and documented experience serve as powerful complements to the diffusion of best practices from formal research studies. The latter carry some limitations of credibility by themselves because community practitioners view the experimentally controlled study circumstances from which best practices or evidence-based practices are derived as unrepresentative of their own circumstances (Green 2008; Green and Mercer 2001).

KEEPING PERSPECTIVE ON PARTICIPATION
AND PARTNERSHIP

Broad participation through a representation process should be sought in the diagnosis of needs, because some of the people least technically "skilled" or formally trained in planning or "making policy" will bring other valuable assets to the planning table.

Although professional health practitioners and planners can take great pride in working collaboratively and responsively with their patients and communities, they should not lose sight of the technical insights and scientific data and skill they can share with communities. Counsel offered in the 1983 WHO Expert Committee Report remains valid even today:

> While health care workers should not compel communities to accept the health technologies they propose, they should also not allow themselves to be forced into a situation where they have to abdicate their views on technical matters. The common ground between the two groups should serve as a basis for fruitful dialogue, which may lead to change . . . (WHO 1986, 17; see also Green and Mercer 2001)

Professionals should take care not to abdicate their responsibilities while engaging the community in dialogue. In working hard to avoid being manipulative, health professionals can go too far and be so fearful of falling into Freire's "cultural invasion" trap of imposing their own agenda that they fail to offer constructive assistance.

As a planner, you can do two things to avoid this situation. First, keep in mind the fact that you, the lay community, and your collaborators in other agencies and sectors are *partners*. Each can contribute technical or cultural experience and capacities to the task of making a difference. Second, make every effort to ensure that all the partners understand what you do and whom you represent. People are more willing to collaborate with you when they know what agency or group you represent and what its mission or agenda is. They need to understand what you can and cannot do—the technical capacities you have to offer as well as the limitations placed on you by your agency or employer. An understanding of these issues, which at first glance may seem irrelevant, helps all parties clarify boundaries and roles and to set realistic expectations.

Partnership implies complementary roles and contributions. Each partner can magnify the contribution of others and, through the partnership, can **leverage** their own capabilities and resources. In the end, the partnership should evolve into delegated power, relinquished by the outside helping agencies, and eventually into full control by the community and its own professional and lay leadership. This will not happen easily if the partnership starts out with a senior partner from the outside, with the community in the role of junior partner.

SUMMARY: PARTICIPATION AND COMMUNITY ENGAGEMENT

The social and behavioral sciences have played important roles in addressing many of the leading causes of death, including injuries, heart disease, cancer, stroke, and infectious diseases (Bauer et al. 2014). One increasingly important aspect of this contribution has been the use of methods and strategies to engage community members in personal health and public health intervention and prevention efforts (Lavery 2018). For instance, this line of participatory health education and support for behavioral and social change has been accelerated in recent years with m-health, the use of portable cell phones and handheld computing and tracking devices (Gold 2022). Moreover, the tools and rationales for population and community engagement have increased in variety and social or theoretical support (Campbell and Jovchelovitch 2000; Rowe and Frewer 2005):

1. Social justice holds that people have the right to be involved in decisions, settings, and processes that affect them.

2. Participation strengthens the opportunity for individuals to participate in the broader society through increased social capital and strengthened democracy.

3. Engagement of intended audiences and affected individuals in the planning, implementation, and evaluation of public health interventions strengthens our interventions by providing a broader range of perspectives on the nature of the problem, its importance, and possible solutions, which can help make our interventions more acceptable and relevant to the intended audience(s).

4. Population and community engagement in interventions may strengthen the ability of individuals, families, and communities to address other health and community issues by building community capacity. (Goodman et al. 1998)

Many mechanisms for population and community engagement have been identified in the literature (Rowe and Frewer 2005). These range from data collection strategies that capture information on population preferences and attitudes to the use of citizen advisory panels and review boards and community-based participatory research (CBPR). This suggests considerable variation in participation, from simply providing information on preferences to actual degrees of control in multiple stages of problem identification, intervention development, evaluation, and dissemination of outcomes (Burke et al. 2013; Rifkin 2014).

A critical issue with engagement and participation is the extent to which participation, however defined, affects program outcomes and improves population health. Numerous efforts to address participation outcomes have been noted in a recent systematic review (Chuah et al. 2018), indicating that much of the work has focused on specific health conditions or specific target populations and settings. Moreover, as noted in other systematic reviews of community participation, the outcomes from participation may hinge upon the extent or intensity of participation (Chuah et al. 2018; Rifkin 2014).

Among several models of participatory practice, an important approach receiving particular attention in recent years is the inclusion of individuals from targeted communities as outreach and program delivery professionals. Frequently referred to as "community health workers," the use of community members in health-related interventions has increased dramatically over the past fifty years, and there is compelling evidence of their effectiveness and efficiency in both developing and developed countries and settings (Chuah et al. 2018; Jeet et al. 2017; Kim et al. 2016; Perry et al. 2014).

A second model of participatory practice is CBPR, in which community members are actively engaged in stages of the research and intervention processes from assessment to design, evaluation, and dissemination (Burke et al. 2013). Community members may also participate in a wide range of research-related activities, including data collection, analysis, interpretations, and dissemination. While there are numerous examples of CBPR in the literature, it may be sufficient to note that in 2004 the US Agency for Healthcare Quality and Research completed a systematic review of the evidence for CBPR (Viswanathan et al. 2004) in which the researchers concluded that, done properly, CBPR can "assist in developing culturally appropriate measurement instruments . . . and establishing a level of trust that enhances both the quantity and the quality of data collected."

In summary, health program planning should begin with more than token participation from community members. It should begin with a level of engagement warranted by a community's concern, readiness, and capacity. Public health and other helping agencies should provide information and technical assistance as requested by the community, and it should lead ideally toward as much community control of the process as the technical complexity of the program's interventions warrant.

─────────────── EXERCISES ───────────────

1. Using the population you selected at the end of chapter 1, what types of questions would you want to pose to community members about the health issues that concern them? How closely would you expect these to align with official agency determinations of community needs?

2. What are methods you would consider for gaining the insights of your community members?

3. What types of partners could you rely on to serve as trusted intermediaries to your community, if you do not already have those relationships yourself?

Notes

1. Health is an instrumental value, not a terminal value. We avoid the misnomer "healthy" in describing actions, policies, or programs conducive to health (e.g., "healthy behavior" or "healthy public policy") because these objects of the adjectives are means, not ends; they are not living organisms that can be healthy. At best they can enhance health, and thus may be healthful, health-promoting, health-protecting, or disease-preventing. Similarly, health can be instrumental in achieving other values associated with quality of life, such as feeling energetic and attractive, being able to cope, being a good partner, neighbor, or colleague, etc.

2. For more on participatory research to assess a population's ultimate values and quality of life, see Green and Mercer (2001); Wallerstein et al. (2018). Internet resources for participatory research approaches to community assessment and development are listed and linked guidelines are online at http://lgreen.net/guidelines.html.

3. For further literature on technical assistance, see Minkler (1997). For classics on participatory approaches in health, see Nyswander (1942); Steuart (1965). *The Guide to Community Preventive Services* (The Community Guide) is a CDC collection of all the evidence-based findings and recommendations of the Community Preventive Services Task Force. For a Canadian source, go to https://www.hc-sc.gc.ca/hppb/healthcare/Building.htm.

4. For discussions contrasting PRECEDE, andragogical, and Freire's approaches, see Freire (1970, 181); see also Marsick (1987), in which PRECEDE was "interpreted from a viewpoint of technical rationality even though it does not have to be so construed. Interpreted narrowly, PRECEDE would emphasize an accurate technical diagnosis of the problem . . . [consulting] with clients and community leaders in the problem setting, but the primary purpose would be to discuss the problem in order to develop the best professional solution" (19). We would argue that the best technical or professional solution *is* one that addresses the felt needs of the community. For other applications of Freirean concepts in health, see Minkler (2000); Wallerstein et al. (2018).

5. See also Wallerstein et al. (2018) for examples of contrasting, contradicting, and paradoxical perspectives in community-based participatory research depending on levels of participation in community, socioeconomic variables, and inherent cultural, economic, and infrastructure needs and capacities of a community. During the height of federal initiatives emphasizing "maximum feasible participation" in health planning, much was said and written about the limitations, misunderstandings, and diluting of community participation efforts, such as Moynihan's (1969) expression of frustration with the undermining of legislation requiring participation as *Maximum Feasible Misunderstanding*," by

making citizen participation a source of volunteer labor rather than a check on professional decision-making. Cooke and Kothari's 2001 book, *Participation: The New Tyranny?*, and two Johns Hopkins professors of political science, Crenson and Ginsberg (2002), saw a government operated by and for elites who preferred a passive, uninvolved citizenry.

6. As a caveat, we would temper some of the sentiments for giving greater autonomy to lay groups in areas of environmental health protection such as water and food safety, as well as health services such as immunizations, or fluoridation, where whole populations may be at extreme risk if the values and misunderstandings of a small but vocal group were to override scientific evidence. This is not, however, to suggest that participatory approaches are more appropriate to health promotion and less important to health protection or health services. Indeed, two of the most significant contemporary initiatives in federal support for participatory research have come from the National Institute of Environmental Health Sciences (O'Fallon and Dearry 2002; Shepard et al. 2002; and the whole issue in which these articles appear; see also the projects supported by the National Institute of Environmental Health, NIEHS). The Indian Health Service and the Health Resources and Services Administration have applied participatory methods in community-oriented primary care (COPC). Brown and Fee (2002) reviewed the history of COPC and noted that some initiatives sought "to jettison a prescriptive, stepwise COPC model in favor of a more fluid and dynamic understanding that emphasizes community engagement and embraces sociopolitical objectives" (1712).

7. On the provenance of the concepts of "indigenous capacity" and "assets of communities": McKnight and Kretzmann (2012) developed the concept and approach to measuring "community assets" rather than focusing on "needs and deficiencies." The National Association of County and City Health Officials' (NACCHO) Assessment Protocol for Excellence in Public Health and Community-Based Environmental Assessments (formerly APEX*PH*) guide local health departments through an organizational capacity assessment and a community health assessment process. Go to https://www.naccho.org/tools.cfm (accessed Nov 17, 2018) to view the instruments and the Protocol for Assessment of Community Excellence in Environmental Health (PACE-EH) at the same website. Each of these CDC-sponsored community health assessment models builds on the previous one. MAPP and PACE-EH are elaborations or special applications of APEX*PH,* which was an extension of the Planned Approach to Community Health (PATCH, Kreuter 1992), which was based largely on the PRECEDE model. During the same time, PRECEDE has evolved as PRECEDE-PROCEED to build on the experience of PATCH and the Kaiser Family Foundation experience of applying a "social reconnaissance" approach to community needs and asset assessment (Green and Kreuter 1999), and on subsequent experience with all of the assessment and planning models and instruments. Many of the assessment procedures in PRECEDE-PROCEED were illustrated in an interactive tutorial software package and manual called Expert Methods of Planning and Organizing Within Everyone's Reach *(EMPOWER,* Gold et al. 1997, now out of print; see Lovato et al. 2003).

8. "Competent community" was a term conceptualized generically by Iscoe in 1974. Its applications in the health field have tended increasingly toward the use of the terms **"community capacity"** (e.g., Kalnins et al. 2002) and **"social capital"** or "community capital" (e.g., Kreuter and Lezin 2002). For a review on the potential negative effects of social capital, see Villalonga-Olives and Kawachi (2017).

9. For further tools and methods for asset identification and development, see Frattaroli et al. (2012); Minkler and Hancock (2003); National Civic League (1999; 2000); Puntenney (2000); Sharpe et al. (2000); Wang (2003).

10. The notion of capacity building as being able to use the lessons of one program planning experience to solve other problems, rather than the once-popular notion of institutionalizing the funded program as the measure of success (Green 1989), is consistent with Senge's (1994) concept of the "learning organization." The most thorough review of

stakeholders and organizational partnerships in the conceptual development of community capacity building in health is Riley and Best (2014).

References

Adler, N.E., & Rehkopf, D.H. (2008). U.S. disparities in health: Descriptions, causes, and
mechanisms. *Annual Review of Public Health, 29*, 235–52. https://doi.org/10.1146
/annurev.publhealth.29.020907.090852

Bandura, A. (2004). Health promotion by social cognitive means. *Health Education and
Behavior, 31*(2), 143–64. https://doi.org/10.1177/1090198104263660

Bauer, U.E., Briss, P.A., Goodman, R.A., & Bowman, B.A. (2014). Prevention of chronic disease
in the 21st century: elimination of the leading preventable causes of premature death
and disability in the USA. *The Lancet, 384*(9937), 45–52. https://doi.org/10.1016/S0140
-6736(14)60648-6

Berkman, L.F., Kawachi, I. & Glymour, M. (2014). *Social Epidemiology* (2nd ed.). Oxford
University Press.

Biglan, A., Ary, D.V., Smolkowski, K., Duncan, T., & Black, C. (2000). A randomised controlled
trial of a community intervention to prevent adolescent tobacco use. *Tobacco Control,
9*(1), 24–32. https://doi.org/10.1136/tc.9.1.24

Blankertz, L., & Hazem, D. (2002). Assessing consumer program needs: advantages of a brief
unstructured format. *Community Mental Health Journal, 38*(4), 277–86. https://doi.org
/10.1023/a:1015951524232

Brosseau, L.M., Parker, D.L., Lazovich, D., Milton, T., & Dugan, S. (2002). Designing intervention effectiveness studies for occupational health and safety: The Minnesota wood
dust study. *American Journal of Industrial Medicine, 41*(1), 54–61. https://doi.org/10.1002
/ajim.10029

Brown, T.M., & Fee, E. (2002). "Palliatives will no longer do": The deep roots and continuing
dynamic of community-oriented primary care. *American Journal of Public Health, 92*,
1711–12. https://doi.org/10.2105/AJPH.92.11.1711

Bunker, J.P. (2001). The role of medical care in contributing to health improvements within
societies. *International Journal of Epidemiology, 30*(6), 1260–63. https://doi.org/10.1093
/ije/30.6.1260

Burke, J.G., Hess, S., Hoffmann, K., Guizzetti, L., Loy, E., Gielen, A.C., Bailey, M., Walnoha, A.,
Barbee, G., & Yonas, M. (2013). Translating community-based participatory research
(CBPR) principles into practice. *Progress in Community Health Partnerships, 7*(2), 115–22.
https://doi.org/10.1353/cpr.2013.0025

Buta, B., Brewer, L., Hamlin, D.L., Palmer, M.W., Bowie, J., & Gielen, A.C. (2011). An innovative
faith-based healthy eating program: From class assignment to real-world application
of PRECEDE/PROCEED. *Health Promotion Practice, 12*(6), 867–75. https://doi.org/10.1177
/1524839910370424

Butler, M.O., Abed, J., Goodman, K., Gottlieb, N., Hare, M., & Mullen, P. (1996). *A case-study
evaluation of the Henry J. Kaiser Family Foundation's Community Health Promotion Grants
Program in the southern states: Phase 2 final report.* Battelle Centers for Public Health
Research and Evaluation, Henry J. Kaiser Family Foundation, and Centers for Disease
Control.

Campbell, C., & Jovchelovitch, S. (2000). Health, community and development: towards a
social psychology of participation. *Journal of Community and Applied Social Psychology,
10*(4), 255–70. https://doi.org/10.1002/1099-1298(200007/08)10:4<255::AID-CASP582
>3.0.CO;2-M

Centers for Disease Control and Prevention (2000). *Measuring healthy days: Population
assessment of health-related quality of life.* Health Care and Aging Studies Branch,
Division of Adult and Community Health, National Center for Chronic Disease Prevention and Health Promotion, CDC.

Chapman, S., & Lupton, D. (1995). *The fight for public health: Principles and practice of media advocacy.* BMJ Publishing Group.

Chuah, F.L.H., Srivastava, A., Singh, S.R., Haldane, V., Koh, G.C.H., Seng, C.K., McCoy, D., & Legido-Quigley, H. (2018). Community participation in general health initiatives in high and upper middle income countries: A systematic review exploring the nature of participation, use of theories, contextual drivers and power relations in community participation. *Social Science and Medicine, 213,* 106–22. https://doi.org/10.1016/j.socscimed.2018.07.019

Cooke, B., & Kothari, U. (2001). *Participation: The New Tyranny?* Zed Books Ltd.

Crenson, M.A., & Ginsberg, B. (2002). *Downsizing Democracy: How America Sidelined Its Citizens and Privatized Its Public.* Johns Hopkins University Press. https://doi.org/10.1353/book.72712

Fetterman, D.M. (2000). *Foundations of Empowerment Evaluation: Step by Step.* SAGE Publishing.

Fielding, J.E., & Teutsch, S.M. (Eds.) (2012). *Public Health Practice: What Works.* Oxford University Press. https://doi.org/10.1093/acprof:oso/9780199892761.001.0001

First International Conference on Health Promotion. (1986). Ottawa Charter for Health Promotion. *Health Promotion International, 1*(4), 405. https://doi.org/10.1093/heapro/1.4.405

Foster-Fishman, P.G., Berkowitz, S.L., Lounsbury, D.W., Jacobson, S., & Allen, N.A. (2001). Building collaborative capacity in community coalitions: A review and integrative framework. *American Journal of Community Psychology, 29*(2), 241–61. https://doi.org/10.1023/A:1010378613583

Frankish, C.J., Lovato, C., & Poureslami, I. (2015). Models, theories, and principles of health promotion and their use with multicultural populations. In Huff, R.M., Kline, M.V., & Peterson, D.V. (Eds.), *Health Promotion in Multicultural Populations: A Handbook for Practitioners and Students* (3rd ed., pp. 41–72). SAGE Publishing. http://dx.doi.org/10.4135/9781483368771

Frattaroli, S., DeFrancesco, S., Gielen, A.C., Bishai, D.M., & Guyer, B. (2006). Local stakeholders' perspective on improving the urban environment to reduce child pedestrian injury: implementing effective public health interventions at the local level. *Journal of Public Health Policy, 27*(4), 376–88. https://doi.org/10.1057/palgrave.jphp.3200103

Frattaroli, S., McDonald, E.M., Tran, N.T., Trump, A.R., O'Brocki, R.C. 3rd, & Gielen, A.C. (2012). Igniting interest in prevention: using firefighter focus groups to inform implementation and enhancement of an urban canvassing program. *Journal of Public Health Management and Practice, 18*(4), 382–9. https://doi.org/10.1097/PHH.0b013e31823e96e9

Freire, P. (1970). *Pedagogy of the Oppressed.* The Seabury Press.

Geiger, H.J. (2002). Community-oriented primary care: A path to community development. *American Journal of Public Health, 92*(11), 1713–16. https://doi.org/10.2105/ajph.92.11.1713

Gielen, A.C., Bishai, D.M., Omaki, E., Shields, W.C., McDonald, E.M., Rizzutti, N.C., Case, J., Stevens, M.W., & Aitken, M.E. (2018). Results of an RCT in two pediatric emergency departments to evaluate the efficacy of an m-health educational app on car seat use. *American Journal of Preventive Medicine, 54*(6), 746–55. https://doi.org/10.1016/j.amepre.2018.01.042

Gielen, A.C., McDonald, E.M., Omaki, E., Shields, W., Case, J., & Aitken, M. (2015). A smartphone app to communicate child passenger safety: an application of theory to practice. *Health Education Research, 30*(5), 683–92. https://doi.org/10.1093/her/cyv035

Gold, R.S. (2022). Applications of the PRECEDE-PROCEED model in communication technologies. In Green, L.W., Gielen, A.C., Ottoson, J.M., Peterson, D., & Kreuter, M.W. (Eds.), *Health Program Planning* (5th ed.). Johns Hopkins University Press.

Gold, R.S., Green, L.W., & Kreuter, M.W. (1997). *EMPOWER: Enabling Methods of Planning and Organizing Within Everyone's Reach.* Jones & Bartlett Learning.

Gold, R.S., & N.L. Atkinson. (2005). Imagine this, imagine that: A look into the future of technology for health educators. *The Health Education Monograph Series, 23*(1), 44–48.

Goodman, R.M., Speers, M.A., McLeroy, K., Fawcett, S., Kegler, M., Parker, E., Smith, S.R., Sterling, T.D., & Wallerstein, N. (1998). Identifying and defining the dimensions of community capacity to provide a basis for measurement. *Health Education and Behavior, 25*(3), 258–78. https://doi.org/10.1177/109019819802500303

Green, L.W. (1989). Comment: is institutionalization the proper role of grantmaking? *American Journal of Health Promotion, 3*(4), 44. https://doi.org/10.4278/0890-1171-3.4.44

Green, L.W. (2004). Introduction of Albert Bandura to Receive the Healthtrac Foundation Health Education Award and to Present the Healthtrac Lecture at SOPHE Annual Conference. *Health Education and Behavior, 31*(2), 141–2. https://doi.org/10.1177/109019 8104263659

Green, L.W. (2008). Making research relevant: if it is an evidence-based practice, where's the practice-based evidence? *Family Practice, 25*(Suppl. 1), i20–4. https://doi.org/10.1093 /fampra/cmn055

Green, L.W, & Allegrante, J.P. (2011). Healthy people 1980–2020: raising the ante decennially or just the name from public health education to health promotion to social determinants? *Health Education & Behavior, 38*(6), 558–62. https://doi.org/10.1177/1090198111429153

Green, L.W., George, A., Daniel, M., Frankish, C.J., Herbert, C.P., Bowie, W., & O'Neill, M. (1995). *Study of participatory research in health promotion: review and recommendations for the development of participatory research in health promotion in Canada.* The Royal Society of Canada.

Green, L.W., & Gielen, A.C. (2015). Evidence of ecological theory in two public health successes for health behavior change. In Kahan, S., Gielen, A.C., Fagan, P., & Green, L.W. (Eds.). *Health Behavior Change in Populations* (pp 26–43). Johns Hopkins University Press.

Green, L.W., & Kreuter, M.W. (1999). Health education's contributions to public health in the twentieth century: A glimpse through health promotion's rear-view mirror. *Annual Review of Public Health, 20*, 67–88. https://doi.org/10.1146/annurev.publhealth.20.1.67

Green, L.W., & Mercer, S.L. (2001). Can public health researchers and agencies reconcile the push from funding bodies and the pull from communities? *American Journal of Public Health, 91*(12), 1926–9. https://doi.org/10.2105/ajph.91.12.1926

Green, L.W., Murphy, R.L., & McKenna, J.W. (2002). New insights into how mass media works for and against tobacco. *Journal of Health Communication, 7*(3), 245–8. https://doi.org/10.1080 /10810730290001710

Hawe, P. (1996). Needs assessment must become more change-focused. *Australian and New Zealand Journal of Public Health, 20*, 473–478.33. https://doi.org/10.1111/j.1467-842X.1996 .tb01624.x

Hawe, P., Noort, M., King, L., & Jordens, C. (1997). Multiplying health gains: The critical role of capacity-building within health promotion programs. *Health Policy, 39*(1), 29–42. https://doi.org/10.1016/s0168-8510(96)00847-0

Hawe, P., & Shiell, A. (2000). Social capital and health promotion: A review. *Social Science and Medicine, 51*(6), 871–85. https://doi.org/10.1016/s0277-9536(00)00067-8

Huff, R.M., Kline, M.V., & Peterson, D.V. (Eds.). (2015). *Health Promotion in Multicultural Populations: A Handbook for Practitioners and Students* (3rd ed.). SAGE Publishing. http://dx .doi.org/10.4135/9781483368771

Iscoe, I. (1974). Community psychology and the competent community. *American Psychologist, 29*(8), 607–13. https://doi.org/10.1037/h0036925

Jeet, G., Thakur, J.S., Prinja, S., & Singh, M. (2017). Community health workers for non-communicable diseases prevention and control in developing countries: Evidence and implications. *PLoS One, 12*(7), 1–21: e0180640. https://doi.org/10.1371/journal.pone .0180640

Johnson, S.L., Burke, J.G., & Gielen, A.C. (2012). Urban students' perceptions of the school environment's influence on school violence. *Children and Schools, 34*(2), 92–102. https://doi.org/10.1093/cs/cds016

Kahan, S., Gielen, A., Fagan, P., & Green, L.W. (Eds.) (2014). *Health Behavior Change in Populations.* Johns Hopkins University Press.

Kalnins, I., Hart, C., Ballantyne, P., Quartaro, G., Love, R., Sturis, G., & Pollack, P. (2002). Children's perceptions of strategies for resolving community health problems. *Health Promotion International, 17*(3), 223–33. https://doi.org/10.1093/heapro/17.3.223

Kim, K., Choi, J.S., Choi, E., Nieman, C.L., Joo, J.H., Lin, F.R., Gitlin, L.N., & Han, H.R. (2016). Effects of community-based health worker interventions to improve chronic disease management and care among vulnerable populations: A systematic review. *American Journal of Public Health, 106*(4), e3–e28. https://doi.org/10.2105/AJPH.2015.302987

Kreuter, M.W., Lezin, N., Kreuter, M.W., & Green, L.W. (2003). *Community Health Promotion Ideas That Work* (2nd ed.). Jones & Bartlett Learning.

Kreuter, M.W., & Lezin, N. (2002). Social capital theory: implications for community-based health promotion. In DiClemente, R.J., Crosby, R.A., & Kegler, M.C. (Eds.), *Emerging theories in health promotion practice and research: Strategies for improving public health* (pp. 228–54). Jossey-Bass.

Kreuter, M.W. (1992). PATCH: Its origin, basic concepts, and links to contemporary public health policy. *Health Education Journal, 23*(3), 135–9. https://doi.org/10.1080/10556699.1992.10616276

Last, J. (2000). *Dictionary of Epidemiology* (4th ed.). Oxford University Press.

Last, J. (2002). Health. In Breslow, L., Goldstein, B.D., Green, L.W., Keck, C.K., Last, J.M., & McGinnis, M. (Eds.), *Encyclopedia of Public Health* (Vol. 2, pp. 519–26). Macmillan Reference USA, Gale Group.

Lavery, J.V. (2018). Building an evidence base for stakeholder engagement. *Science, 361*(6402), 554–6. https://doi.org/10.1126/science.aat8429

Lipskey, M. (1980). *Street-Level Bureaucracy.* Russell Sage Foundation.

Lovato, C., Potvin, L., Lehoux, P., Proulx, M., Chiasson, M., Milligan, D., Tremblay, M., Gariépy, E., Dingwell, G., & Green, L.W. (2003). Software to assist with programme planning: two community-based cases. *Promotion and Education, 10*(3), 120–6.

Mabry, P.L., Olster, D.H., Morgan, G.D., & Abrams, D.B. (2008). Interdisciplinarity and systems science to improve population health: A view from the NIH Office of Behavioral and Social Sciences Research. *American Journal of Preventive Medicine, 35*(Suppl. 2), S211–24. https://doi.org/10.1016/j.amepre.2008.05.018

Marsick, V.J. (1987). Designing health education programs. In Lazes, P.M., Kaplan, L.H., & Gordon, K.A. (Eds.), *Handbook of Health Education* (2nd ed., pp. 3–30). Aspen.

Marmot, M. (2000). Social determinants of health: From observation to policy. *Medical Journal of Australia, 172*(8), 379–82. https://doi.org/10.5694/j.1326-5377.2000.tb124011.x

Marmot, M., & Wilkinson, R. (Eds.) (2006). *Social Determinants of Health* (2nd ed.). Oxford University Press.

Martin, N. et al. (2017). *Advancing the Anchor Mission of Healthcare* (p. 10). The Democracy Collaborative. https://democracycollaborative.org/sites/default/files/downloads/han-final-for-achi_0.pdf

McDonnell, K.A., Gielen, A.C., Burke, J.G., O'Campo, P., & Weidl, M. (2011). Women's perceptions of their community's social norms towards assisting women who have experienced intimate partner violence. *Journal of Urban Health, 88*(2), 240–53. https://doi.org/10.1007/s11524-011-9546-9

McDowell, I. (2002). Social health. In Breslow, L. (Ed.), *Encyclopedia of Public Health* (Vol. 4, pp. 1123–4). Macmillan Reference USA.

McKnight, J.L., & Kretzmann, J.P. (2012). Chapter 10: Mapping community capacity. In Minkler, M. (Ed.), *Community Organizing and Community Building for Health* (3rd ed., pp. 171–86). Rutgers University Press.

McLoughlin, E., & Fennell, J. (2000). The power of survivor advocacy: making car trunks escapable. *Injury Prevention, 6*(3), 167–70. https://doi.org/10.1136/ip.6.3.167

Mindell, J. (2001). Lessons from tobacco control for advocates of healthy transport. *Journal of Public Health, 23*(2), 91–7. https://doi.org/10.1093/pubmed/23.2.91

Minkler, M., Thompson, M., Bell, J., Rose, K., & Redman, D. (2002). Using community involvement strategies in the fight against infant mortality: Lessons from a multisite study of the national Healthy Start experience. *Health Promotion Practice, 3*(2), 176–87. https://doi.org/10.1177/152483990200300213

Minkler, M. (2000). Using participatory action research to build healthy communities. *Public Health Reports, 115*(2–3), 191–7.

Minkler, M., & Hancock, T. (2003). Community-driven asset identification and issue selection. In Minkler, M. & Wallerstein, N. (Eds.), *Community-Based Participatory Research for Health* (pp. 135–54). Jossey-Bass.

Minkler, M. (Ed.) (1997). *Community Organizing and Community Building for Health*. Rutgers University Press.

Moynihan, D.P. (1969). *Maximum Feasible Misunderstanding: Community Action in the War on Poverty*. Free Press.

National Civic League. (1999). *The Civic Index: Measuring your community's civic health*. National Civic League.

National Civic League and Staff of the St. Louis County Department of Health. (2000). *A Guide to a Community-Oriented Approach to Core Public Health Functions*. National Civic League.

Nyswander, D. (1942). *Solving School Health Problems*. Oxford University Press.

O'Fallon, L.R., & Dearry, A. (2002). Community-based participatory research as a tool to advance environmental health sciences. *Environmental Health Perspectives, 110*(Suppl. 2), 155–9. https://doi.org/10.1289/ehp.02110s2155

Parsons, T. (1964). The superego and the theory of social systems. In Coser, R.L. (Ed.), *The Family: Its Structure and Functions* (pp. 433–49). St. Martin's Press.

Perry, H.B., Zulliger, R., & Rogers, M.M. (2014). Community health workers in low-, middle-, and high-income countries: An overview of their history, recent evolution, and current effectiveness. *Annual Review of Public Health, 35*, 399–421. https://doi.org/10.1146/annurev-publhealth-032013-182354

Puntenney, D. (2000). *A Guide to Building Sustainable Organizations from the Inside Out: An Organizational Capacity Building Toolbox from the Chicago Foundation for Women*. Institute for Policy Research, Northwestern University and Chicago Foundation for Women.

Raeburn, J.M., & Rootman, I. (1998). *People-Centred Health Promotion*. John Wiley & Sons.

Rifkin, S.B. (2014). Examining the links between community participation and health outcomes: A review of the literature. *Health Policy and Planning, 29*(Suppl. 2), ii98–ii106. https://doi.org/10.1093/heapol/czu076

Riley, B., & Best, A. (2014). Extending the ecological model: Key stakeholders and organizational partnerships. In Kahan, S., Gielen, A.C., Fagan, P.J., & Green, L.W. (Eds.), *Health Behavior Change in Populations* (pp. 44–63). Johns Hopkins University Press.

Rose, G. (1992). *The Strategy of Preventive Medicine*. Oxford University Press.

Rowe, G., & Frewer, L.J. (2005). A typology of public engagement mechanisms. *Science, Technology, and Human Values, 30*(2), 251–90. https://doi.org/10.1177/0162243904271724

Senge, P. (1994). *The Fifth Discipline Fieldbook: Strategies and Tools for Building a Learning Organization*. Doubleday.

Sharpe, P.A., Greaney, M.L., Lee, P.R., & Royce, S.W. (2000). Assets-oriented community assessment. *Public Health Reports, 115*(2–3), 205–11.

Shepard, P., Northridge, M.E., Prakash, S., & Stover, G. (2002). Preface: Advancing environmental justice through community-based participatory research. *Environmental Health Perspectives, 110*(Suppl. 2), 139–40. https://doi.org/10.1289/ehp.02110s2139

Shor, I., & Freire, P. (1987). *A Pedagogy for Liberation*. Bergin and Garvey Publishers.

Shoveller, J., & Green, L.W. (2002). Decentralization and public health. In Breslow, L., Goldstein, B.D., Green, L.W., Keck, C.W., Last, J., & McGinnis, M. (Eds.), *Encyclopedia of Public Health*. Macmillan Reference USA.

Stead, M., Hastings, G., & Eadie, D. (2002). The challenge of evaluating complex interventions: A framework for evaluating media advocacy. *Health Education Research, 17*(3), 351–64. https://doi.org/10.1093/her/17.3.351

Steuart, G.W. (1965). Health, behavior and planned change: An approach to the professional preparation of the health education specialist. *Health Education Monographs, 1*(20), 3–26. https://doi.org/10.1177/109019816500102001

Stillman, F.A., Cronin, K.A., Evans, W.G., & Ulasevich, A. (2001). Can media advocacy influence newspaper coverage of tobacco: Measuring the effectiveness of the American stop smoking intervention study's (ASSIST) media advocacy strategies. *Tobacco Control, 10*(2), 137–44. https://doi.org/10.1136/tc.10.2.137

Villalonga-Olives, E., & Kawachi, I. (2017). The dark side of social capital: A systematic review of the negative health effects of social capital. *Social Science and Medicine, 194*, 105–27. https://doi.org/10.1016/j.socscimed.2017.10.020

Viswanathan, M., Ammerman, A., Eng, E., Garlehner, G., Lohr, K.N., Griffith, D., Rhodes, S., Samuel-Hodge, C., Maty, S., Lux, L., Webb, L., Sutton, S.F, Swinson, T., Jackman, A., & Whitener, L. (2004). *Community-Based Participatory Research: Assessing the Evidence*. Agency for Healthcare Research and Quality.

Wallerstein, N., Duran, B., Oetzel, J., & Minkler, M. (Eds.) (2018). *Community-Based Participatory Research: Advancing Social and Health Equity* (3rd ed.). Jossey-Bass, Wiley.

Wandersman, A., & Florin, P. (2000). Citizen participation and community organizations. In Rappaport, J. & Seidman, E. (Eds.), *Handbook of Community Psychology* (pp. 247–72). Academic/Plenum.

Wang, C.C. (2003). Using photovoice as a participatory assessment and issue selection tool. In Minkler, M., & Wallerstein, N. (Eds.), *Community-Based Participatory Research for Health* (pp. 179–96). Jossey-Bass.

World Health Organization. (1986). *New Policies for Health Education in Primary Health Care*. World Health Organization.

Zimmerman, R.K., Nowalk, M.P., Bardella, I.J., Fine, M.J., Janosky, J.E., Santibanez, T.A., Wilson, S.A., & Raymund, M. (2004). Physician and practice factors related to influenza vaccination among the elderly. *American Journal of Preventive Medicine, 26*(1), 1–10. https://doi.org/10.1016/j.amepre.2003.09.020

PART II
PRECEDE-PROCEED
Phases

Planning, Implementation, and Evaluation

CHAPTER 3

Social Assessment: Quality of Life

•

Lawrence W. Green, Marshall W. Kreuter,
and Andrea Carlson Gielen

*The whole of science is nothing more than a refinement
of everyday thinking.*

—Albert Einstein

Learning Objectives

After completing the chapter, the reader will be able to:

- Explain why quality of life concerns should be part of health program planning.
- Describe at least three ways to measure quality of life in a community.
- Identify at least two limitations on your ability to measure quality of life in a community.

INTRODUCTION

Community participation steps were introduced in the previous chapter, even before the first phase of health program planning. As we start Part II of the book, chapters 3 through 9, you will be guided through the various phases of PRECEDE-PROCEED. A you-are-here "map," such as figure 3.1, will begin each chapter with a visual representation of where you are in the work of PRECEDE-PROCEED. To further help you find and keep your place, box 3.1 aligns model phases with book parts and chapters.

With an understanding of the role of community participation, health planners, together with their community participants or partners, can usefully consider the question, "Health for what purpose?" Health, social conditions and **quality of life** are closely intertwined. People seek health to enhance or secure their socioeconomic, social, and physical qualities of life. Quality of life and social conditions affect the achievement and enhancement of health. They co-exist with reciprocal effects on each other.[1]

QUALITY OF LIFE: AN EXPRESSION OF ULTIMATE VALUES

As noted in chapter 2, an ultimate or terminal value (as distinct from an instru-mental value) usually goes beyond health. When people undertake efforts to be healthy, creative, and productive and try to make their conditions of living safe and enjoyable, they are seeking to improve some quality or qualities of life attached to their values. Health *is* one dimension of quality of life, but it usually has other purposes, each of which makes health and the motivation to preserve or enhance it a means to some other end.[2] People seek health in order to be more effective, attractive, productive, a better parent, a better family member; to live lives that are longer, livelier, more independent, comfortable, and respected. Like most concepts, quality of life is measurable to the extent that it can be oper-ationally defined, but unlike most concepts, this one is elusive at the individual level. We define it as the perception of individuals or groups that their needs are

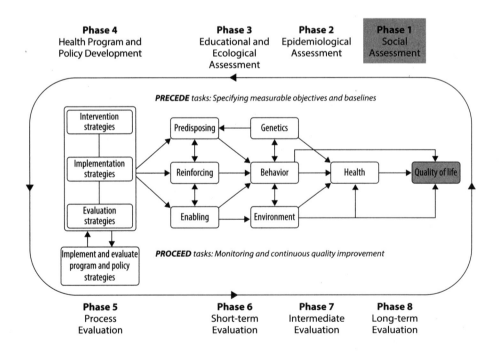

FIGURE 3.1. The first phase of the PRECEDE-PROCEED model, social assessment, focuses on the popula-tion's quality of life relative to health and other factors.

being satisfied and that they have sufficient opportunities to pursue happiness and fulfillment. As figure 3.2 illustrates, quality-of-life measurement for community or population health planning will usually be at the population level as part of the **social assessment**, with comparative indicators that are measurable as quality of life, using rates or percentages for segments of the population.

BOX 3.1

Aligning PRECEDE-PROCEED Phases with Book Parts and Chapters

Chapter #	Content Focus	PRECEDE-PROCEED Phase(s)
Part I: Hallmarks of the PRECEDE-PROCEED Model		
1	A model for population health planning, implementation, and evaluation	All
2	Participation and community engagement in planning	All
Part II: PRECEDE-PROCEED Phases: Planning, Implementation and Evaluation		
3	Social assessment: quality of life	1
4	Epidemiological assessment I: population health	2
5	Epidemiological assessment II: behavioral and environmental factors	2
6	Educational and ecological assessment: predisposing, enabling, and reinforcing factors	3
7	Health program and policy development I: intervention strategies	4
8	Health program and policy development II: implementation strategies	4
9	Health program and policy development III: evaluation strategies	4, 5, 6, 7, and 8
Part III: Application of PRECEDE-PROCEED in Specific Settings		
10–14	Applications in varied settings and technology channels	All

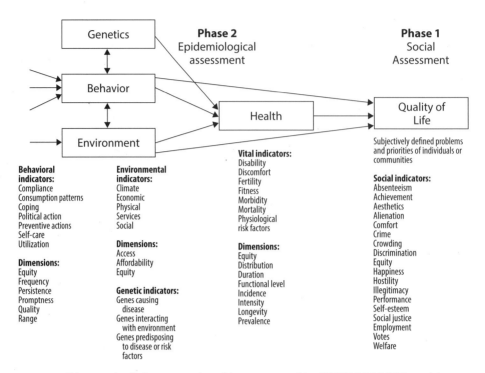

FIGURE 3.2. This more detailed representation of the outcomes of the PRECEDE-PROCEED model (Phases 1 and 2) shows examples of the relationships, indicators, and dimensions of factors that might be identified in a PRECEDE diagnostic assessment and the outcome evaluation phases.

MEASURING QUALITY OF LIFE FOR INDIVIDUALS

Various questionnaires or tools have been used to assess quality of life as it pertains to specific health outcomes, including pain management (Lorig et al. 2002), functional disability and physical therapy outcomes (Gold et al. 2002; Haley et al. 2002; Jette and Keysor 2002), leisure (Burdine et al. 2000), quality-adjusted life years lost or gained after medical procedures (Kaplan and Frosch 2005), unemployment rates, and descriptions of other ecological measures of health (Karpati et al. 2002).

Some quality of life scales are designed for individual assessments, based on the assumption that quality of life can only be determined by each person's unique values and experiences. Ware reported on 20 years of validation studies for the SF-36, a widely used instrument for assessing patients' views of physical and mental well-being and ability to function (Ware and Kosinski 2001). In medical or nursing care, the counterpart of community social indicators or quality of life measures are health outcome measures other than biomedical. These may include the ability to perform the tasks of daily living, tolerance for side effects of medications, energy level, and other indicators of well-being associated with but not identical to the medical condition (Kosinski et al. 2002; Manocchia et al. 2001).

MEASURING QUALITY OF LIFE FOR COMMUNITIES OR POPULATIONS

The Behavioral Risk Factor Surveillance System (BRFSS)[3] of the Centers for Disease Control and Prevention (CDC) contains a set of questions that provide a valid and reliable measure called Health-Related Quality of Life (HRQOL). Based on self-reported responses to the four questions that have been part of the BRFSS since 1993, the National Health and Nutrition Examination Survey (NHANES) incorporated them in 2000. Collected annually by most states in the United States and in some larger population areas within states, HRQOL provides planners with a concrete means to show how health problems in adult populations (age 18 and older) also compromise the quality of life of those populations. "Unhealthy days" are an estimate of the total number of days during the previous 30 days when respondents felt that either their physical or mental health was not good. That number is obtained by combining responses to questions 2 and 3 in box 3.2. Thus, a person who reports three physically unhealthy days and two mentally unhealthy days would be assigned a value of five unhealthy days.

Based on the analysis of national data, here are examples of HRQOL findings (Centers for Disease Control and Prevention 2000):

- Americans said they feel unhealthy (physically or mentally) about five days per month.

- Americans said they feel "healthy and full of energy" about 19 days per month.

- Nearly one-third of Americans said they suffer from some mental or emotional problem every month—including 9 percent who said their mental health was not good for 14 or more days a month.

- Younger American adults, aged 18–24 years, suffered the most mental health distress.

- Older adults suffered the most poor physical health days and activity limitations.

- American Indians and Alaska Natives reported the highest levels of unhealthy days among American race/ethnicity groups.

- Adults with the lowest income or education reported more unhealthy days than did those with higher income or education.

BOX 3.2

Examples of Questions Used to Measure Health-Related Quality of Life

1. Would you say that in general your health is: (a) Excellent? (b) Very good? (c) Fair? (d) Poor?

2. Now thinking about your physical health, which includes physical illness and injury, for how many days during the past 30 days was your physical health not good?

3. Now thinking about your mental health, which includes stress, depression, and problems with emotions, for how many days during the past 30 days was your mental health not good?

4. During the past 30 days, for about how many days did poor physical health keep you from doing your usual activities, such as self-care, work, or recreation?

5. During the past 30 days, for about how many days did poor mental health keep you from doing your usual activities, such as self-care, work, or recreation?

Source: Centers for Disease Control and Prevention. (2018, October 31). *Health-Related Quality of Life (HRQOL).* Retrieved April 7, 2021, from https://www.cdc.gov/hrqol

---

LIMITATIONS OF QUALITY OF LIFE DATA

Some worry that efforts to make explicit and to generalize perceptions of quality of life will necessarily ignore the subtle differences in perceptions among individuals within a population, contending that it is inappropriate to impose one person's perception of wellness and satisfaction on others whose values and priorities may differ. Accordingly, aggregating individual data and reporting averages can seem to ignore or devalue what is most precious in some people's lives. Respect for the diversity inherent in communities justifies seeking greater insight about local values and interests through a social assessment (sometimes referred to as a social diagnosis) phase of planning for health programs and policies, as in the PRECEDE model. At the individual level, we have tools that enable us to identify individual interests and perceived quality of life. At the group or community level, we have access to numerous sources of information and methods that give people opportunities to hear and understand each other. These tools and methods increase the chances of identifying priorities that reflect the common concerns of all and the variability of concerns among individuals and groups. Not all of these, to be described in the last sections of this chapter, produce quantitative data.

METHODS AND STRATEGIES FOR SOCIAL ASSESSMENT

The social assessment phase of PRECEDE-PROCEED is designed to help planners with two tasks:

- to identify and interpret the social conditions, and perceptions of them, shared at the community, professional and organizational levels, and
- to make the connections between those conditions and perceptions of them and the diversity of health program strategies that will be needed to accommodate the diversity of values and needs.

To find specific and innovative methods to plan, implement, and evaluate health programs, planners should look to the continually evolving print and online literature of public health, epidemiology, social and behavioral sciences, community development, community nursing, health services research, health promotion, and public health education. By examining the findings and methods of others, planners will gain techniques and insights to sharpen their thinking on social assessment and quality of life perspectives (Finegood et al. 2014; Gold et al. 2002; Kaplan and Frosch 2005).

The literature illustrates the ways diverse methods of data collection have been used in social assessments and other phases of health program planning, including key informant interviews, community forums, focus groups, nominal group process, and surveys. Because time and resources are precious, it is wise to retrieve existing information whenever possible; most sources of routinely collected health data at the state and national levels are governmental, so most of these are in the public domain (i.e., can be freely reproduced and republished) and relatively accessible on federal or other governmental websites. A thorough local social assessment and health program planning process, however, will usually require at least some new and tailored information (especially in these times of rapid technological and climate change), or their data will tend to reinforce the status quo and fail to reflect changing circumstances. The following descriptions of procedures and methods provide evidence-based options for obtaining such information.

Assessing Community Capacity-Related Social Capital

Studies testing the effectiveness of community-based public health programs reveal that even with the application of sound theory and tested methods that are adequately supported by evidence, some programs may fall short of their expected goals. At least some portion of so-called program failures is likely to be attributable to preexisting social factors that mediate the planning and execution of those programs. One such factor may be a given community's past experience and current resources—its social capital (Burdine et al. 2000; Hawe and Shiell 2000; Kreuter and Lezin 2002; Putnam 2001), a concept that emerged at the turn of the century.

We define community capacity related to **social capital** as the processes and conditions among people and organizations that lead to accomplishing a goal of mutual social benefit. Those processes and conditions are manifested by four interrelated constructs: trust, cooperation, civic engagement, and reciprocity.

The constructs or components of social capital (trust, civic participation, social engagement, and reciprocity) have been independently measured (Kreuter and Lezin 2002; Muntaner et al. 2001). The Civic Index[4] offers a practical approach that gives planners a sense of the level of a community's capacity for undertaking a community-based health program. Devised by the National Civic League and applied in numerous settings, the Civic Index addresses ten categories, each of which has just a few questions or probes designed to elicit information about the community's strengths and weaknesses for that domain (see figure 3.3).

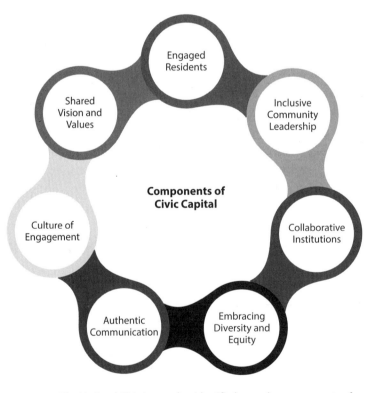

FIGURE 3.3. The National Civic League has identified seven key components of civic capital. For more on these components and a tool for community assessment around the components, see http://www.nationalcivicleague.org.

Asset Mapping

Over the years, social and health policy initiatives have been focused on health problems, with outsiders and professionals calling attention to those needs. For some, especially low-income populations, this problem-oriented approach can be interpreted as too negative. To complement that perspective, McKnight and Kretzmann (2012) advocate a strategy called *asset mapping,* based on the capacities and skills of individuals and the existing assets in a neighborhood or community.[5] The process of asset mapping is divided into three tiers called primary building blocks, secondary building blocks, and potential building blocks. Primary building blocks, the most accessible of them all, can be discovered by assessing individual leadership capacities and those assets *controlled within the neighborhood or community.* Secondary building blocks refer to those assets located in the neighborhood or community but *controlled by those outside that area* (see table 3.1).

Potential building blocks refer to potential assets *located and controlled outside of the community.* Examples include state and federal grant programs, corporate capital investments, and public information campaigns. The lists of specific assets in a community can be visually reflected using an architectural metaphor, as suggested by the notion of building blocks, or as a balance scale showing assets on one side and needs and problems on the other.

TABLE 3.1. Community "building blocks"

Primary building blocks: Assets that are readily available	
Individual assets	**Organizational assets**
• Skills, talents, and experience of residents	• Associations of businesses
• Individual businesses	• Citizens' associations
• Home-based enterprises	• Cultural organizations
• Personal income	• Communication organizations
• Gifts	• Religious organizations

Secondary building blocks: Assets that are not so readily available		
Private and nonprofit organizations	**Public institutions and services**	**Physical resources**
• Institutions of higher education	• Public schools	• Vacant land
• Hospitals	• Police	• Commercial and industrial structures
• Social services agencies	• Libraries	• Housing
	• Fire departments	• Energy and waste resources
	• Parks	

Source: McKnight, J.L., & Kretzmann, J.P. (2012). Mapping community capacity. In Minkler, M. (Ed.), *Community Organizing and Community Building for Health and Welfare* (3rd ed., pp. 171–86). Rutgers University Press.

Note: Community building blocks represent assets that can facilitate planning and should be acknowledged in the planning process to balance the negative connotation sometimes associated with only assessing needs or problems.

Other Assessment Methods

Surveys. Given the diversity of communities and cultures, experienced health program planners may be inclined to devise their own simple surveys to identify community assets and individual abilities within the areas they serve. Before doing so, however, we urge planners to review existing survey instruments such as the Civic Index, mentioned earlier, textbooks (e.g., Gilmore and Campbell 2012), or the myriad tools and guidelines available online, such as the Community Tool Box (Fawcett et al. 2000; Work Group for Community Health and Development [https://ctb.ku.edu/en]).

Health workers or any other group whose work requires a better understanding of the **beliefs**, perceptions, knowledge, and attitudes of the people they serve depend on surveys to fill the gaps in social indicators and health reporting systems such as registries and service reports. The quality of a survey is determined by the validity and reliability of the instrument (Does it accurately and consistently measure what it is supposed to?), how representative the survey sample is (Can you generalize your results to the entire community or group?), and how the survey is administered (Are the questions asked and coded in the same way for all the subjects interviewed?). Various texts offer practical descriptions of the steps and methods used to develop and implement a participatory community-based survey (Fink 2002; Fowler 2001; Green et al. 2003; Minkler 2012).

Some varied examples of using survey methods for social assessments specifically within the context of applying the PRECEDE-PROCEED model include:

- An assessment in El Paso, Texas, on the perception of quality of life for those with bowel dysfunction among Hispanic and non-Hispanic whites (Zuckerman et al. 1996);

- Worksite surveys of employees and managers prior to planning health promotion and disease prevention programs in occupational settings (Bailey et al. 1994; Bertera 1990a; 1990b; 1993; Terry et al. 2020; chapter on worksite applications in this edition);

- An award-winning project in Houston, Texas, that used surveys and focus groups with adolescent patients and their parents concerning their lives with cystic fibrosis in the design and eventually the diffusion of programs (Bartholomew et al. 1989; Bartholomew et al. 2000);

- Surveys of staff nurses in eight British Columbia hospitals and pediatricians in private practice concerning their perceptions of health promotion and disease prevention counseling in their professional roles and of the assets, resources, and needs of hospitals or private practice to support them in these roles (Berland et al. 1995; Cheng et al. 1999);

- Surveys with adolescents in Manaus, on the Amazon in Brazil, and with rural poor African-American residents in North Carolina to assess social and economic aspects of their nutrition (Campbell et al. 1999; Doyle and Feldman 1997); and

- Both the United States and Canada federal governments applying the PRECEDE-PROCEED model in expanding the range of variables included in their first national health promotion surveys beyond the usual health status and health risk factors.[6]

Equity Data. Many jurisdictions are compiling data that highlight both the consequences of structural and social inequities on health and the opportunities to address equity issues to improve quality of life. For example, the National Equity Atlas in the United States compiles a wide variety of equity-related data, with a data-rich equity profile available by locality, state, and region. The city of Dallas, Texas, is one of many local jurisdictions that have created an Equity Index and used it to measure progress in improving various equity-related indicators, such as access to prenatal care (City of Dallas 2019).

Public Service Data. Data on perceived needs and problems are more readily available than one might realize. For example, local broadcast media, often overlooked, can provide rich sources of such data. The US Federal Communications Commission requires television and radio broadcasters to ascertain community needs and concerns on a regular basis and to offer public service programming to address such problems. Members of the print media, along with radio and television broadcasters, have formed coalitions with universities and foundations to conduct public opinion surveys periodically to identify the needs and problems of the population in their service areas (e.g., National Civic League 1999; 2000). When asked to do so, most organizations will share their data unless they have proprietary value that they have not yet exploited or that another organization could use to competitive advantage against them.

MOVING FORWARD BASED ON DATA

When are existing data good enough? Having assessed the community's priority concerns and aspirations for social change, planners come now to a critical junction in deciding which of two or more priorities to pursue. Based on their assessment of the relative urgency of the problems or needs identified and the availability of resources, they can *proceed* immediately to application and action. Or they may see the need and opportunity to continue through a more systematic planning process that would still *precede* action.

Even if a specific route is chosen, key challenges are likely to arise in each of the next three phases of the planning process. Accordingly, conscious decisions have to be made in each phase as to whether the resources, patience, and fortitude of the planners and the community will permit a further refinement as the planning process continues. At each phase, planners need to make assumptions about causation and draw heavily on strategies and methods for interventions that have been tested elsewhere but may or may not be optimal for their particular situation. Each additional phase of the PRECEDE-PROCEED model will further refine and verify the causal assumptions on which the right selection of interventions can be made. But the ideal should not drive out the good or even the adequate and practical actions that have some prospect of addressing priority problems and advancing the community toward its goals.

Communities and populations are complex and differ on virtually any demographic or sociocultural or economic parameters one can think of: population size, ethnicity, culture, history, industry, inequality, employment, geography, and so on. They also vary in their resources and capacities, including past experience with implementing community-based health programs. Together with the highest-priority problems or aspirations of the community and the goals and resources of the planning organization, these constitute the elements of a **situation analysis** (Hallfors et al. 2002), which is an important part of the social assessment process undertaken in this phase of planning. An illustrative example is provided in box 3.3.

An early concern with PRECEDE (before it became PRECEDE-PROCEED) was the time needed to conduct the planning process. For example, an extensive evaluation of the model, applied by the CDC in a Planned Approach to Community Health (PATCH) program in the state of Maine, included the systematic community assessments and local data collection, which took about one year (Goodman et al. 1993).

Some of the authors of that evaluation went on to define dimensions and measures of **community capacity** and community **coalitions**, and to examine more critically the participatory research dimension of the planning process (Goodman 2001; Goodman et al. 1996; Goodman et al. 1998; Green et al. 2001; Green and Kreuter 2002). The CDC and state health departments responded by trying to provide more efficient ways to make state surveillance data available and usable at community levels through technical assistance to communities in compiling and using existing data (Remington and Goodman 1998; Teutsch and Churchill 2000). Support for planning must take into account the practical realities faced by community planning groups, which often include unpaid volunteers who are at the table because they want to see *action* on the problems identified.

A rapidly growing literature analyzes the causes, down to the motivational and enabling factors for change in specific behaviors and environments. It

---

BOX 3.3
Case Example: The North Karelia Project:
Success Built on Social Diagnosis

Analysis of 25 years' worth of data and experience from the North Karelia Cardio-vascular Disease Prevention Project compared to the rest of Finland revealed that the combination of their multiple intervention strategies achieved a 50% decline in cardiovascular mortality among Finnish men. In an early publication describing their methods and strategies, the investigators offered this advice: "To the greatest extent possible, the community analysis ('community assessment') should provide a comprehensive understanding of the situation at the start of the program" (Puska et al. 1985, 164). Forging the principles of social diagnosis, they systematically obtained data to understand the people's perceptions of the problems and how they felt about the possibility of solving those problems, but they did not stop there.

Because the program would depend upon the cooperation of local decision makers and health personnel, these groups were surveyed at the outset. *The community resources, sentiments, and service structure were also considered before deciding on the actual forms of program implementation* (Puska et al. 1985, 165, italics ours).

Sources: Puska et al. (1985); Puska et al. (1998); Vartiainen et al. (2000). See contrast for the neighboring area of Russia: Laatikainen et al. (2002); Farquhar and Green (2015).

---

increasingly provides theory-guided and evidence-based meta-analyses of the best practices identified by research, combined with practice-based evidence that has been shown in systematic evaluations to produce the necessary changes in specific behaviors, environments, or health problems (Vaidya et al. 2017).

We caution planners not to shortcut the planning process too readily, because "best practices" for action derived from studies conducted elsewhere under very different circumstances may not fit the situation of your community or population.[7] The steps outlined in the PRECEDE-PROCEED planning process can help assure you that the causes identified for the highest-priority problems of your community are indeed the ones that lead you to the right selection of best practices. Your planning process can be aided by the situation analysis, which begins with asking the questions posed in table 3.2.

SKIPPING, COMBINING, OR ELABORATING STEPS

When planners take stock of the situation analysis covered in Phase 1, they will be well-positioned to continue the planning process. Depending on your familiarity with the science and the local circumstances, you might readily see a clear path from the social assessment's conclusions about the most important goal

TABLE 3.2. Situation analysis: some key questions to be addressed before planning

Stakeholders (All those who have an investment in the health of the community)	Potential organizational collaborators and key informants	Staff/technical resources	Budget
Who are they?	Who are they?	Are experienced personnel available for this planning?	Have planning costs been estimated?
Are they aware of community health concerns?	Have they been invited to participate?	Will the staff require special training for planning?	Are the facilities and space necessary to conduct the program available?
Are they aware of the program?	Are they supportive or apprehensive?	What existing data and systems resources are available to plan a program or strategy? (Plant the seeds for implementation.)	Are there opportunities to apply for funds to meet staff, equipment, and space needs?
What would count as program "success?" (Plant the seeds for evaluation here.)			What is the timeline for the planning process before the program must begin?
Are they supportive or apprehensive?			

to the next steps required in analyzing the problem. You might even see a clear path to formulating the solutions because the problem has been so thoroughly analyzed before in the scientific and professional literature.

An important question at the end of Phase 1 is whether the social assessment points so clearly to a particular health problem and goal for the focus of Phase 2 that the epidemiological analysis and procedures (chapters 4 and 5) might not be necessary. If this is the case, then one can reasonably skip to Phase 3 (chapter 6). For instance, a social assessment conducted with a low-income community might result in a clear priority health focus on reducing the incidence of untreated opioid use disorder (OUD) because of its negative impact on the quality of life concerns related to employment and educational opportunities. In such a case, the planning team could reasonably skip to Phase 3 with an agreed-upon measurable health objective (e.g., to reduce the incidence of untreated OUD in the community by x% in x years).

The question one can ask upon entering Phase 3 is whether the **etiology** (i.e., the behavioral and environmental determinants of the clearly defined health problem or objective) is so well established that one can simply draw down from the epidemiological literature. For example, if the health problem is malaria or West Nile fever, mosquitoes and their breeding places are clearly the environmental causes. People's use of protective clothing, netting, screening, and insect repellants and their actions to eliminate standing water are very well established as the behavioral and environmental determinants of the problem and the objectives that need to be achieved to reduce the incidence of malaria or West Nile fever. Thus, one can skip planning Phase 3 for this health problem/objective, except to write clear objectives for one or more of these behavioral and environmental outcomes to sharpen the focus in Phase 4.

Skipping phases in the planning process hastens the movement toward formulating the solutions and program or policy action. Such skipping carries with it, however, the liability of not establishing actual baseline data on the community or population for later use in evaluation. It also risks mistaking generalized scientific knowledge as being applicable in circumstances where the populations and social circumstances are extremely diverse or the research on which the scientific knowledge is based is out of date. It will be more difficult to satisfy local constituents that your assumptions for their community, based on data from other populations, are locally appropriate (Green 2001). Local populations will naturally tend to be more skeptical that their community is like others. This is understandable because social assessments of quality of life and health concerns are embedded within the heterogeneous territory of beliefs, attitudes, and cultural norms. Participatory planning can help to minimize these concerns and help determine when skipping from Phase 1 to Phase 3 is possible.

Finally, there will be the temptation in Phase 4 to pull off-the-shelf packaged programs, commercially advertised products, and especially the scientifically verified best practices or evidence-based practices into a program design to streamline that phase. We encourage the use of these, especially the latter, and then especially as they become increasingly well founded in evidence that has grown out of multiple trials in widely varied communities or settings. The data and the tools for making the goodness-of-fit decisions at this stage have become more thoroughly delineated since our previous edition of this book.[8] They remain, however, part of an inexact science of matching and mapping often incompletely tested strategies to local circumstances and population characteristics that differ from those in which the research was done. The science often applies to interventions isolated from their embedding in more complex programs, tested in relatively controlled studies that are uncharacteristic of the real circumstances in which they would be applied locally. Thus, decisions about skipping steps or importing existing programs require careful consideration by the planning group.

SUMMARY

Working jointly with community leaders and residents to identify social and economic problems, the community's existing assets, and quality of life aspirations important to them are essential first steps in thorough health program planning. Health is not an ultimate value in itself except insofar as it relates to social benefits, quality of life, or an organization's bottom line. Health takes on greater importance—both to those who must support the program and those expected to participate in it—when they can see clearly the connection between the health objective and some broader or more compelling social or quality of life objective. This chapter has described a series of steps and a variety of strategies and techniques the planner can use to gather and analyze information about social problems and perceived quality of life, as well as to seek out maximum feasible participation and mobilize community assets.

One can summarize the objectives of social assessment (Phase 1 of health program planning) as follows:

1. To *engage* the community as active partners in the social assessment processes;

2. To *identify* ultimate values and subjective concerns with quality of life or conditions of living in the target population;

3. To *verify* and clarify these subjective concerns, either through existing data sources or new data from surveys or interviews;

4. To *demonstrate* how social concerns and ultimate values can serve to heighten awareness of and motivation to act on health problems;

5. To *assess* the resources, capacities, and assets of a community;

6. To *make explicit* the rationale for the selection of priority problems; and, ultimately,

7. To use the documentation and rationale from social assessment as one of the variables on which to *evaluate* the program.

The social assessment, combined with an analysis of the knowledge available in the literature on the issues identified by it, can produce a situation analysis that leaps over one or more of the other phases of planning in the chapters just ahead. Getting as expeditiously as possible to action and ultimately to outcomes is, after all, what planning is for. But the trade-offs between expediency and quality or effectiveness of the actions, and potential sacrifices in equity of the outcomes, must be weighed carefully before omitting steps in the systematic series of assessments that make up the additional planning processes in the chapters to follow.

EXERCISES

We suggest that these exercises be carried out on a real population accessible to the student or practitioner, in consultation with members of that population and service providers in that community. If this is not possible, the exercises can be applied to a more distant population using published census data, vital statistics, and data from surveys and other online sources to construct a hypothetical case example.

1. List three ways you would or could (or did) involve the members of the population you selected in exercise 3 of chapter 2 in identifying their quality of life concerns and their resources or assets for addressing them. Justify your methods in terms of their feasibility and appropriateness for the population you are trying to help.

2. How did (or would) you verify the subjective data gathered in exercise 1 with objective data on social problems or quality of life concerns, and on assets or resources?

3. Display and discuss your real or hypothetical data as a quality of life diagnosis, justifying your selection of social, economic, and health problems to become the highest priority for a new program.

Notes

1. On cultural considerations in ultimate values: the phrase in the US Constitution protecting "life, liberty, and the pursuit of happiness" acknowledges that the pursuit of happiness and fulfillment are highly individualized concepts and the right to pursue them is a matter of choice. The wisdom of most philosophical systems suggests that we can help other people find the freedom and capacity to pursue those elusive states, but we cannot expect to achieve them for other people. Furthermore, happiness and fulfillment are *states* of being, not permanent *traits*. As states, they are variable and, therefore, can serve as positive and appropriate goals for health promotion. The Canadian variation on the theme of "life, liberty, and the pursuit of happiness" is "peace, order, and good government." This phrase reflects a cultural difference in ultimate values that conditions how the people of neighboring countries might judge their quality of life, civic harmony, and social conditions differently. For examples of community research on the differences in citizens' and scientists' perceptions of policy issues in public health matters, see Pederson et al. (1994) for Canada; Wallerstein et al. (2018) for US and international; Huff et al. (2015) for health promotion in multicultural populations.

2. On measuring personal health-related quality of life: Quality of life measures taken specifically within social assessments and studies using the PRECEDE-PROCEED model are reviewed by McGowan and Green (1995). The notion originally articulated by Fries and Crapo (1981) of adding life to years rather than merely years to life, or "compression of morbidity," is discussed in the context of using theory and models such as PRECEDE-PROCEED in patient education planning by Fries et al. (1989) and Prochaska and Lorig (2001). Jambroes et al. (2016) reviewed the implications for public health policy of

defining health as 'the ability to adapt and self-manage." Holley (1998) provides applications of quality of life measures in mental health.

3. On the Behavioral Risk Factor Surveillance System: CDC's website contains details on the 15 health-related quality of life measures that have been used selectively in BRFSS surveys since 1995; see more at https://www.cdc.gov/brfss/index.html.

4. A copy of the Civic Index can be obtained from the National Civic League, 1445 Market Street, Suite 300, Denver, CO 80202, or online at http://nationalcivicleague.org.

5. For further information on asset mapping, see also Painter (2002).

6. For more background on national health surveys incorporating quality of life measures, see also Green et al. (1983) and Rootman (1988). The Behavioral Risk Factor Surveillance System, a common survey conducted now by all 50 states, with coordination from the CDC, has increasingly incorporated health-related quality of life and social health indicators in the telephone surveys (Centers for Disease Control and Prevention 2000; and http://www.cdc.gov/brfss/, accessed September 17, 2021, or http://www.cdc.gov /hrqol. See also community-level indicators, Karanek et al. 2000. These measures have been used also at the community level, such as in Canada, by Ounpuu et al. (2000) and https://doi.org/10.1007/BF03404258.

7. For more caveats on "best practices" research as a sole guide to interventions appropriate for communities other than those in which the research was conducted, see Cohen et al. (2008); Fidelity versus flexibility: translating evidence-based research into practice (Brownson et al. 2018); Reconciling the pulls of practice and the push of research (Green and Nasser 2018).

8. For further information on the growing science of aligning theory and research on "best practices" to population and community characteristics, see Bartholomew-Eldredge et al. (2016); Centers for Disease Control and Prevention (2000); Fiore et al. (2000); Gilbert and Sawyer (2000); Gregory (2002); Wandersman et al. (2000); World Health Organization (2001; 2002); Zaza et al. (2001). For an alternative approach to the synthesis of quantitative evidence in arriving at "what works" for neighborhoods and communities, see Schorr (1997).

References

Bailey, P.H., Rukholm, E.E., Vanderlee, R., & Hyland, J. (1994). A heart health survey at the worksite: The first step to effective programming. *AAOHN Journal, 42*(1), 9–14.

Bartholomew, L.K., Czyzewski, D., Swank, P.R., McCormick, L., & Parcel, G.S. (2000). Maximizing the impact of the cystic fibrosis family education program: Factors related to program diffusion. *Family and Community Health, 22*(4), 27–47. https://doi.org/10.1097 /00003727-200001000-00005

Bartholomew-Eldredge, L.K., Markham, C.M., Ruiter, R.A.C., Fernández, M.E., Kok, G., & Parcel, G.S. (2016). *Planning Health Promotion Programs: An Intervention Mapping Approach* (4th ed.). Jossey-Bass, Wiley.

Bartholomew, L.K., Seilheimer, D.K., Parcel, G.S., Spinelli, S.H., & Pumariega, A.J. (1989). Planning patient education for cystic fibrosis: Application of a diagnostic framework. *Patient Education and Counseling, 13*(1), 57–68. https://doi.org/10.1016/0738-3991 (89)90070-0

Berland, A., Whyte, N.B., & Maxwell, L. (1995). Hospital nurses and health promotion. *Canadian Journal of Nursing Research, 27*(4), 13–31.

Bertera, R.L. (1990a). The effects of workplace health promotion on absenteeism and employment costs in a large industrial population. *American Journal of Public Health, 80*(9), 1101–5. https://doi.org/10.2105/ajph.80.9.1101

Bertera, R.L. (1990b). Planning and implementing health promotion in the workplace: A case study of the Du Pont Company experience. *Health Education Quarterly, 17*(3), 307–27. https://doi.org/10.1177/109019819001700307

Bertera, R.L. (1993). Behavioral risk factor and illness day changes with workplace health promotion: Two-year results. *American Journal of Health Promotion, 7*(5), 365–73. https://doi.org/10.4278/0890-1171-7.5.365

Brownson, R.C., Fielding, J.E., & Green, L.W. (2018). Building capacity for evidence-based public health: Reconciling the pulls of practice and the push of research. *Annual Review of Public Health, 39*, 27–53. https://doi.org/10.1146/annurev-publhealth-040617-014746

Burdine, J.N., Felix, M.R., Abel, A.L., Wiltraut, C.J., & Musselman, Y.J. (2000). The SF-12 as a population health measure: an exploratory examination of potential for application. *Health Services Research, 35*(4), 885–904. https://www.ncbi.nlm.nih.gov/pmc/articles/PMC1089158

Campbell, M.K., Demark-Wahnefried, W., Symons, M., Kalsbeek, W.D., Dodds, J., Cowan, A., Jackson, B., Motsinger, B., Hoben, K., Lashley, J., Demissie, S., & McClelland, J.W. (1999). Fruit and vegetable consumption and prevention of cancer: The Black Churches United for Better Health Project. *American Journal of Public Health, 89*(9), 1390–6. https://doi.org/10.2105/ajph.89.9.1390

Centers for Disease Control and Prevention. (2000). *Measuring healthy days: Population assessment of health-related quality of life.* Health Care and Aging Studies Branch, Division of Adult and Community Health, National Center for Chronic Disease Prevention and Health Promotion, CDC. https://www.cdc.gov/hrqol/pdfs/mhd.pdf

Cheng, T.L., DeWitt, T.G., Savageau, J.A., & O'Connor, K.G. (1999). Determinants of counseling in primary care pediatric practice. *Archives of Pediatrics & Adolescent Medicine, 153*(6), 629–35. https://doi.org/10.1001/archpedi.153.6.629

City of Dallas. (2019). *Dallas Equity Indicators: Measuring Change Toward Greater Equity in Dallas: 2019 Report.* https://dallascityhall.com/departments/pnv/dallas-equity-indicators/DCH%20Documents/equity-indicators-booklet-2019.pdf

Cohen, D.J., Crabtree, B.F., Etz, R.S., Balasubramanian, B.A., Donahue, K.E., Leviton, L.C., Clark, E.C., Isaacson, N.F., Stange, K.C., & Green, L.W. (2008). Fidelity versus flexibility: translating evidence-based research into practice. *American Journal of Preventive Medicine, 35*(Suppl. 5), S381–9. https://doi.org/10.1016/j.amepre.2008.08.005

Doyle, E.I., & Feldman, R.H.L. (1997). Factors affecting nutrition behavior among middle-class adolescents in urban area of northern region of Brazil. *Revista de Saúde Pública, 31*(4), 342–50. https://doi.org/10.1590/s0034-89101997000400003

Farquhar, J. & Green, L.W. (2015). Community intervention trials in high-income countries. In Detels, R., Gulliford, M., Abdool Karim, Q., and Tan, C.C. (Eds.), *Oxford Textbook of Public Health* (6th ed., Vol. 2, pp. 516–27). Oxford University Press. https://doi.org/10.1093/med/9780199661756.003.0112

Fawcett, S.B., Francisco, V.T., Schultz, J.A., Nagy, G., Berkowitz, B., & Wolff, T.J. (2000). The Community Tool Box: A Web-based resource for building healthier communities. *Public Health Reports, 115*(2–3), 274–8.

Finegood, D.T., Johnston, L.M., Steinberg, M., Matteson, C.L., & Deck, P. (2014). Complexity, systems thinking, and Health Behavior Change. In Kahan, S., Gielen, A., Fagan, P.J., & Green, L.W. (Eds.), *Health Behavior Change in Populations* (pp. 435–58). Johns Hopkins University Press.

Fink, A. (Ed.). (2002). *The survey kit: Ten volume set* (2nd ed.). SAGE Publishing.

Fiore, M.C., Bailey, W.C., Cohen, S.J., Dorfman, S.F., Goldstein, M.G., Gritz, E.R., Heyman, R.B., Jae, C.R., Kottke, T.W., Lando, H.A., et al. (2000). *Treating tobacco use and dependence: Quick reference guide for clinicians.* US Department of Health and Human Services. Public Health Service.

Fowler, F.J. (2001). *Survey research methods* (3rd ed.). SAGE Publishing.

Fries, J.F., & Crapo, L.M. (1981). *Vitality and aging.* W.H. Freeman and Company.

Fries, J., Green, L.W., & Levine, S. (1989). Health promotion and the compression of morbidity. *The Lancet, 1*(8636), 481–3. https://doi.org/10.1016/s0140-6736(89)91376-7

Gilbert, G., & Sawyer, R. (2000). *Health education: Creating strategies for school and community health* (2nd ed.). Jones & Bartlett Learning.

Gilmore, G.D., & Campbell, M.D. (2012). *Needs and Capacity Assessment Strategies for Health Education and Health Promotion* (4th ed.). Jones & Bartlett Learning.

Gold, M.R., Stevenson, D., & Fryback, D.G. (2002). HALYs and QALYs and DALYs, oh my: Similarities and differences in summary measures of population health. *Annual Review of Public Health, 23,* 115–34. https://doi.org/10.1146/annurev.publhealth.23.100901.140513

Goodman, R.M. (2001). Community-based participatory research: Questions and challenges to an essential approach. *Journal of Public Health Management & Practice, 7*(5), v–vi. https://doi.org/10.1097/00124784-200107050-00001

Goodman, R.M., Speers, M.A., McLeroy, K., Fawcett, S., Kegler, M., Parker, E., Smith, S.R., Sterling, T.D., & Wallerstein, N. (1998). Identifying and defining the dimensions of community capacity to provide a basis for measurement. *Health Education and Behavior, 25*(3), 258–78. https://doi.org/10.1177/109019819802500303

Goodman, R.M., Steckler, A., Hoover, S., & Schwartz, R. (1993). A critique of contemporary community health promotion approaches: based on a qualitative review of six programs in Maine. *American Journal of Health Promotion, 7*(3), 208–20. https://doi.org/10.4278/0890-1171-7.3.208

Goodman, R.M., Wandersman, A., Chinman, M., Imm, P., & Morrisey, E. (1996). An ecological assessment of community-based interventions for prevention and health promotion: Approaches to measuring community coalitions. *American Journal of Community Psychology, 24*(1), 33–61. https://doi.org/10.1007/BF02511882

Green, L.W. (2001). From research to "best practices" in other settings and populations. American Journal of Health Behavior, 25(3), 165–78. https://doi.org/10.5993/ajhb.25.3.2

Green, L.W., Daniel, M., & Novick, L. (2001). Partnerships and coalitions for community based research. Public Health Reports, 116(Suppl. 1), 20–31. https://doi.org/10.1093/phr/116.S1.20

Green, L.W., George, A., Daniel, M., Frankish, C.J., Herbert, C.P., Bowie, W., & O'Neill, M. (2003). Guidelines for participatory research, reproduced from *Study of participatory research in health promotion in Canada.* Ottawa, Royal Society of Canada, 1996. In Minkler, M., & Wallerstein, N. (Eds.). *Community-based participatory research for health* (2nd ed., pp. 135–54). Jossey-Bass.

Green, L.W., & Kreuter, M,W. (2002). Fighting back, or fighting themselves? Community coalitions against substance abuse and their use of best practices. *American Journal of Preventive Medicine, 23*(4), 303–6. https://doi.org/10.1016/S0749-3797(02)00519-6

Green, L.W., & Nasser, M. (2018). Furthering dissemination and implementation research: The need for more attention to external validity. In Brownson, R., Colditz, G., & Parker, E. (Eds.), *Dissemination and Implementation Research: Translating Science to Practice* (2nd ed., pp. 305–26). Oxford University Press.

Green, L.W., Wilson, R.W., & Bauer, K.G. (1983). Data required to measure progress on the objectives for the nation in disease prevention and health promotion. *American Journal of Public Health, 73*(1), 18–24. https://doi.org/10.2105/ajph.73.1.18

Gregory, S. (2002). *Guidelines for comprehensive programs to promote healthy eating and physical activity.* Human Kinetics.

Haley, S.M., Jette, A.M., Coster, W.J., Kooyoomjian, J.T., Levenson, S., Heeren, T., & Ashba, J. (2002). Late Life Function and Disability Instrument: II. Development and evaluation of the function component. *The Journals of Gerontology Series A Biological Sciences and Medical Sciences 57*(4), M217–22. https://doi.org/10.1093/gerona/57.4.m217

Hallfors, D., Cho, H., Livert, D., & Kadushin, C. (2002). Fighting back against substance abuse: are community coalitions winning? *American Journal of Preventive Medicine, 23*(4), 237–45. https://doi.org/10.1016/s0749-3797(02)00511-1

Hawe, P., & Shiell, A. (2000). Social capital and health promotion: A review. *Social Science and Medicine 51*(6), 871–85. https://doi.org/10.1016/s0277-9536(00)00067-8

Holley, H. (Ed.). (1998). Quality of life measurement in mental health. *Canadian Journal of Community Mental Health*(Special Suppl. 3), 9–20, 9–21.

Huff, R.M., Kline, M.V., & Peterson, D.V. (Eds.). (2015). *Health Promotion in Multicultural Populations: A Handbook for Practitioners and Students* (3rd ed.). SAGE Publishing.

Jambroes, M., Nederland, T., Kaljouw, M., van Vliet, K., Essink-Bot, M.-L., & Ruwaard, D. (2016). Implications of health as 'the ability to adapt and self-manage' for public health policy: a qualitative study. *The European Journal of Public Health, 26*(3), 412–16. https://doi.org/10.1093/eurpub/ckv206

Jette, A.M., & Keysor, J.J. (2002). Uses of evidence in disability outcomes and effectiveness research. *The Milbank Quarterly, 80*(2), 325–45. https://doi.org/10.1111/1468-0009.t01-1-00006

Kaplan, R.M., & Frosch, D.L. (2005). Decision making in medicine and health care. *Annual Review of Clinical Psychology, 1*, 525–56. https://doi.org/10.1146/annurev.clinpsy.1.102803.144118

Karanek, N., Sockwell, D., Jia, H., & CDC. (2000). Community indicators of health-related quality of life—United States, 1993–1997. *Morbidity and Mortality Weekly Report, 49*(13), 281–5. https://www.cdc.gov/mmwr/preview/mmwrhtml/mm4913a4.htm

Karpati, A., Galea, S., Awerbuch, T., & Levins, R. (2002). Variability and vulnerability at the ecological level: Implications for understanding the social determinants of health. *American Journal of Public Health, 92*(11), 1768–72. https://doi.org/10.2105/ajph.92.11.1768

Kosinski, M., Kujawski, S.C., Martin, R., Wanke, L.A., Buatti, M.C., Ware, J.E. Jr., & Perfetto, E.M. (2002). Health-related quality of life in early rheumatoid arthritis: impact of disease and treatment response. *American Journal of Managed Care, 8*(3), 231–40.

Kreuter, M.W., & Lezin, N. (2002). Social capital theory: implications for community-based health promotion. In DiClemente, R.J., Crosby, R.A., & Kegler, M.C. (Eds.), *Emerging theories in health promotion practice and research: Strategies for improving public health* (pp. 228–54). Jossey-Bass.

Laatikainen, T., Delong, L., Pokusajeva, S., Uhanov, M., Vartiainen, E., & Puska, P. (2002). Changes in cardiovascular risk factors and health behaviours from 1992 to 1997 in the Republic of Karelia, Russia. *European Journal of Public Health, 12*(1), 37–43. https://doi.org/10.1093/eurpub/12.1.37

Lorig, K.R., Laurent, D.D., Deyo, R.A., Marnell, M.E., Minor, M.A., & Ritter, P.L. (2002). Can a back pain e-mail discussion group improve health status and lower health care costs? A randomized study. *JAMA Internal Medicine, 162*(7), 792–6. https://doi.org/10.1001/archinte.162.7.792

Manocchia, M., Keller, S., & Ware, J.E. (2001). Sleep problems, health-related quality of life, work functioning and health care utilization among the chronically ill. *Quality of Life Research, 10*(4), 331–45. https://doi.org/10.1023/a:1012299519637

McGowan, P., & Green, L.W. (1995). Arthritis self-management in native populations of British Columbia: An application of health promotion and participatory research principles in chronic disease control. *Canadian Journal on Aging, 14*(1, Suppl. 1), 201–12. https://doi.org/10.1017/S0714980800005511

McKnight, J.L., & Kretzmann, J.P. (2012). Mapping community capacity. In Minkler, M. (Ed.), *Community Organizing and Community Building for Health* (3rd ed., pp. 171–86). Rutgers University Press.

Minkler, M. (Ed.). (2012). *Community Organizing and Community Building for Health and Welfare* (3rd ed.). Rutgers University Press.

Muntaner, C., Lynch, J., & Smith, G.D. (2001). Social capital, disorganized communities, and the third way: Understanding the retreat from structural inequalities in epidemiology and public health. *International Journal of Health Services, 31*(2), 213–37. https://doi.org/10.2190/NVW3-4HH0-74PX-AC38

National Civic League. (1999). *The Civic Index: Measuring your community's civic health.* National Civic League. https://www.nationalcivicleague.org.

National Civic League and Staff of the St. Louis County Department of Health. (2000). *A Guide to a Community-Oriented Approach to Core Public Health Functions.* National Civic League.

Ounpuu, S., Kreuger, P., Vermeulen, M., & Chambers, L. (2000). Using the U.S. Behavior[al] Risk Factor Surveillance System's health related quality of life survey tool in a Canadian city. *Canadian Journal of Public Health, 91*(1), 67–72. https://doi.org/10.1007/BF03404258

Painter, S.B. (2002). *Community health education and promotion manual* (2nd ed.). Aspen Publishers.

Pederson, A., O'Neill, M., & Rootman, I. (Eds.). (1994). *Health Promotion in Canada.* WB Saunders Canada.

Prochaska, T.R., & Lorig, K. (2001). What do we know about what works? The role of theory in patient education. In Lorig, K., *Patient Education: A Practical Approach* (3rd ed., pp. 21–55). SAGE Publishing.

Puska, P., Nissinen, A., Tuomilehto, J., Salonen, J.T., Koskela, K., McAlister, A., Kottke, T.E., Maccoby, N., & Farquhar, J.W. (1985). The community-based strategy to prevent coronary heart disease: Conclusions from the ten years of the North Karelia Project. *Annual Review of Public Health, 6*, 147–93. https://doi.org/10.1146/annurev.pu.06.050185.001051

Puska, P., Vartiainen, E., Tuomilehto, J., Salomaa, V., & Nissinen, A. (1998). Changes in premature deaths in Finland: successful long-term prevention of cardiovascular diseases. *Bulletin of the World Health Organization, 76*(4), 416–25.

Putnam, R.D. (2001). *Bowling Alone: The Collapse And Revival Of American Community.* Simon & Schuster.

Remington, P.L., & Goodman, R.A. (1998). Chronic disease surveillance. In Brownson, R.C., Remington, P.L., & Davis, J.R. (Eds.), *Chronic Disease Epidemiology and Control* (2nd ed., pp. 55–76). American Public Health Association.

Rootman, I.R. (1988). Canada's Health Promotion Survey. In Rootman, I., Warren, R., Stephens, T., & Peters, L. (Eds.), *Canada's Health Promotion Survey: Technical Report.* Minister of Supply and Services.

Schorr, L.B. (1997). *Common Purpose: Strengthening Families and Neighborhoods to Rebuild America.* Anchor Books, Doubleday.

Teutsch, S.M., & Churchill, R.E. (2000). *Principles and Practice of Public Health Surveillance* (2nd ed.). Oxford University Press.

Vaidya, N., Thota, A.B., Proia, K.K., Jamieson, S., Mercer, S.L., Elder, R.W., Yoon, P., Kaufmann, R., & Zaza, S. (2017). Practice-based evidence in Community Guide Systematic Reviews. *American Journal of Public Health, 107*(3), 413–20. https://doi.org/10.2105/AJPH.2016.303583

Vartiainen, E., Jousilahti, P., Alfthan, G., Sundvall, J., Pietinen, P., & Puska, P. (2000). Cardiovascular risk factor changes in Finland, 1972-1997. *International Journal of Epidemiology, 29*(1), 49–56. https://doi.org/10.1093/ije/29.1.49

Wallerstein, N., Duran, B., Oetzel, J.G., & Minkler, M. (Eds.). (2018). *Community-Based Participatory Research for Health: Advancing Social and Health Equity.* Jossey-Bass/John Wiley & Sons, Inc.

Wandersman, A., Imm, P., Chinman, M., & Kafterian, S. (2000). Getting to outcomes: A results-based approach to accountability. *Evaluation and Program Planning, 23*(3), 389–95. https://doi.org/10.1016/S0149-7189(00)00028-8

Ware, J.E., & Kosinski, M. (2001). Interpreting SF-36 summary health measures: a response. *Quality of Life Research, 10*(5), 405–13; 415–20. https://doi.org/10.1023/a:1012588218728

Work Group on Health Promotion and Community Development, The Community Toolbox. (n.d.) *A Model for Getting Started.* University of Kansas. https://ctb.ku.edu/en/get-started

World Health Organization. (2001). *International classification of functioning, disability and health*. World Health Organization.

World Health Organization. (2002). *The World Health Report 2002: Reducing risks, promoting healthy life*. World Health Organization.

Zaza, S., Sleet, D.A., Thompson, R.S., Sosin, D.M., Bolen, J.C., & Task Force on Community Preventive Services. (2001). Reviews of evidence regarding interventions to increase use of child safety seats. *American Journal of Preventive Medicine, 21*(Suppl. 4), 31–47. https://doi.org/10.1016/s0749-3797(01)00377-4

Zuckerman, M.J., Guerra, L.G., Drossman, D.A., Foland, J.A., Gregory, G.G. (1996). Health-care-seeking behaviors related to bowel complaints—Hispanics versus non-Hispanic whites. *Digestive Diseases and Sciences, 41*(1), 77–82. https://doi.org/10.1007/BF02208587

CHAPTER 4

Epidemiological Assessment I: Population Health

•

Lawrence W. Green, Andrea Carlson Gielen,
and Marshall W. Kreuter

Learning Objectives

After completing the chapter, the reader will be able to:

- Understand the community or population health components of an epidemiological assessment.
- Describe epidemiology concepts of prevalence, incidence, and adjusted rates.
- Use these and other problem indicators to create program objectives.

INTRODUCTION

Mindful of the reciprocal relationship between quality of life and health status, we now turn to the analytic tasks that will help planners focus their health programs on issues that are both *important* and *amenable to change*. Specifically, those tasks include (1) identifying the health problems or community challenges deserving of priority program focus, (2) uncovering the behavioral and environmental factors most likely influencing the priority health issues that emerged from the first task, and (3) translating those priority problems and factors into measurable objectives to enable program evaluation.

We refer to this phase of the PRECEDE-PROCEED model as the **epidemiological assessment** (see figure 4.1), because the problem-solving principles and the subject matter of epidemiology provide a sound and credible foundation to guide planners as they undertake those three tasks. The epidemiological assessment includes three factors: health, behavioral, and environmental. Here we start with the population's *health* assessment; chapter 5 will continue with the *behavioral* and *environmental* assessments and discuss genetics.

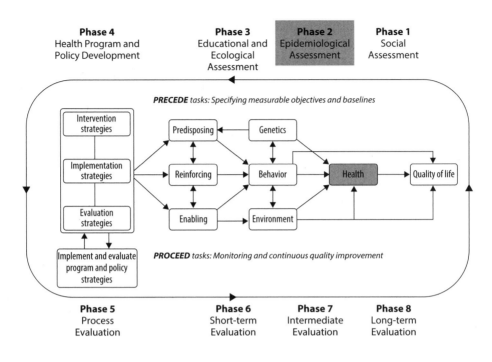

Phase 4
Health Program and
Policy Development

Phase 3
Educational and
Ecological
Assessment

Phase 2
Epidemiological
Assessment

Phase 1
Social
Assessment

PRECEDE tasks: Specifying measurable objectives and baselines

Intervention strategies

Implementation strategies

Evaluation strategies

Implement and evaluate program and policy strategies

Predisposing

Reinforcing

Enabling

Genetics

Behavior

Environment

Health

Quality of life

PROCEED tasks: Monitoring and continuous quality improvement

Phase 5
Process
Evaluation

Phase 6
Short-term
Evaluation

Phase 7
Intermediate
Evaluation

Phase 8
Long-term
Evaluation

FIGURE 4.1. The second phase of the PRECEDE-PROCEED model, epidemiological assessment, begins with a focus on the incidence, prevalence, and distribution of health conditions.

STARTING IN THE MIDDLE: A REALITY FOR PRACTITIONERS

Before examining the methods and procedures for carrying out the process of epidemiological assessment, we need to clarify what we mean by "starting in the middle." As a logic model, the PRECEDE-PROCEED process ideally begins with a social assessment that (1) yields insight into the quality of life for a given population, and (2) promotes collaborative actions designed to foster local participation in the planning and implementation process (see chapters 2 and 3).

That assessment is followed by a delineation of the priority health problems relevant to the findings of the social assessment. For a majority of practitioners and organizations, however, the health issue is the starting point, rather than the second phase of planning, as the PRECEDE-PROCEED logic model would imply with the placement of "social problem" or "quality of life" as the ultimate outcome. Thus, for many, the planning task is undertaken in a context in which a health problem or issue is predetermined by a sponsoring agency's mission. For example, such would be the case for a nurse in the office of maternal and child health at a local health agency; a health educator in the injury prevention and control division in a state or provincial health department; the tobacco control director for the American Cancer Society; and the fitness coordinator for a worksite wellness program. Because the general health goal is settled in each of these cases, further planning will logically start with an analysis of the various environmental and behavioral factors that are determinants of the pre-determined health problem, as in, starting in the middle. One may ask, "If starting in the middle is so often the norm, why bother having a command of both the social assessment and epidemiologic assessment phases of the PRECEDE-PROCEED model?" We offer three very important and practical reasons.

THREE REASONS WHY PLANNERS SHOULD KNOW AND USE THE WHOLE MODEL

Reason 1

First, there will be circumstances when community or organizational health program planning efforts are initiated precisely for the purpose of establishing program priorities based on the unique social or economic needs and circumstances of a given population. An example of this would be a vaccination program for newly arrived immigrant children needing to enroll in school in the United States. In those instances, the planning process is used to clarify and sort out multiple health and social issues and concerns and to establish mutually agreed-upon priorities for program and policy action. These are ideal circumstances for the application of both the social and epidemiological assessments of PRECEDE. A COVID-19 example comes from the experience of the early months of the immunization campaign. Epidemiological analyses in many states and communities showed that ethnic and racial minority and other low-income groups had low rates of vaccination compared with their community rates. Social and behavioral analyses provided insight into reasons for distrust of the vaccines and the procedures for the vaccination, which led to adjustments in the communications and neighborhood intervention strategies across communities.

Reason 2

Sometimes, when the health problem is predetermined by a policy or funding agency, or by an epidemic, solving that problem is viewed as the end, not as a means to some other end. To avoid the mistake of casting health as an ultimate, rather than instrumental, value (as discussed in chapter 3), planners will find it useful to understand why this health problem or issue matters—to affirm the connection between the health status of a population and its ability to cope with the demands and quality of life or social conditions shaping their lives (Huber et al. 2011). The World Health Organization (WHO) definition of health has been challenged on these grounds (Green 2017; Johnson et al. 2014). This connection has been formally established in the international public health community through the International Classification of Functioning, Disability, and Health (ICF). Developed by the WHO (2001), the ICF clarifies the interconnected and dynamic relationships between a given health condition and important quality of life concerns of individuals, including functional and structural impairments, activity limitations, and social and participation restrictions.

When planners explore the potential benefits that might accrue to the population if a program or policy accomplished its health improvement goals, they will be simultaneously addressing broader social concerns and issues. Sensitivity on the part of decision makers and the general public to these potential social benefits can be instrumental in sustaining support for a program. For example, programs and policies that are effective in reducing youth violence will create a safer environment. In turn, safer communities will make it more likely that residents will walk in their neighborhoods and perhaps even create and promote the use of recreational facilities in those neighborhoods. Commercial enterprises are more apt to make investments in those places deemed to be safe.

Reason 3

In cases where a given health problem or issue has been declared the focal point for a program, planners can get a head start on the evaluation process by thoroughly familiarizing themselves with any baseline data on the program's focal point. Over time, evaluation strategies and program direction will be influenced by a working knowledge of the baseline indicators that were used to determine the health priority. That same working knowledge can help planners make program adjustments based on changes in demographic trends or technological advances. For example, categorical programs and surveillance systems focusing on the early detection and treatment of breast and cervical cancer have served as the foundation for a more comprehensive approach to cancer prevention and control as the technical capacity to screen and treat other cancers has developed and improved. Evaluation, as the middle part of the word implies, involves "valuing." The values placed on health are related to the social, economic, and emotional consequences of specific health outcomes—accordingly, evaluation has to take these into account and can do so more systematically if it can follow and build on a social assessment. This will be the case regardless of whether that assessment is done before or after identifying the priority health problem.

RECIPROCITY, SOCIAL DETERMINANTS, AND PARTICIPATION

By definition, the reciprocal, ecological nature of health and social problems means that causation is multidirectional (see also chapters 2 and 3). Thus, the planner should consider how social determinants and quality of life concerns influence the priority health problem, especially from the perspective of those who are living with the health condition and will be participating in the program, and how the health problem is influencing the social or quality of life concerns.

The relationships in figure 4.2 are supported by growing scientific evidence documenting the powerful influence that social, economic, and environmental factors have on health status (Frank 1995). The figure illustrates how poverty, health, lifestyle, and environmental factors can be viewed in an ecological perspective of reciprocal relationships. This categorization of factors can help planners gather relevant information that will provide the rationale, if not a mandate, for crafting programs directed at health-related factors that are framed within a broader social and ecological context. For example, migrant workers and their

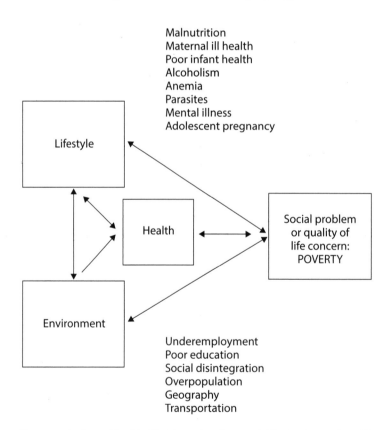

FIGURE 4.2. The examples here of health, lifestyle, and environmental factors interacting with poverty in reciprocal relationships support an ecological approach to assessment that cannot be rigidly linear or unidirectional in addressing causes and effects.

families might suffer from poor access to organized social support systems such as education and welfare. Poor roads or geographic isolation might contribute to poverty, as might a lack of jobs. In addition, research indicates biases regarding racial or ethnic minority status frequently contribute to social and health problems (Stewart and Nápoles-Springer 2003; Whaley and Geller 2003; Zuvekas and Taliaferro 2003).

Health programs undertaken by governmental health agencies are sometimes criticized for not placing greater emphasis on social and economic factors and their inequities. This lack of emphasis is due, in part, to the way public health programs are funded. Planners are informed that their programs must focus on tightly defined categorical imperatives (i.e., specific diseases or risk factors), the appropriations for which have been made by federal or state legislators or local commissioners. Those mandates, coupled with the reality that the expenditure of tax dollars will be carefully audited, inhibit planners from using health agency resources to address social issues, even though evidence of a connection to health may have been documented.

Effective planners can maintain the spirit of those regulatory realities and address the social dimensions connected to health problems by acting on one of the main points emphasized in chapter 2: that planning health programs inevitably requires the active participation and input from partners outside the traditional health sector. Many of those partners will be associated with public, private, or philanthropic organizations whose missions and mandates focus on critical social or economic issues, particularly those social determinants of health that the health agency would find difficult to tackle alone (see box 4.1).

BOX 4.1

Case Example: Seattle Partners for Healthy Communities

Seattle Partners for Healthy Communities (SPHC) is a multidisciplinary collaboration of community agencies and interest groups that carries out **participatory research** aimed at improving the health of socioeconomically marginalized communities (Krieger et al. 2002). The stated goal of the SPHC is "to identify promising approaches through which communities and professionals can collaboratively address the social determinants of health" (362). One of the SPHC projects focused on the problem of childhood asthma. Here is the list of collaborative partners with a key stake in the outcomes of that project:

- American Lung Association
- Center for Multicultural Health
- Community Coalition for Environmental Justice
- League of Women Voters

(continued)

- Odessa Brown Children's Clinic
- Parent and Child Development Center
- Seattle Housing Authority
- Seattle Tenants Union
- Washington Toxics Coalition
- Seattle-King County Health Department
- University of Washington School of Public Health

The organizational diversity of this coalition creates the potential for leveraging resources, data, and support not only from the public and nonprofit health sector, but also from other key sectors, including justice, child development and education, cultural diversity, parent groups, political advocacy, and housing. It is evident that sustained and committed engagement of these partners in a health program will depend on the extent to which they can see that the health goals of the program also contribute to and complement the goals of their respective agencies and organizations. They will see that more clearly if they have participated in the formative research and evaluation process as part of the planning process.

EPIDEMIOLOGY

Key Principles and Terms of Descriptive Epidemiology

For planners, the process of assessment is informed as they seek and obtain answers to five epidemiological questions:

1. What is the problem (according to whom)?

2. Who has the problem?

3. Why do those with the problem have it?

4. What are we going to do about it?

5. How will we know if our programmatic **actions** are having the intended effect?

Evaluation is at the heart of the fifth question, and it is addressed in detail in chapter 9.

Epidemiology is the study of the distribution and causes of health-related conditions or events in defined populations and the application of this study to control health problems.[1] The questions above are at the core of the epidemiological analysis needed for this phase of PRECEDE. Problem definition is critical. In the past, there have been areas, due to economic or organizational limitations, where certain data elements were not available for a population. Yet when credible community surveys have been undertaken, problems deemed important and serious by residents can be detected, and possibly incorporated, as part of the problem identification process (see box 4.2).

A closer examination of the components of this definition reveals why the principles of epidemiology are relevant for all phases of the PRECEDE-PROCEED planning process.

First, the word "study" implies a planned examination of health problems through a combination of methods: (1) observation and surveillance, and (2) interpretive analysis.

"Distribution" is an important concept because it highlights the reality that health problems are not distributed equally within or across populations. Not everyone is at the same risk of having, or eventually developing, a given health problem.

"Determinants" refer to those factors and conditions that influence health or cause disease, disability, or death. Over time, we have come to use adjectives such as physical, biological, social, economic, environmental, structural, cultural, behavioral, and emotional to distinguish among a variety of different categories of determinants. These multiple determinants, many of which interact with one another, provide key insights for those responsible for health program planning and evaluation.

These two dimensions, distribution and determinants, distinguish the two major parts of this chapter, the first addressing descriptive epidemiology and the second addressing the etiological analyses needed to identify relevant causes or determinants of the health problems.

"Health-related conditions" refers to specific, measurable events. Examples include diseases, injuries, disabilities, and causes of death, behavior such as the use of tobacco, and the provision and use of health services.

"Specified populations" refers to those who either have or are at risk for having one or more health-related conditions. An example would be a population or subpopulation living in or around areas where environmental conditions may put them at risk (e.g., living in areas with high sun exposure increases the chances for skin cancers, or children with asthma living in roach-infested housing increases the likelihood of asthma attacks).

Finally, the phrase "application to control" refers to the ultimate aim of epidemiology—using the information gathered as the basis for developing programs and policies to promote, protect, and restore health. In the examples that follow in this chapter, we will see that epidemiology provides planners with rich descriptive insights that will help them not only as they sift and sort through various health indicators, but also in their efforts to explain the relevance of those indicators to others.

BOX 4.2
Case Example: The Importance of Community Input in Planning

Atlanta, Georgia, is organized into 25 neighborhood planning units (NPUs). Each NPU has volunteer resident leaders whose goals are to (1) enhance relevant social and economic conditions that influence the quality of life in their neighborhood, and (2) use their local experience as the basis for formal recommendations presented to the mayor and city council on zoning, land use, and other issues in those neighborhoods. Georgia State University received a three-year grant from the National Institute on Minority Health and Health Disparities to identify effective approaches to addressing priority health problems in one of those areas (NPU-V), which had 17,000 mostly low-income African-American residents in five contiguous neighborhoods.

An initial step in the grant was to create a team of community health workers (CHWs) recruited from each of the five NPU-V neighborhoods. An initial task of the CHWs was to help neighborhood residents answer these key questions linked to the PRECEDE-PROCEED model: What's the leading health problem? Who has it? Why them? And what can we do about it?

As a part of that process, the CHWs provided each neighborhood group with the current health priorities based on data from Fulton County and the Southside Medical Center (which provided primary health services across NPU-V). Those data were shared in "listening sessions," during which residents were asked to identify the health problems that were "most critical" and should be a community priority.

The priority problem they chose (which did not show up in the county health data or Southside medical data) came from a CDC Behavioral Risk Factor question used in a local survey: "Thinking about mental health (which includes stress, depression, and problems with emotions), for how many days in the last 30 days was your mental health not good? (Frequent mental distress is defined as having 14 or more days per month.)"

In the five NPU-V neighborhoods, 26% of participants indicated that they experienced 14 or more days of mental distress per month—that was more than 2.5 times higher than the national average of 9.4%. Although previously unaware of those data, *NPU-V residents selected mental health and depression as their top priority.* The CEO of the Southside Medical Center indicated that those findings

> "are a reflection of the reality that mental health and depression were not among those health conditions our primary care center screened for . . . that doesn't mean that depression and mental health were not problems, it meant we weren't collecting those data!"

Southside Medical Center and other health nonprofits serving NPU-V residents subsequently changed their approach to behavioral health screening and treatment.

Source: Kreuter, M.W., Kegler, M.C., Joseph, K.T., Redwood, Y.A. & Hooker, M. (2012). The impact of implementing selected CBPR strategies to address disparities in urban Atlanta: a retrospective case study. *Health Education Research, 26*(4), 729–41. https://doi.org/0.1093/her/cys053

In sum, the epidemiological analysis of health data is essential to the planning process because it:

- Establishes the relative importance and prevalence or incidence of various health problems in the target population as a whole and in population subgroups;

- Provides evidence for setting program priorities among the various health problems and subgroups;

- Identifies the relative importance and prevalence or incidence of various determinants or factors that are influencing the health problems in the environment and in people's behaviors; and

- Establishes markers and indicators essential for program evaluation, with data that represent before-program baseline measures compared with data collected post-program or during implementation of the program. These data are used to assess progress toward or the accomplishment of program objectives.

PROBLEM INDICATORS

The classic indicators of health problems are **mortality** (death), **morbidity** (disease or injury), and disability (dysfunction). Sometimes, discomfort and dissatisfaction are added, making a list of "five Ds" extending into quality of life measures, which might be labelled "desires" to round out the alphabetic continuity. In addition, there are positive indicators of health status, such as health-related quality of life, life expectancy, and fitness. Since 1982, mortality has been expressed as the years of potential life lost (YPLL) to give greater weight to deaths at younger ages.[2] This measure is more sensitive to the preventable mortality in children, youth, and adults in their "productive" years. Fertility measures among the vital statistics collected in virtually every jurisdiction in the world provide another measure commonly used in health planning.

Data on these indicators are available from a variety of sources, all of which have online websites. These include the National Center for Health Statistics (NCHS) of the Centers for Disease Control and Prevention (CDC), and other agencies of the Department of Health and Human Services in the United States or the ministries of health in other countries. Local and state or provincial health departments and ministries, the Census Bureau (see the annual Statistical Abstract of the United States) and Statistics Canada, some professional journals and associations, voluntary health associations, and the World Health Organization all have websites with accessible data. One can easily search these for statistical information on specific diseases, injuries, vital statistics, and survey data. Many of these sources include charts and graphs one can download to create PowerPoint presentations, use in planning meetings, and bring the data to life for community groups.[3]

Surveillance systems provide another source for health problem indicator data. The word "surveillance" is derived from the French term *surveiller*, which means "to watch over." Mowat and Hockin (2002) define health surveillance as the "ongoing, systematic use of routinely collected health data to guide public health action in a timely fashion." In the United States, surveillance began with, and continues to depend heavily upon, the National Vital Statistics System (NVSS). State health agencies have the responsibility for maintaining a system that correctly documents the cause of death for every resident. Through cooperative activities of the states and the NCHS, which is part of the CDC, standard forms and model procedures are developed and recommended for state use. Federal and state health agencies share the costs incurred by the states in providing vital statistics data for national use. Thanks to continuous advances in epidemiological research into the etiology of health problems, combined with parallel advances in communications technology and the Internet, today's planners have ready access to sophisticated sources of health information and problem-specific surveillance data.

RATES

One can make data comparisons only between like data—apples with apples, oranges with oranges. For example, expressing rates of death and disease uniformly as "number per thousand population per year" allows direct comparisons between populations of different sizes within the same period and over time. It does not mean much to say, "In 2001, County Z had 48 fatal injuries, and its state [or another state] had 1,712." Because the state is much bigger than the county (or the other state is smaller) and the size of neither is given, one cannot compare the numbers. One must first turn them into rates. A rate is the number of events (in this case, fatal injuries) for some common base population, usually per 1,000 or 100,000 population.

To generate rates for comparison between the county and the state in our example, here are the core steps:

- First, divide the number of deaths in the county by the population of the county.
- Then, divide the number of deaths in the state by the population of the state.
- Finally, multiply each of the results by a multiple of 10 to obtain the final values, preferably between 1 and 100 or 1,000.

This calculation enables one to compare data with common properties: The injury death rate in County Z within the United States is 55.8 deaths per 100,000, and that of the state is 36.4 deaths per 100,000. Because the county has a higher *rate* of fatal injuries than does the state as a whole, further examination is warranted to determine what factors might explain the differences. For example, knowing that fatal injuries are more common among younger age groups, planners might want to see whether the age distribution of the county might explain a portion of the difference observed. Summary descriptions of the epidemiological rates commonly used to support planning are presented in table 4.1.

TABLE 4.1. Common epidemiological measures of comparison purposes; their numerators, denominators, and multipliers for standardized expression of number at risk

Natality measure	Numerator	Denominator	Expressed per number at risk
Crude birth rate	Number of live births reported during a given time interval	Estimated total population at mid-interval	Per 1,000
Crude fertility rate	Number of live births reported during a given time interval	Estimated number of women aged 15–44 at mid-interval	Per 1,000

Morbidity measure	Numerator	Denominator	Expressed per number at risk
Incidence rate	Number of new cases of a specified disease reported during a given time interval	Average or midpoint population during time interval	Variable: $10x$, where $x = 2,3,4,5,6$
Attack rate	Number of new cases of a specified disease reported during an epidemic period of time	Population at the start of the epidemic period	Variable: $10x$, where $x = 2,3,4,5,6$
Point prevalence	Number of current cases, new and old, of a specified disease at a given point in time	Estimated population at the same point in time	Variable: $10x$, where $x = 2,3,4,5,6$
Period prevalence	Number of current cases, new and old, of a specified disease identified over a given time interval	Estimated population at mid-interval	Variable: $10x$, where $x = 2,3,4,5,6$

(continued)

TABLE 4.1. (*continued*)

Mortality measure	Numerator	Denominator	Expressed per number at risk
Crude death rate	Total number of deaths reported during a given time interval	Estimated mid-interval population	Per 1,000 or Per 100,000
Cause-specific death rate	Number of deaths assigned to a specific cause during a given time interval	Estimated mid-interval population	Per 100,000
Neonatal mortality rate	Number of deaths under 28 days of age during a given time interval	Number of live births during the same time interval	Per 1,000
Infant mortality rate	Number of deaths under one year of age during a given time interval	Number of live births reported during the same time interval	Per 1,000

Source: Adapted from Centers for Disease Control and Prevention: Office of Workforce and Career Development. (2012). *Self-Study Course SS1978: Principles of Epidemiology in Public Health Practice* (3rd ed.) Centers for Disease Control and Prevention. Available at https://www.cdc.gov/csels/dsepd/ss1978/SS1978.pdf.

SPECIFIC AND ADJUSTED RATES

Rates may need other kinds of statistical control or adjustment to make them equivalent for comparison. For example, data from different years or locations may need to be age-specific or **age-adjusted** to account for different age distributions in the populations across years and locations.

The **age-specific obesity** rates for youth and for adults per 100 population in United States from 1999–2016 are shown in figure 4.3. Because the rates are age-specific for a broader range of ages in the adults (20–74), they must also be age-adjusted to a population standard so that changes in the distribution of ages during the 17-year span of this chart are taken into account. With these statistical controls on age, the trends for increasing obesity must be ascribed to some factor or factors other than the changing age structure of the nation. If you were looking for the leading causes of death for white males, ages 18 to 24, you would ask for an age-race-sex-specific rate. Comparing the rates of different groups can provide a clearer picture of the relative importance of health problems among or between those groups. If we examine the differences in cause-specific death rates among socioeconomic groups, we can identify causes of death that are more important for the poor or for the affluent.

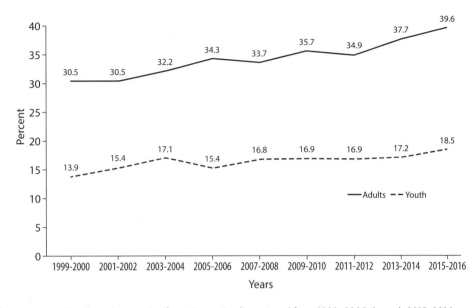

FIGURE 4.3. The chart shows a significant increasing linear trend from 1999–2000 through 2015–2016. Note: All estimates for adults are age-adjusted by the direct method to the 2000 US census population using the age groups 20–39, 40–59, and 60 and over. *Source:* NCHS, National Health and Nutrition Examination Survey, 1999–2016. Accessible from https://www.cdc.gov/nchs/nhanes/index.htm.

INCIDENCE AND PREVALENCE

Two rates deserve particular discussion: **incidence** and **prevalence**. Though both measure morbidity (disease or injury) in the population, they have important differences. Incidence measures new cases of the disease within a certain period, whereas the prevalence of a disease (or a risk factor) is a measure of that portion of the population that represents cases at a particular point in time.

Incidence. Although incidence rates for population groups are hard to find, especially for chronic diseases, they can reveal important insights for planners. For example, the annual or other period of age-standardized incidence rates for selected cancer sites among US men and women for 2017 are shown in figure 4.4. Such rates are based on the year each case or group of cases were detected in screening programs or diagnosed in medical care settings, or both. The age-standardized mortality among men and women for the same cancer sites over the same period of time are shown in figure 4.5. Increasing incidence rates for breast cancer coincide with public health screening efforts to enhance the detection of breast cancer. The declining breast cancer mortality rates are at least in part a manifestation of early treatment of breast cancer thanks to the effectiveness of those early screening and detection efforts.

Prevalence. Prevalence rates and incidence rates give health planners complementary, but different, information. Prevalence reflects both the incidence and the *duration* of disease. Suppose that Diseases A and B have equal incidence rates, but Disease A is mild and unlikely to be life-threatening, while B is severe and causes early death. Disease A will have a higher prevalence in the population, because those who died from Disease B are no longer around to be counted when the prevalence survey is done. Just looking at the prevalence rates could mislead you in determining which disease affects a population most.

This is illustrated by comparing common allergies with AIDS. Because of both a higher incidence and a much milder disease course, allergies have a much

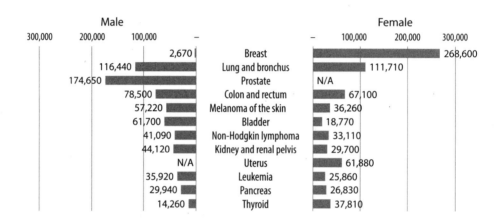

FIGURE 4.4. The top 12 most common cancer sites will account for more than three-quarters of all new cancer cases (Incidence). *Source:* National Institutes of Health (NCI) (2020). *Cancer Stat Facts: Common Cancer Sites.* https://seer.cancer.gov/statfacts/html/common.html

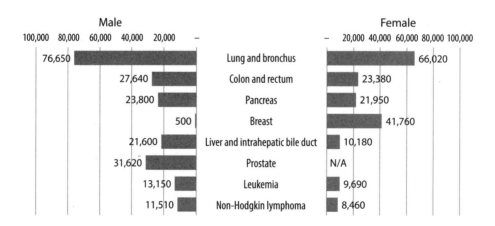

FIGURE 4.5. The eight deadliest cancer sites will account for almost two-thirds of all expected cancer deaths (Mortality). *Source:* National Institutes of Health (NCI) (2020). *Cancer Stat Facts: Common Cancer Sites.* https://seer.cancer.gov/statfacts/html/common.html

higher prevalence than does AIDS. It would certainly be incorrect to deduce from the higher prevalence that allergies are more important, because here the one with the low prevalence causes more serious illness and death. When drug therapies proved effective in prolonging the lives of people with AIDS, the prevalence of the disease increased even though the incidence was declining.

MAKING COMPARISONS TO GAIN INSIGHT

Throughout this section, we have made the point that comparisons serve as one of the primary criteria used to determine the relative importance among several health problems, and the use of rates enables one to compare data with common properties. Planners can compare the data of interest in the community they are serving with those of other communities, or their county, state, province, or the nation. They can also compare data for different health problems within those same areas, as well as for various subgroups of the community, based on age, race, or gender. Comparing data is as fundamental to evaluation as it is to planning, a point that is emphasized in the evaluation chapter.

SETTING PRIORITIES AND OBJECTIVES FOR HEALTH PROGRAMS

In setting sound program priorities, skilled planners exercise their skills in facilitating a process that balances the perceptions of stakeholders with objectively constructed descriptions of prevailing health problems and how they are distributed in the target population. The process of selecting one problem or a cluster of related problems for the focus of a program will be informed as members of a planning team use the data and information they have gathered to seek answers to a series of questions (see box 4.3). The process of working through the health data and information enables planners to establish priority program targets. It has the added benefit of representing the community's need for support from state or national agencies to fund an innovative program to solve the problem and to demonstrate the effectiveness of the solution for other communities.

An emergency medical services program (EMS) provides immediate emergency medical services (including the transportation of injury victims to the appropriate facility). A rehabilitative effort would deal with disabilities resulting from injuries and with increasing the number of victims who regain productive lives and the speed at which they do so. Epidemiological information will provide insights on which facets of the problem will or will not yield to intervention and the extent to which preventive, curative, or rehabilitative services are priorities.

BOX 4.3
Key Questions for Setting Priorities and Objectives
for Health Programs

1. Which problems have the greatest impact in terms of death, disease, days lost from work, rehabilitation costs, disability (temporary and permanent), family disorganization, and cost to communities and agencies for damage repair or loss and cost recovery?

2. Are certain subpopulations, such as children, mothers, ethnic minorities, refugees, or Indigenous populations, at special risk?

3. Which problems are most amenable to intervention?

4. Which problem is not being addressed by other organizations in the community?

5. Which problem, when appropriately addressed, has the greatest potential for yielding measurable improvements in health status, economic savings, or other benefits?

6. Are any of the health problems also highly ranked as a regional or national priority? (State health agencies develop priorities among health problems, often based on local epidemiological data, and they may allocate state resources to the communities able to give priority to reducing the health problem.)

7. To what extent does the problem(s), as manifested in the community, constitute a disproportionately high burden compared to other communities or the rest of the state?

DEVELOPING HEALTH OBJECTIVES

When the health problem has been specifically defined, the next step is to develop the program **objectives**.[4] This vital phase in program planning is crucial to program evaluation; too often it is treated quite superficially, which too often leads to unfortunate consequences for program implementation and evaluation (see chapters 8 and 9).

Objectives are crucial. They form a fulcrum for converting diagnostic data into program direction and resource allocation over time. *Health objectives should be cast in the language of epidemiological or medical outcomes and should answer the four questions of who will attain how much of what, by when?* At each of the phases of the PRECEDE model, the questions take a slightly different form on the "what," but at this stage it is specifically in relation to *health* benefits that should be achieved by the nascent program:

- Who will benefit from the program?
- What health benefit should they receive?
- How much of that benefit should be achieved?
- By when should it be achieved, or how long should it take for the program to produce a benefit?

Consider box 4.4, containing data from the Grafton County Maternal and Child Health Planning Team. The following program objective could be developed, based on those diagnostic data and consonant with the mission or resources of the given agency:

> The infant mortality rate in Grafton County will be reduced by 10 percent within the first two years and an additional 25 percent over the next three years, continuing to decline until the state average is reached.

The target population (who) is demographically implied (pregnant women) and geographically explicit (within Grafton County). What is reduced is specified (infant mortality). How much benefit is to be achieved, and by when, is stated in stages: a 10% reduction in two years, then a 25% reduction over three years, then the decline will continue until the state average rate is achieved. (Note that the average rate for the state will probably go down concurrently, though more slowly, so the evaluation of the program will have to compare itself against a moving target.)

In developing program objectives, the planner should strive to set up the plan so that (1) progress in meeting objectives can be measured; (2) objectives are based on relevant, reasonably accurate data; and (3) objectives are in harmony across topics as well as across levels. The third of these conditions implies consistency. It means that objectives dealing with various aspects of a health problem (for example, the objectives of a maternity program to improve nutrition, prenatal appointment compliance, weight and blood pressure control, and percentage of hospital deliveries) should be consistent with, and complement, each other in a hierarchy of objectives related to the presumed cause-and-effect relationships among them. The causal hierarchy will unfold more clearly as the logic model for the program plan unfolds in the diagnostic planning phases ahead.

Objectives should also be coherent across levels, with those objectives becoming successively more refined and more explicit and usually multiplied from one level to the next. In the usual language of health planners, goals are considered to be more general than are objectives. For example, the maternal and child health program objective just presented serves a broader program *goal* of improved quality of life or social conditions caused by poor perinatal or infant health. It is in reality part of a hierarchy of concordant objectives all pointing to the achievement of an overall program goal, a set of more specific program objectives, and several even more specific objectives stated in behavioral, environmental, educational, administrative, and organizational terms (as described in subsequent chapters). So far, we have covered the first two:

1. Program goal: for example, the well-being of mothers, infants, and children will be raised through the healthy birth and optimal growth and development of children.

2. Health objectives: for example,

   a. The infant mortality rate within Grafton County will be reduced by 10% within the first two years and an additional 25% over the next three years, with reductions continuing until the state average rate is reached.

BOX 4.4

Case Example: Grafton County Maternal and Child Health Planning Team

A planning team for a maternal and child health unit in a predominately rural county agency is grappling with a range of issues related to the quality of infant care in their county. They have at hand the following information:

- The area of interest is populated mainly by a low-income minority agricultural group with a high rate of teenage pregnancy.
- The infant mortality rate in this area has remained at 24.9/1,000 live births while there has been an overall decline in the state rate to 14.6/1,000.
- The identified pregnancy outcome problems include premature birth, low birth weight, respiratory distress at delivery, and failure to thrive.
- The visiting nurse service also reports a high prevalence of maternal anemia and a high incidence of gastrointestinal infection and respiratory diseases in infants.
- Many mothers are at risk because of age (a disproportionate number between ages 14 and 17), poor nutrition, lack of medical care, multiple pregnancies, and pre-eclampsia during pregnancy.
- Childhood health is poor: injuries are common, children look malnourished and report for school with handicapping conditions and no immunizations.

While some observers feel that these problems reflect inadequate hospital equipment and facilities to care for neonates, the planning team believes that the data suggest that the real causes probably lie in poor prenatal care, poor maternal and infant nutrition, and lack of infant immunizations.

b. The perinatal mortality rate will be reduced by 94%.

c. Fetal death rate will be reduced from x percent to y percent in the same period.

National health objectives have been the mainstay of the planning and evaluation of the US National (and for many states) Disease Prevention and Health Promotion initiative, with published objectives decennially since the 1980s, under the departmental "Healthy People" initiative. This was developed by Michael McGinnis and his staff and other federal agencies, prominently the CDC, in consultation with the 50 states (McGinnis 1990). It was launched with a Surgeon General's Report and the setting of 10-year consensus goals and objectives for each of the health priorities by the then Department of Health, Education, and Welfare (Green and Fielding 2011). It provided for evaluating progress periodically with state and combined national surveillance data (Green 2011; Green et al. 1983). These decennial objectives have become a touchstone for planning and evaluating national, state, and local disease prevention and health programs.

Besides national and state programs with legislated or negotiated objectives and standards, health, environmental, policy, and behavioral objectives have been developed at the local level with guidance from scientific reviews of research. These have been guided by "what works" conclusions from so-called evidence-based practice guidelines for interventions. The planning, implementation, and evaluation of programs has been guided increasingly by scientific research producing what has become guidelines for practice, and often enforced by professional associations controlling certification, accreditation, and licensure of organizations, programs and practitioners.

At the program level, global systematic reviews of scientific research studies on the effectiveness of specific program components, such as the Community Preventive Services Task Force (https://www.thecommunityguide.org/), are adapted at state levels with websites such as http://whatworksforhealth.wisc.edu/. These have become the gold standard for selecting interventions and programs. But these have also produced a controversy over the limitations of "evidence-based practices," which are based on highly controlled, usually experimental research designs that may not represent the circumstances in which the program is to be implemented. Too often, the program designers and practitioners are caught between the so-called "best practices" from systematic reviews of science on one side, and the advice of the community leaders and participants recommending other interventions or modifications of the "best practice" interventions. This has led some of us to argue that "if we want more evidence-based practice, we need more practice-based evidence" (Green and Mercer 2001; Green and Ottoson 2004; Truswell et al. 2012).

The more specific behavioral and environmental objectives will emerge from the epidemiological **assessment**, through which we address the behavioral and environmental assessments in the next chapter.

─── EXERCISES ───

1. List the health problems related to the quality of life concerns identified in your population in exercise 3 of chapter 2.

2. Rate (low, medium, high) each health problem in the inventory according to

   a. its relative importance in affecting the quality of life concerns, and

   b. its potential for change.

3. Discuss the reasons for giving high-priority ratings to health problems in exercise 2a in terms of their prevalence, incidence, cost, virulence, severity, or other relevant dimensions. Extrapolate from national, state, or regional data when local data are not available.

4. Cite the evidence supporting your ratings of health problems in exercise 2b. Refer to the success of other programs and to the availability of medical or other technology to control or reduce the high-priority health problems you have selected.

5. Cite two uses for data generated by epidemiological assessments other than for program planning, and give an example of each.

6. Write a program objective for the highest-priority health problem, indicating who will achieve how much of what benefit by when.

Notes

1. Last (2007). The definition and explanation of epidemiology has been paraphrased in Last (2007, 111). For variations on this definition, see Green and Ottoson (1999, 70); Timmerick (1998, 2–3). See also Krieger (1994).

2. In use since 1982, years of potential life lost (YPLL) measures the impact of diseases and injuries that kill people before the customary age of retirement. It is computed as the sum of products over all age groups up to age 65, sometimes 75, each product being an annual number of deaths in an age group multiplied by the average number of years remaining before the age of 65 (or 75) for that age group. See Centers for Disease Control (1986); McDonnell and Vossberg (1998).

3. The National Center for Health Statistics issues an annual publication, in addition to its detailed tables comparing health status and health behavior statistics among regions, states, and demographic groups, which contains a detailed description of the sources and limitations of vital and health data systems of the federal government and various other national organizations, as well as a glossary of social and demographic terms used in health statistics. The text and tables of all *Vital and Health Statistics* reports can be

viewed and downloaded from https://www.cdc.gov/nchswww/. For sources and examples particularly relevant to health promotion, see also Green and Lewis (1986, 128–45).

4. Some applications of PRECEDE illustrating epidemiological assessments and setting of health objectives include Antoniadis and Lubker (1997); Gielen (1992); Green et al. (1983); Green et al. (1986); Green et al. (1991); Livingston (1985); Simons-Morton et al. (1988); Stevenson et al. (1996); Timmerick (1998, 338–40); Walter et al. (1985). The bibliography of over 1,200 published applications of the PRECEDE-PROCEED model at http://www.lgreen.net also includes many helpful examples.

References

Antoniadis, A., & Lubker, B.B. (1997). Epidemiology as an essential tool for establishing prevention programs and evaluating their impact and outcome. *Journal of Communication Disorders, 30*(4), 269–83; quiz 283–4. https://doi.org/10.1016/s0021-9924(97)00003-8

Frank, F.W. (1995). Why "population health"? *Canadian Journal of Public Health, 86,* 162–4.

Gielen, A.C. (1992). Health education and injury control: Integrating approaches. *Health Education Quarterly, 19*(2), 203–18. https://doi.org/10.1177/109019819201900205

Green, L.W. (2017). Definition of health. *Oxford Bibliographies Online—Public Health.* Oxford University Press. https://www.oxfordbibliographies.com

Green, L.W. (2011). Population health objectives and targets. *Oxford Bibliographies Online—Public Health.* Oxford University Press. https://www.oxfordbibliographies.com

Green, L.W., & Fielding, J. (2011). The Healthy People initiative: Its genesis and its sustainability. *Annual Review of Public Health, 32,* 451–70. https://doi.org/10.1146/annurev-publhealth-031210-101148

Green, L.W., & Gielen, A.C. (2015). Evidence of ecological theory in two public health successes for health behavior change. In Kahan, S., Gielen, A.C., Fagan, P., & Green, L.W. (Eds.). *Health Behavior Change in Populations* (pp 26–43). Johns Hopkins University Press.

Green, L.W., & Lewis, F.M. (1986). *Measurement and Evaluation in Health Education and Health Promotion.* Mayfield Publishing Company.

Green, L.W., & Mercer, S.L. (2001). Community-based participatory research: Can public health researchers and agencies reconcile the push from funding bodies and the pull from communities? *American Journal of Public Health, 91*(12), 1926–9. https://doi.org/10.2105/ajph.91.12.1926

Green, L.W., Mullen, P.D., & Friedman, R.B. (1986). An epidemiological approach to targeting drug information. *Patient Education and Counseling, 8*(3), 255–68. https://doi.org/10.1016/0738-3991(86)90004-2

Green, L.W., & Ottoson, J.M. (1999). *Community and Population Health* (8th ed.). WCB/McGraw-Hill.

Green, L.W., & Ottoson, J.M. (2004). From efficacy to effectiveness to community and back: Evidence-based practice vs practice-based evidence. In Green, L., Hiss, R., Glasgow, R., et al. (Eds.), *From Clinical Trials to Community: The Science of Translating Diabetes and Obesity Research* (pp. 15–18). National Institutes of Health.

Green, L.W., Wilson, R.W., & Bauer, K.G. (1983). Data requirements to measure progress on the objectives for the nation in health promotion and disease prevention. *American Journal of Public Health, 73*(1), 18–24. https://doi.org/10.2105/ajph.73.1.18

Huber, M., Knottnerus, A.J., Green, L.W., van der Horst, H., Jadad, A.R., Kromhout, D., Leonard, B., Lorig, K., Loureiro, M.I., van der Meer, J.W.M., Schnabel, P., Smith, R., van Weel, C., & Smid, H. (2011). How should we define health? *The BMJ, 343,* d4163. https://doi.org/10.1136/bmj.d4163

Johnson, N.B., Hayes, L.D., Brown, K., Hoo, E.C., & Ethier, K.A. (2014). CDC National Health Report: leading causes of morbidity and mortality and associated behavioral risk and protective factors—United States, 2005-2013. *Morbidity and Mortality Weekly Report, Suppl.63*(4), 3–27. https://www.cdc.gov/mmwr/preview/mmwrhtml/su6304a2.htm

Kreuter, M.W., Kegler, M.C., Joseph, K.T., Redwood, Y.A. & Hooker, M. (2012). The impact of implementing selected CBPR strategies to address disparities in urban Atlanta: A retrospective case study. *Health Education Research, 27*(4), 729–41. https://doi.org/10.1093/her/cys053

Krieger, J.W., Allen, C., Cheadle, A., Ciske, S., Schier, J., Senturia, K., & Sullivan, M. (2002). Using community-based participatory research to address social determinants of health: Lessons learned from Seattle Partners for Healthy Communities. *Health Education and Behavior, 29*(3), 361–82. https://doi.org/10.1177/109019810202900307

Krieger, N. (1994). Epidemiology and the web of causation: Has anyone seen the spider? *Social Science & Medicine, 39*(7), 887–903. https://doi.org/10.1016/0277-9536(94)90202-x

Last, J.M. (2007). *A Dictionary of Public Health.* Oxford University Press. https://doi.org/10.1093/acref/9780195160901.001.0001

Livingston, I.L. (1985). Hypertension and health education intervention in the Caribbean: A public health appraisal. *Journal of the National Medical Association, 77*(4), 273–80.

McGinnis, J.M. (1990). Setting objectives for public health in the 1990s: Experience and prospects. *Annual Review of Public Health, 11*, 231–49. https://doi.org/10.1146/annurev.pu.11.050190.001311

Mowat, D.L., & Hockin, J. (2002). Building capacity in evidence-based public health practice. *Canadian Journal of Public Health, 93*(1), 19–20. https://doi.org/10.1007/BF03404411

Simons-Morton, B., Parcel, G., Brink, S., et al. (1988). *Promoting physical activity among adults: A CDC Physical activity community intervention handbook.* Centers for Disease Control and Prevention.

Stevenson, M., Jones, S., Cross, D., Howat, P., & Hall, M. (1996). The child pedestrian injury prevention project. *Health Promotion Journal of Australia, 6*(3), 32–6.

Stewart, A.L., & Nápoles-Springer, A.M. (2003). Advancing health disparities research: Can we afford to ignore measurement issues? *Medical Care, 41*(11), 1207–20. https://doi.org/10.1097/01.MLR.0000093420.27745.48

Timmerick, T.C. (1998). *An Introduction to Epidemiology* (2nd ed.). Jones & Bartlett Learning.

Truswell, A.S., Hiddink, G.J., Green, L.W., Roberts, R., & van Weel, C. (2012). Practice-based evidence for weight management: Alliance between primary care and public health. *Family Practice, 29*(Suppl 1), i6–i9. https://doi.org/10.1093/fampra/cmr058

Walter, H.J., Hofman, A., Connelly, P.A., Barrett, L.T., & Kost, K.L. (1985). Primary prevention of chronic disease in childhood: Changes in risk factors after one year of intervention. *American Journal of Epidemiology, 122*(5), 772–81. https://doi.org/10.1093/oxfordjournals.aje.a114160

Whaley, A.L., & Geller, P.A. (2003). Ethnic/racial differences in psychiatric disorders: A test of four hypotheses. *Ethnicity and Disease, 13*(4), 499–512.

World Health Organization. (2001). *International Classification of Functioning, Disability and Health (ICF).* WHO. http://www.who.int/classifications/icf/en/

Zuvekas, S.H., & Taliaferro, G.S. (2003). Pathways to access: Health insurance, the health care delivery system, and racial/ethnic disparities, 1996-1999. *Health Affairs (Millwood), 22*(2), 139–53. https://doi.org/10.1377/hlthaff.22.2.139

CHAPTER 5

Epidemiological Assessment II: Behavioral and Environmental Factors

•

Lawrence W. Green, Marshall W. Kreuter, and Andrea Carlson Gielen

The important thing is not to stop questioning.
—Albert Einstein

Learning Objectives

After completing the chapter, the reader will be able to:

- Understand three interactive levels of influence on health that move from the more proximal to distal and that can be affected by population health programs and policy interventions.
- Recognize the interventions and influential elements of at least two great public health success stories, as exemplified in tobacco control and injury control experiences.
- Understand the four steps of a community behavioral assessment for at least two contrasting health-risk factors.

INTRODUCTION

"**Behavior**," in the PRECEDE-PROCEED model, surfaces and resurfaces as an important influence on health at three levels—(1) *proximal,* the direct actions or inactions of individuals that influence their own health; (2) *interpersonal,* the actions or inactions of others that can directly influence the health behavior and related actions of an individual at risk; and (3) the more *distal* policy and enforcement actions, individually or collectively, on or by people acting in the organizational or policy environment (as shown in figure 5.1).

Similarly, "**environment**" arises as a balancing influence, in which it can have an independent, *direct* effect on health that comes through locations and

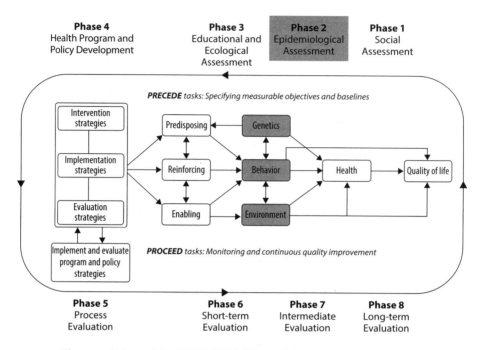

FIGURE 5.1. The second phase of the PRECEDE-PROCEED model continues the epidemiological assessment with a focus on the population's health relative to behavior, the environment, and genetics.

circumstances beyond the control or effort of individuals; it can also have an *indirect* effect on health through the behavioral habits or efforts of an individual or population to promote, protect, or manage health by building, modifying, or regulating the public and private use of environments. This leads to a distinction seen increasingly in the population health and climate change literature between the "built environment," the "regulated environment," and the "natural environment." Smoking, obesity, and injury prevention provide the best evidence of successful interventions on such environments and behavioral changes.

The combined influence of these several risk factors (smoking and their consequent influence on lung cancer deaths, for example) was dramatically illustrated by the statewide California Tobacco Control Program before and after the passage of the state ballot initiative, Proposition 99, as shown in figure 5.2. That popular voter initiative set in motion the authority and funding for a comprehensive program aimed at individuals, schools, and worksites; increased tobacco taxes and restrictions on advertising, sales to minors, and smoking in public places; and instituted a multifaceted program of research and evaluation to strengthen these and other programs (Barnoya and Glantz 2004; Fichtenberg and Glantz 2000).

Planners can draw on good evidence showing the strength of a given *behavioral* risk (e.g., not wearing a mask) and a specific health problem (e.g., COVID-19)

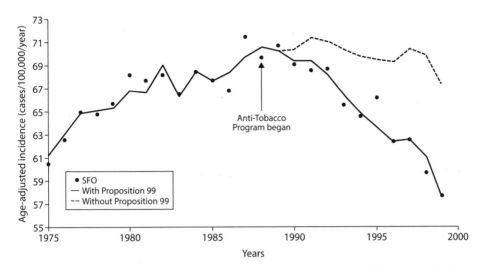

FIGURE 5.2. Lung cancer rates for the San Francisco area increasing before 1988 and decreasing after the beginning of the California statewide voter Initiative on Comprehensive Tobacco Control. *Source:* Barnoya, J., & Glanz, S. (2004). Association of the California Tobacco Control program with declines in lung cancer incidence. *Cancer Causes and Control, 15*(7), 689–95. https://doi.org/10.1023/B:CACO.0000036187.13805.30

for many pressing public health issues. Risk behaviors like failure to wear face masks, smoking, diet, being sedentary, or not wearing seat belts are more *proximal* to the health problems respectively of COVID-19, lung cancer, obesity, and automobile-related injuries than actions at the other two levels (*interpersonal* and *distal*). But behavior change usually requires support from these other levels, including organizational and regulatory policies and their enforcement (Crawford and Jeffrey 2006; Gielen and Green 2015; Gielen et al. 2006; Golden et al. 2015; Green and Gielen 2014; Mukherjea and Green 2014; Richard et al. 1996). This multiplicity of behaviors and environments, which are implicated in most complex health conditions and trauma events, is what makes Albert Einstein's quote, "The important thing is not to stop questioning," an important and practical reminder for practitioners engaged in program planning, implementation, and evaluation.

THREE LEVELS OR CATEGORIES OF BEHAVIOR

During a behavioral assessment, the focus is first on the *proximal level* of actions taken by individuals, or groups of individuals, that are known to have a direct effect on the health problem or issue in question. In some instances, this definition may also include the actions of others, such as parents' behaviors that influence their children's health and over which the child has limited or no control (e.g., breastfeeding to promote infant health), or clinicians' actions that directly influence their patients' health (e.g., clinicians' handwashing to prevent clinic-acquired infections).

The second level of behaviors includes those actions, or inactions, taken by others that can directly influence the actions of an individual at risk. This *interpersonal* level of behavior can have a major impact on the social or physical environment of the individuals at risk. In turn, this can result in the support of (or deterrence from) efforts to modify the individuals' health-risk behaviors. Examples include the actions of parents to influence their adolescent children's decision-making and risk behaviors (e.g., teaching teens safe driving skills and restricting them from driving at night) or caregivers' interactions with their patients (e.g., encouraging patient compliance by offering supportive services).

A third level of behaviors is represented by those actions taken by individuals or groups that could influence some dimension of the physical, social, or political environment and are thus the most *distal*. These, in turn, could influence a specific risk behavior or even the health problem directly. It is important to realize that, because they are more distal from the health problem than behaviors in the first two categories, this third level of behavior is manifested by those in positions where their actions and decisions can influence or directly shape the social norms, policies, regulations, and laws that influence the physical and organizational environments of homes, institutions, neighborhoods, communities, states, and nations. Examples that fit the most distal category of behaviors that influence policies, and environmental controls that ultimately promote health, include the organized actions taken by individuals or advocacy groups, such as actions taken by:

- city planners to create user-friendly walking environments;
- legislators passing a clean indoor act to prevent indoor smoking;
- the board of a corporation instituting an employee wellness program;
- engineers to design roads and vehicles that make them safer.

These are realistic examples that fit the most distal category of behaviors that influence policies and environmental controls that ultimately promote health and protect whole populations.

The second and third levels of behavior described above most often have indirect effects on the ultimate health problem. These effects are featured prominently in the process of educational and ecological assessment and the health program and policy development phase. These are also described in subsequent chapters (10–14) on the settings or channels in which the PRECEDE-PROCEED model can be applied with maximum effect.[1] If planners focus only on the most proximal behaviors—individual risk behaviors—and ignore the importance of behaviors in the other two categories and nonbehavioral causes (exposure to hazards in the environment, genetic predisposition, age, gender, congenital disease, physical and mental impairment, and social or economic disadvantage), the policies and programs they develop are likely to have two serious flaws.

First, such an approach will inevitably place all the responsibility for health improvement on the individuals whose health is threatened. Programs limited to that narrow focus are likely to yield modest and temporary effects and potentially add to the burden of those at risk. Second, programs that focus only on the behavioral actions of those at risk will not only be vulnerable to the charge of "blaming the victim," but will also be missing the opportunity to address other powerful determinants of health. By keeping an eye on all three levels of behavior (as well as relevant nonbehavioral factors), planners acknowledge the ecological reality that most human health problems can be linked to the interaction among behaviors, environmental conditions, genetic variation, and other nonbehavioral factors. It is important to recognize that most of these factors are amenable to change through strategic interventions in varied settings such as schools and worksites and mass media, as well as clinical settings, which will be described in the later chapters of this book.

GENETICS AND BEHAVIORAL INTERACTIONS

The interactions of genes with behavior and the environment are inherently complex; consequently, genes will seldom be treated as independent effects on health, except in a few genetic diseases such as phenylketonuria (PKU), sickle cell anemia, cystic fibrosis, and Tay-Sachs disease. Applications of genetics to public health practice in areas like diet and obesity will become more useful as our understanding of the human genome and its complex interaction with the environment grows.

The purpose of the diagnostic phases of PRECEDE-PROCEED is to help detect valid and accessible information that can be used by planners in their efforts to tailor programs designed to meet the health needs of a given population. Insights into potential individual genetic variations will enable local-level planners to develop programs and policies that consider those variations. For example, the uniform dietary guidelines highlighted in the United States Department of Agriculture's (USDA) food pyramid constitute a national recommendation. While those guidelines do not, *per se*, infer that all Americans are the same culturally, socioeconomically, physiologically, and genetically, they leave little room for variability. Data from the Human Genome Project and other studies show that genetic variation among individuals alters interactions among dietary chemicals that can lead to health improvement or to increased susceptibility to specific diseases.

Obesity has emerged as a serious global health problem that illustrates the interactions of genetic, behavioral, and environmental determinants and the range of interventions that encompass these (Koplan et al. 2010; Kumanyika et al. 2010). Not only has it reached epidemic proportions in the United States, obesity rates have increased threefold or more since 1980 in some areas of the United Kingdom, China, Eastern Europe, the Middle East, the Pacific Islands, and Australia (WHO 2000). The global obesity epidemic appears to be the result of modern lifestyles, which combine access to and consumption of high-calorie foods with decreasing levels of physical activity. Many people appear to respond to this modern life environment by an imbalance that favors energy input over the expenditure of energy and results in overweight, while others do not. What accounts for these differences? Genetic research offers strong evidence for a genetic component to obesity. However, genes interact with one another (polygenic) and, collectively, those interactions work in combination with other factors like nutrients, physical activity, and smoking (Froguel and Boutin 2001).

Developed by the CDC, box 5.1 summarizes some of the important knowledge that has been accumulated about genetics and obesity, as well as some of the unanswered questions. Rapid strides are being made in the pursuit of a better understanding of how variations in our genetic makeup influence various illnesses, risk factors, and biological conditions. The capacity of health program planners will be greatly enhanced as they gain access to answers to questions about genetic variability like those raised regarding obesity in box 5.1.

While the science for most of the gene-gene, gene-environment, and gene-behavior interactions is well underway, at this stage, however, it has not been

---

BOX 5.1
Public Health Genomics and Obesity
Behavior, Environment, and Genetic Factors All Have a Role in Causing People to Be Overweight and Obese

Do Genes Have a Role in Obesity?
In recent decades, obesity has reached epidemic proportions in populations whose environments promote physical inactivity and increased consumption of high-calorie foods. However, not all people living in such environments will become obese, nor will all obese people have the same body fat distribution or suffer the same health problems. These differences can be seen in groups of people with the same racial or ethnic background and even within families. Genetic changes in human populations occur too slowly to be responsible for the obesity epidemic. Nevertheless, the variation in how people respond to the same environment suggests that genes do play a role in the development of obesity.

How Could Genes Influence Obesity?

Genes give the body instructions for responding to changes in its environment. Studies of resemblances and differences among family members, twins, and adoptees offer indirect scientific evidence that a sizable portion of the variation in weight among adults is due to genetic factors. Other studies have compared obese and non-obese people for variations in genes that could influence behaviors (such as a drive to overeat, or a tendency to be sedentary) or metabolism (such as a diminished capacity to use dietary fats as fuel, or an increased tendency to store body fat). These studies have identified variants in several genes that may contribute to obesity by increasing hunger and food intake.

Rarely, a clear pattern of inherited obesity within a family is caused by a specific variant of a single gene (monogenic obesity). Most obesity, however, probably results from complex interactions among multiple genes and environmental factors that remain poorly understood (multifactorial obesity).

Any explanation of the obesity epidemic has to consider both genetics and the environment. One explanation that is often cited is the mismatch between today's environment and "energy-thrifty genes" that multiplied in the distant past, when food sources were unpredictable. In other words, according to the "thrifty genotype" hypothesis, the same genes that helped our ancestors survive occasional famines are now being challenged by environments in which food is plentiful year-round. Other hypotheses have been proposed, including a role for the gut microbiome as well as early life exposures associated with epigenetic changes.

Can Public Health Genomics Help?

With the exception of rare genetic conditions associated with extreme obesity, currently, genetic tests are not useful for guiding personal diet or physical activity plans. Research on genetic variation that affects the body's response to changes in diet and physical activity is still at an early stage. Doing a better job of explaining obesity in terms of genes and environmental factors could help encourage people who are trying to reach and maintain a healthy weight.

Excerpted from https://www.cdc.gov/genomics/resources/diseases/obesity/index.htm

developed sufficiently for widespread application. This section on genetics is, therefore, essentially a placeholder for the anticipated opportunities likely to surface for health program planners, implementors, and evaluators in the not-too-distant future. The interaction of genetics with the other two classes of health determinants—behavior and the environment—are indicated by the vertical arrows in figure 5.1, with Phase 2 connecting these three sets of determinants. Most controls on the gene-environment interactions depend on the behavior of individuals and populations, their access to and use of genetics counseling, and personal or genealogical data. In addition, they also depend on the behavior of community, national, and international decision makers, in the exposure of people to environmental risks. Therefore, we have placed behavior between genetics and the environment as a practical matter. This is also consistent with the inclusion of behavior within the use of the term "environment" in most of the genetics literature.

FOUR STEPS OF A BEHAVIORAL ASSESSMENT

For instructional purposes, the process of behavioral assessment (as well as the environmental assessment) has been delineated into four steps to highlight important nuances that help keep the process focused on the program's goal. As planners have used the steps in practice, however, they have discovered that the process is indeed more than the sum or sequence of its parts; one step seamlessly merges with the next, but next steps often send the planners back to revisit and revise previous steps.

Step 1: Listing Potential Behavioral Risks Related to the Health Problem

Keep an eye on the literature. The primary task for this step is to list those behaviors that are known to account for some portion of the specific health problem you are addressing. Experienced practitioners, especially those who work on a given health topic over time, are likely to have a good working knowledge of those risk behaviors. Regardless of experience, however, it is prudent to review the literature and current scientific reports of known risk factors for the disease or health problem in question.[2] The risk factors and conditions associated with the leading causes of death in the United States, shown in table 5.1, can serve as pathways to prevention. Some of the risk factors under the heart disease category in table 5.1—including smoking, alcohol abuse, high-fat diet, and sedentary lifestyle—immediately fall into the behavioral category and are clearly behavioral. Although not strictly or only behavioral, other risk factors—those associated with high cholesterol, obesity, and high blood pressure—serve as signposts calling our attention to behaviors like eating habits and inactivity.

Systems thinking. Further review of the behaviors listed in table 5.1 reminds us that some of the risk factors and their implicit behaviors are dependent on prior behaviors and on their interaction with environmental circumstances. For example, suppose a blood test reveals that a person, even after efforts to increase levels of physical activity and control intake of fat, is found to have an elevated level of serum cholesterol. After an assessment, the physician prescribes a given medication and informs the patient that they need to return after one month to get another test to confirm whether the initial prescription or dosage was working properly with no side effects. "Taking a prescribed medication,"

Table 5.1. The most common priorities for public health and other population-based prevention, health promotion, and health protection programs

Risk factors and conditions	Leading causes of death										
	Heart disease	Cancers	Stroke	Injuries (non-vehicular)	Influenza, pneumonia	Injuries (vehicular)	Diabetes	Cirrhosis	Suicide	Homicides	AIDS
Behavioral risk factors											
Smoking	•	•		•	•						
High blood pressure	•		•								
High cholesterol	•										
Diet	•	•					•				
Obesity	•	•					•				
Sedentary lifestyle	•	•	•				•				
Stress	•		•	•		•					
Alcohol abuse		•		•		•		•	•	•	
Drug misuse	•		•	•		•			•	•	•
Seat belt nonuse						•					
Handgun possession				•					•	•	
Sexual practices											•
Biological risk factors (e.g., genetics)	•	•	•				•	•			
Environmental risk factors											
Radiation exposure		•									
Workplace hazards		•		•		•					
Environmental contaminants		•									
Infectious agents		•			•						
Home hazards				•							
Auto/road design						•					
Speed limits						•					
Medical care access	•	•	•		•		•	•	•	•	
Product design				•							
Social risk factors[a]	•		•	•		•	•		•	•	

Source: Adapted from unpublished material from the Centers for Disease Control and Prevention, US Department of Health and Human Services.

[a]This category of social determinants of health includes a variety of less well-defined or circumscribed conditions of living related to social relationships, social support, social pressures, early childhood experiences, and socioeconomic status.

while a relatively discrete behavior, is logically influenced by other discrete behaviors such as seeking medical care, obtaining a prescription, and seeing that the medication is modified as necessary, as in the control of high blood pressure *in addition to* the cholesterol.

This cycle of actions and interactions is an example of what is meant by the statement "health behavior is best understood as part of an ecological system." Experienced planners who work in clinical settings understand that this cycle could be undermined at many points along the way. For example, a patient may fail to keep an appointment at which prescriptions might be renewed or changed. Failure to keep an appointment could be the result of a variety of possibilities. One can create this kind of systems picture quite simply by asking, as Einstein would ask at each juncture, "But why?"

Many of the answers can be linked to behaviors that might be added to the list you are compiling or could be deferred as a category of behavior taken by others.

- Appointments aren't being kept.

    But why?

- Patients are dissatisfied.

    But why?

- In some instances, they had a bad relationship with the caregiver; in other instances, they had to wait 30–45 minutes after the scheduled appointment time.

    But why did they have to wait too long?

- The clinic had to adjust the schedule to compensate for broken appointments.

A "systems" view of the broken-appointment cycle example is provided in figure 5.3. This kind of systems-level thinking helps planners identify and isolate concrete behavioral events, in the context of nonbehavioral and environmental factors, that enable them to more precisely target program strategies. Training staff, adjusting appointment schedules, and making childcare or transportation arrangements all could become relevant interventions identified by the behavioral assessment reflected in the broken-appointment cycle.

Roseville case example. Suppose you were assigned to coordinate the planning of a health program focused on the prevention of heart disease for the hypothetical community of Roseville. As a first step in your behavioral diagnosis, you share the risk factors listed for the leading causes of death with the other members of the planning team. For example, in the heart disease column in table 5.1, risk factors include smoking, high blood pressure, diet, and so on.

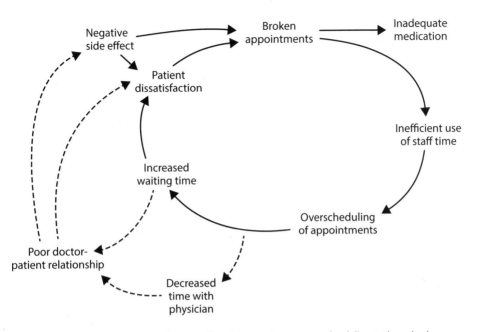

FIGURE 5.3. A systems view of the behavior of keeping appointments can be delineated as a broken-appointment cycle with a sequence of actions and reactions, decisions and choices, branching toward or away from further broken appointments.

Based on their collective experiences in Roseville, the planning team thinks that five risk factors and conditions are especially relevant and prevalent: smoking, high blood pressure, high cholesterol, obesity, and physical inactivity. After further discussion, members of the team want to add low fruit and vegetable consumption because of its possible connection to weight reduction. Thus, the starting list included more specific risk-reduction behaviors embedded in the more general list of risk factors:

- Reduce weight (fewer foods high in saturated fat; more fruits and vegetables);
- Get a cholesterol screening test;
- Get blood pressure screening for hypertension;
- Increase physical activity (reduce sedentary lifestyle); and
- Eliminate smoking.

Step 2: Rating Behaviors on Importance

From a realistic perspective, few programs have enough resources to do everything that might be done. So, the extensive list of behaviors identified in Step 1 now needs to be reduced to a manageable number. This is done first by determining which behaviors are the most important and eliminating (or at least deferring) the least important. The broad criteria for determining the **importance** of a given behavior include evidence that it (1) is clearly linked to the health problem, and (2) is present (you can document that it occurs) and prevalent in the population of interest. The latter point becomes especially critical in those situations where a given risk factor, although universally acknowledged to be important, has an unusually low prevalence rate in the target population in question. For example, smoking or drinking alcohol behaviors are not likely to surface as important factors in cultures where they are prohibited or highly restrained.

Continuing the Roseville case. To help planning team members weigh the importance of the behavioral factors they have identified, you call their attention to the information in table 5.2. You point out that relative risk estimates for five of six risk factors (not including diabetes) on their current list fall within a range of 2.4 to 1.9, telling you that a person with one of those risks essentially has twice the chance of developing coronary heart disease (CHD).

You then introduce the team to some additional Roseville-specific risk-factor information from two sources. The first source provides data from a behavioral risk factor survey of adults aged 18 to 64 and gathered semi-annually over the past decade. Those data reveal the following trends:

- There has been a steady decline in smoking from 36.8% to a current level of 17.8%.

- The percentage of those who were not screened for hypertension in the last two years has declined and is now stable at 5%.

- The percentage of those who have had their cholesterol checked in the past five years is 81%, exceeding the current objectives for the nation.

- The percentage of the population reported to be overweight rose from 27% to 39%.

- The percentage of persons reporting no leisure time activity increased from 21% to 30%.

The second source includes information and data gathered the year before in a joint effort carried out by the Roseville School District and the Roseville Health Department. It includes two school-based surveys (one of high school students and one of elementary students) and a short community survey and tobacco policy assessment.

- In the survey of students in grades 9–12, they found:
  - 40% of students surveyed indicated that they had used tobacco at least once in the last 30 days.
  - 11% of male and 8% of female students were overweight.

TABLE 5.2. Relative risk for each of the major risk factors for coronary heart disease in middle-aged men, compiled from various US government sources

Risk factor	Relative risk
Smoking	2.0
Hypertension	2.4
Elevated serum cholesterol	2–3 (depending on level of elevation)
Diabetes	2.5
Obesity	2.1
Physical inactivity	1.9

Source: With thanks to Denise Simons-Morton, MD, then-postdoctoral fellow, for the compilation from various sources and years.

- In a companion survey of elementary schools:
    - 13% of male sixth-grade students answered yes to the question: "Have you used tobacco in the last 30 days?"
    - 24% percent of male seventhgrade students answered yes to the same question.

Based on those local risk factor prevalence rates, the planning team concludes that in Roseville, behaviors related to overweight and obesity constitute important problems, especially considering data showing declines in the levels of physical activity. Since the word "overweight" describes a condition rather than a behavior, the team decides to delineate three specific behaviors known to be associated with the problem of overweight: (1) consumption of food high in saturated fats, (2) low consumption of fruits and vegetables, and (3) low levels of physical activity.

Although there is a very promising decline in smoking among adults, the planning team finds the data on vaping or the use of electronic cigarettes among youth troubling and views it as a harbinger of things to come. They are aware of some literature indicating that the earlier one initiates smoking or the use of electronic cigarettes, the more likely one is to become a smoker as an adult—a clear sign that postponing the onset of smoking among youth will reduce addiction to nicotine and will decrease tobacco use among adults (Brownson et al. 2018; Glantz and Bareham 2018; Jacobsen et al. 2001). The planning team is unanimous that smoking or vaping among youth should be specified as important. They also note that the preventive behaviors associated with screening for cholesterol and hypertension are moving in the right direction and, for Roseville, may not need to be focal points for program intervention. So, the behavioral risk factors deemed to be important for the emerging heart disease prevention program in Roseville are:

- Consumption of foods high in saturated fat;
- Low consumption of fruits and vegetables;
- Physical inactivity; and
- Smoking or vaping among youth.

The absence of the behaviors related to cholesterol and hypertension screening from this list provides planners with valuable information as they move forward in the planning process. The positive trend in screening sends a signal that prevention is working. It implies that those providing preventive services are doing a good job, and that benefits Roseville. When such assets are built into health programs as complementary components, they strengthen the program's comprehensive nature and its political support.

Step 3: Rating Behaviors on Changeability

Having established the level of *importance* of selected behaviors among the intended audience for the program, the next step in this phase is to determine whether there is reasonable evidence that the behaviors in question can be changed in that group. Estimates of the relative **changeability** of perceived attributes of selected behaviors can be found in table 5.3. It is not possible to provide valid, reliable, and up-to-date estimates of the changeability of a given risk behavior that will apply with "external validity" across different populations and cultures (Green and Gielen 2014). For this reason, planners must take the responsibly to stay abreast of the current literature on evidence-based intervention strategies. They need also to use the latest practice-based evidence, such as evaluation of ongoing programs, as a complementary source of their rationale for making professional judgments about changeability (Green et al. 2009; Green and Ottoson 2004).

With those caveats in mind, here are a few practical rules of thumb that will help planners continue the analytical process. A given behavior has a higher probability for change when:

- It is still in the developmental stages or has been established only recently;
- It is not deeply rooted in cultural patterns or lifestyles; or
- There is a compelling theoretical rationale for its changeability.

Most resistant to change, or subject to the highest relapse rates, are those behaviors that have an addictive component (tobacco, alcohol, drug misuse), those with deep-seated compulsive elements (compulsive eating, compulsive work), and those with strong family patterns or routines surrounding them

TABLE 5.3. Relative changeability based on perceived attributes of selected preventive health behaviors, as illustrated here for heart-health behaviors[a]

Health behavior	Relevance	Social approval	Advantages	Complexity	Compatibility with values, experiences, and needs	Divisibility or trialability	Observability
Quitting smoking	+	+	+	-	-	+	+
Controlling weight	+	+	+	-	+	+	+
Controlling blood pressure	+	+	-	-	-	+	-
Taking medication	+	+	-	-	-	+	-
Maintaining a low-sodium diet	+	+	-	-	-	+	-
Maintaining a low-sodium, low-cholesterol diet	+	+	+	-	+	+	+
Exercising	+	+	+	-	+	+	+
Having preventive medical examinations	+	+	+	-	+	-	+

Sources: Adapted from Green, L.W. (1975). Diffusion and adoption of innovations related to cardiovascular risk behavior in the public. In Enelow, A., & Henderson, J.B. (Eds.), *Applying Behavioral Sciences to Cardiovascular Risk* (pp. 84–108). American Heart Association; and Farquhar, J. & Green, L.W. (2015). Community intervention trials in high-income countries. In Detels, R., Gulliford, M., Abdool Karim, Q., and Tan, C.C. (Eds.), *Oxford Textbook of Public Health* (6th ed., Vol. 2, pp. 516–27). Oxford University Press. https://doi.org/10.1093/med/9780199661756.003.0112

[a] + = positive, - = negative. Changes since the first edition in 1980 reflect changes in social norms and technologies. The only change in a negative direction has been in the complexity dimension of having preventive medical examinations. This is a manifestation of disparities in accessibility of health services to the rural and disadvantaged segments of the population in the United States.

(eating patterns, work, and leisure). Also, judgments about changeability should include careful consideration of the time factor. What expectations are being held as to when a change in each risk factor will be manifested? Deeply rooted and widespread behaviors are likely to take a while to change, making the time factor important.

By testing behaviors for changeability, we come closer to an informed decision on which behaviors we should slate or recommend for intervention, or decisions about the resources it will require to achieve program objectives for change in the intended audience. In table 5.4, the behavior generated by the Roseville cardiovascular disease prevention program planning team is among those listed in the rows. The four "rules of thumb" are expanded in the column headings of the table to include more specific attributes of health practices or technologies that predict their rate of adoption. Planners will find this kind of simple analysis helpful as they attempt to estimate the changeability of the risk factors being considered for program intervention.

Table 5.4. Assessing the changeability of risk behaviors

Health behavior	Documented evidence for change	Still in developmental stages	Not deeply rooted in culture/lifestyle	Strong supporting theory
Consumption of foods high in saturated fat	Variable	Variable	Deeply rooted for some in Roseville	Modest
Consumption of fruits/vegetables	Variable	Variable	Deeply rooted for some in Roseville	Modest
Physical activity	Trends promising, especially related to environmental strategies	For many, no	Not deeply rooted	Strong
Smoking among youth	Good evidence	Yes	Varies by gender and cultural and ethnic factors	Strong

After reviewing table 5.4, the planning team concluded that: (1) smoking and physical activity were deemed changeable based jointly on findings from the literature as well as positive estimates on the matters of development stage and theory, and (2) the changeability rating of the two eating-related behaviors stimulated considerable discussion and debate.

Some members of the planning team indicated that the dramatic changes in the dietary habits documented in the famous North Karelia Cardiovascular Disease Prevention Project and the Stanford Five-City Project (Farquhar and Green 2015) provide adequate assurance that these are changeable. Specific evidence from this project has shown that the consumption of high-fat foods could be reduced and that the consumption of fruits and vegetables could be increased through community-based interventions. While acknowledging that evidence, others called attention to advice from the CDC's online guidelines (from the Community Preventive Services Task Force, updated regularly from their systematic reviews of the evidence) and a report from the National Academy of Medicine (Green et al. 2013). These sources indicated that even though behavioral research was being conducted to test numerous dietary interventions in a variety of populations, no consistent understanding had emerged regarding which interventions are universally more efficacious in influencing dietary change. Thoughtful exchanges of this kind indicated that planners engaged in a serious and caring examination of options. Such discussions also characterize a key element of effective health program planning work—*the continuous struggle to strike a prudent balance among scientific certitude, consultation with the community and specific groups, and good judgment among scientists and professionals.*

Step 4: Choosing Behavioral Targets

With the behaviors ranked on importance and changeability, the planning team is ready to select those risk behaviors that will constitute one of several strategic focal points in the total health program. To facilitate the selection process, we recommend that the ratings for importance and changeability be arranged in a simple fourfold table, as shown in figure 5.4.

Depending on the program objectives, the behavioral objectives will most likely originate in Quadrants 1 and 2. Evaluation is crucial when one is uncertain about whether change will occur. Behaviors in Quadrant 3 will be unlikely candidates. Two exceptions to this might arise. One involves a political need to address a lower-priority behavior. For instance, a community group representing the taxpayers who support the agency might insist on their preference for a behavior that scientific review has deemed less important. The other exception might arise when an administrator or steering committee needs to see "evidence" of some change before investing in more costly behavioral interventions. When such a need exists, the behaviors should be given priority on a temporary basis only, and *only if the planner can proceed with assurance that no harm will be done.* In some instances, it is possible that no behaviors will surface in Quadrant l; this is most likely to occur because of limited evidence on changeability. If the health problem

	More important	**Less important**
More changeable	High priority for programs focus (Quadrant 1)	Low priority except to demonstrate change for political purposes (Quadrant 3)
Less changeable	Priority for innovative program; evaluation crucial (Quadrant 2)	No program (Quadrant 4)

FIGURE 5.4. The rankings of behaviors on the two dimensions of importance and changeability leads to at least four categories of possible action.

is urgent, then extensive educational and behavioral research and experimental or pilot program evaluation are justified. These procedures merely make explicit and systematic what most good practitioners and planners, agencies, and foundations do intuitively and implicitly in determining their own research and program priorities and their decisions on funding of program proposals.

Using figure 5.4 as a template, the Roseville example would likely place smoking and physical activity in Quadrant 1 and the two eating behaviors in Quadrant 2. Even though all those actions are deemed important in preventing cardiovascular disease, the team was divided on the matter of whether sufficient evidence supports the idea that both are amenable to sustained change.

Step 5: Stating Behavioral Objectives

Once target behaviors have been identified, the final step in this stage is stating behavioral objectives. In this step, specificity is vital. Such objectives are foundational to program evaluation (see chapter 9). The efficiency and effectiveness of health promotion efforts are jeopardized when behavioral objectives are too vague or generic. Given the scarcity of health promotion resources, vagueness is a luxury one cannot afford. Instances of "intangible" and claims of "unmeasurable" target behaviors generally reflect inadequacy in how the behavioral components of the health problem have been delineated. Well-intended phrases such as "improve health habits" and "increase the use of health services" cannot stand as useful behavioral objectives. Program efforts aimed at such diffuse targets will likely be scattered, with too little effort directed at any one behavior to make a difference for the individuals reached or with too few individuals reached to make a difference on the population level. For this reason, when behavioral change is possible and appropriate, one must take the utmost care in stating the objectives with *specificity*. Each behavioral objective should answer the following question: "Who is to show how much of what change, by when?"

- Who? The people (e.g., individuals, groups, or organizations) expected to change.
- What? The action or change in behavior or health practice to be achieved.
- How much? The extent of the condition to be achieved.
- When? The time in which the change is expected to occur.

In the hypothetical Roseville cardiovascular disease prevention program example, one of the behaviors that surfaced was smoking among youth. As they considered crafting a behavioral objective, the planning team concluded that that the term "youth" is too general and imprecise. Based on the survey data available, tobacco or electronic cigarette use was initiated sometime around or before the sixth grade and continued to accelerate through to high school. They decided that:

- "Who" (for at least part of the program) would consist of all sixth-grade students in Roseville.
- "What" would be a reduction in the incidence of the onset of smoking.
- "How much" was established as a 38% reduction, which would be a decrease from the baseline rate of 13% to 8%. The planning team arrived at that estimate based on a report that in a recent three-year period, the rate of tobacco and electronic cigarette use among sixth-graders in Massachusetts dropped from 16.5% to 7%. The team determined that it would be reasonable to achieve a 38% reduction to 8%, getting Roseville closer to the state average.
- "When" is defined as the proposed time of follow-up evaluation, which the planning team set as three years.

Concisely stated, then, the behavioral objective would read as follows:

> "Sixth-grade students in Roseville will show a 38% reduction in the onset of tobacco and electronic cigarette smoking within three years of program implementation."

Such an objective might be seen as misplaced precision, but the process of developing it makes it defensible and operational.

FOUR STEPS OF AN ENVIRONMENTAL ASSESSMENT

As has been emphasized repeatedly, risk behaviors constitute one among a complex array of multiple factors that influence health status. We now turn our attention to the examination of the social and environmental factors that influence the health and behavioral priorities already identified. Regardless of the health problem, the environment around us greatly affects our health status. The places where we live and work, the air we breathe and the water we drink, the physical terrain and climate, and the sources of transportation can all be healthful or pose potential risks. Similarly, our health is also affected by social and structural factors that surround us (Green and Ottoson 1999). There is growing scientific evidence supporting what we know intuitively: that individuals' health and well-being are likely to be enhanced when people are surrounded by social support in their families and communities, and when policies support equity in the fundamentals of health (e.g., education, employment, care, etc.).

A model of health determinants taken from the CDC's National Center for Health Statistics' *Shaping a Vision of Health Statistics for the 21st Century* is presented below in figure 5.5. Although designed to illustrate the various indicators that are needed to assess the wide range of social and environmental factors that influence health and require attention in a national health statistics system, you will see the parallels with the diagnostic process discussed earlier. The health problem of interest is anchored in the center of the model; this is consistent with the task of epidemiologic assessment. The various determinants of that health problem are positioned in successive concentric circles. In the two outer concentric circles ("Community Attributes" and "Context"), factors in the subcategories entitled "social characteristics," "biological characteristics," "health services, "collective lifestyle and health practices," and "cultural context" are directly addressed by either the health or behavioral assessment. Regarding the latter, recall the broken-appointment cycle example cited previously.

The subcategories of "population-based health programs," "economic resources," "natural environment," "political environment," and "built environment" contain many factors that are likely to surface during an environmental assessment. The "built environment" refers to that aspect of the physical environment that is manmade and is often the source of factors that surface in the

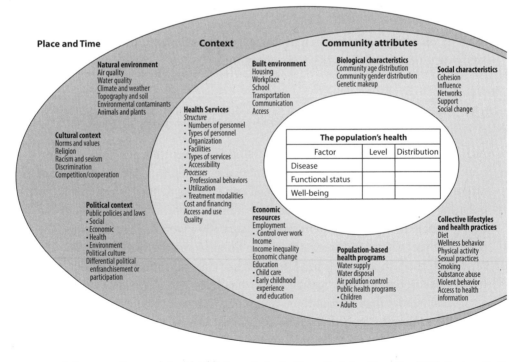

FIGURE 5.5. Influence on the population's health. *Source:* Centers for Disease Control and Prevention. (2002). *Shaping a Health Statistics Vision for the 21st Century*. Department of Health and Human Services, National Center for Health Statistics.

environmental assessment. Our homes, schools, and workplaces; our sidewalks, streets, and freeways; our waterpipes, sewers, and parks—these make up the built environment. From a public health perspective, the way we go about building and shaping our environment has a direct and powerful effect on health (Dannenberg et al. 2003; Killingsworth et al. 2003). Strategies designed to enhance the built environment include those that (1) foster recreational and physical activity; (2) provide and promote safe, affordable housing; (3) provide safe, reliable, and affordable means of transportation; (4) ensure safe, clean water, soil, air, and building materials; and (4) ensure a well-maintained, aesthetically appealing environment.

The physical environment makes its greatest impact on living conditions as well as risk factors for disease brought about by exposures ranging from air, water, soil, and housing to transportation and an absence of safe modes for walking and recreation. For example, the demographic shift from a rural to an urban lifestyle has led to some compounding of risks. Work has become primarily an indoor activity to the point where the average person spends over 90% of their time indoors. Those indoor areas, built "airtight" to conserve energy, reduce the infiltration of fresh air that, in turn, can lead to an increase in indoor air contamination and transmission of infectious diseases.

If the scope of environmental determinants on health becomes so encompassing and complex as to be impractical for the scope of the health program you are planning, we recommend concentrating attention on those aspects of the environment that are:

1. More social than physical (e.g., organizational and economic);

2. Interactive with behavior in their impact on health; and

3. Changeable by social action and health policy.

Much of health promotion concerns the passage of laws and organizational changes to regulate or constrain behavior that threatens the health of others. We consider the initial stimulation of public interest and support for such legislation to be, in large part, a function of the third category of behavior discussed in the previous chapter: those planned behaviors and acts of advocacy taken by individuals or groups that influence some dimension of the physical, social, or political environments. Of particular note in recent decades have been initiatives in pursuit of gun control, automobile safety design features, vaccine development, and school and recreational or occupational restraints on exposure to infectious diseases and air or water contaminants.

Step 1: Identifying Environmental Factors

This first step parallels Step 1 in the behavioral assessment: list those environmental factors known to contribute to the health problem or goal directly or indirectly (through a high-priority behavioral factor). Continuing with the Roseville example, recall that the planning team established the following as one of its behavioral objectives:

> "Sixth-grade students in Roseville will show a 38% reduction in the onset of tobacco and electronic cigarette smoking within three years of program implementation."

What factors in the social or physical environment are likely to have an influence on the attainment of that objective? After pondering that question, the planning team agreed on a short answer: nicotine. That, of course, is the obvious priority now that vaping must also be considered in the mix. Both electronic cigarettes and tobacco cigarettes contain nicotine, and vaping can result in youth later turning to tobacco cigarettes to fulfill their need for nicotine. The team's selection of tobacco and electronic cigarettes use by youth was in large part based on the compelling evidence indicating that earlier initiation of either vaping or smoking leads to becoming an adult smoker who is likely to be addicted.

In the United States, the federal minimum age of sale of any tobacco products is 21 years as of March 2020. While this law makes it more difficult for young people to obtain these products, access to them remains an important environmental factor, as evidenced by the prevalence of their use among youth. Recall that during the behavioral assessment, the planning team used findings from surveys jointly carried out by the Roseville School District and the Roseville Health Department. That same effort included a brief community survey and tobacco policy assessment. Information combining findings from that community survey and policy assessment with two items from the youth surveys is presented in table 5.5.

Step 2: Rating Environmental Factors on Relative Importance

The planning team concluded from these data that they may be able to achieve a substantial effect by focusing attention on the following as potential environmental factors related to the onset of vaping and smoking among sixth-grade students in Roseville:

- Merchants selling tobacco and vaping products to youth;
- Merchants verifying age prior to selling tobacco and vaping products; and
- School policy banning tobacco use and vaping on school grounds.

TABLE 5.5. Summary of findings from Roseville community survey

Percentage of current smokers (middle school) who bought cigarettes at gas stations or convenience stores	63%[a]
Percentage of current smokers (middle school) who purchased cigarettes but were not asked to show proof of age	72%[a]
Number of restaurants that are entirely smoke-free	46% (17/37)[b]
Number of Roseville merchants (clerks) who ask for verification of age before selling	62% (34/55)[b]
A formal program to train merchants about minors' access to tobacco	None[b]
School policy calling for a uniform ban on tobacco use for students, teachers, and staff, not only on school grounds but at all school-related functions	None[b]
Enforcement-related activities reported by the police department:	
• Inspections for signs?	No[b]
• Periodic compliance checks?	Yes[b]
• Citations?	No[b]
• Awards/letters of compliance?	No[b]
• Volunteers in tobacco enforcement?	No[b]

[a] Hypothetical data for Roseville case study, reflective of those in Youth Tobacco Survey. Centers for Disease Prevention and Control.

[b] Hypothetical interview data for Roseville case study. (Numbers in parentheses = number interviewed from total available)

As with the behavioral assessment, the broad criteria for determining the importance of a given environmental factor include evidence that it (1) is clearly linked to the health problem, and (2) is present (you can document that it occurs) and prevalent in the population of interest. Some of the factors will matter more than others because of one or both of the following criteria: (1) the strength of the relationship of the environmental factor to the health or quality of life goal or problem; and (2) the incidence, prevalence, or number of people affected by the environmental factor. Based on the information they have in hand, the Roseville planning team judged all three of the previously cited environmental factors identified to be important.

Step 3: Rating Environmental Factors on Changeability

With a list of important factors in hand, the task in this step is to select those that are most likely to yield to intervention through policy, regulation, or organizational change strategies. As was the case for assessing the changeability of specific risk behaviors, planners are urged to consult relevant literature for evidence that environmental factors can be modified. But even if there is compelling scientific evidence indicating that certain strategies are effective in creating environmental change, the implementation of those strategies may be impossible without public or political support. This reality provides further re-inforcement for the ongoing need for planners to act on the critical principles of *participation*, *stakeholder involvement*, and *situational analysis* discussed in previous chapters. We will return to these questions when we reach the health program and policy development in Phase 4.

Assessing the political will to make changes is essential to changeability anal-ysis, because environmental factors, like lifestyle factors, will often prove to be important to the community for purposes other than health. For example, a common dilemma is the occupational hazard that can only be eliminated at the risk of losing the industry that supplies jobs for the community. Recall the West Virginia mining example. The lung disease might be largely attributable to the mining work, and so there might not be a way to eliminate that hazard without eliminating the jobs. When the hazard cannot be eliminated, it is critical to im-plement behavioral solutions, such as wearing protective equipment, stopping smoking, and going for periodic screening.

Consultation by risk assessors (you, the planner) with risk managers (prac-titioners, policy makers, company officials, and others responsible for the en-vironmental or ecological risks) and with stakeholders (the employees and community) should occur at least at two points in the assessment and planning process, as suggested by figure 5.6. At the early point of formulating the prob-lem or issue (upper left in figure) and at the point of analyzing the results (lower center), discussion should assess views of changeability as a matter of assessing political will and costs associated with change. Views of importance as a matter of subjective quality of life concerns and lifestyle priorities can be factored into these discussions, but most of the analysis of importance is part of the technical ecological risk assessment itself (center of figure) (Green and Mercer 2001).

Here are some questions planners should consider as they assess the *change-ability* of important environmental factors.

- Is there evidence that this factor is amenable to change? (This is not quite the same as a later step, in which the question becomes, "Is there evidence that specific interventions have worked to change this factor?")

- Is there public and political support for the proposed environmental change? If not, can that support be gained?

As the Roseville planning team discussed the issue of changeability, they once again agreed that merchants selling tobacco to youth, verification of age prior to selling vaping paraphernalia or tobacco, and school policy banning vaping or tobacco use on school grounds were all changeable. However, they also concluded that the behavior of the merchants was not likely to change with-out periodic compliance checks by law enforcement authorities. Members of the

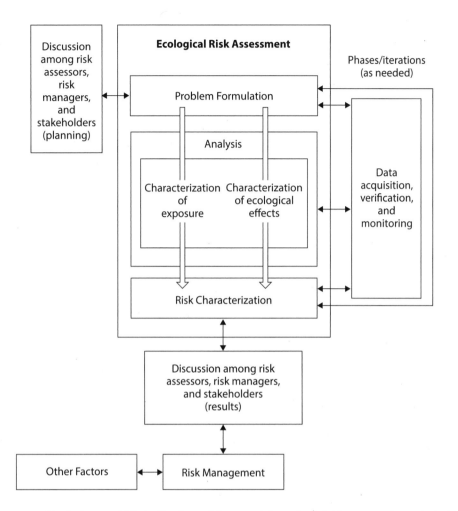

FIGURE 5.6. The Environmental Protection Agency's framework for ecological risk assessment was adapted by the Commission on Risk Assessment and Risk Management for the US Congress to include the particular points at which public consultation or community "stakeholders" would be most important.

planning committee met with Roseville law enforcement officials, who indicated that they would be willing to add periodic merchant checks to their workload contingent on their budget not being cut by the city council. Accordingly, the list of environmental factors then included:

- Merchants selling tobacco and vaping products to youth;
- Verification of age by merchants prior to selling tobacco and vaping products;
- Formal compliance checks by law enforcement, including issuing citations when not in compliance and letters of recognition when in compliance; and
- School policy banning vaping and tobacco use on school grounds.

Note that the environmental changes often needed to involve, as in this case, changes in the behavior of people who control the environment. We will return to this layering of behavioral changes in later chapters.

Step 4: Choosing the Environmental Targets

The analytic method for selecting behavioral targets, previously illustrated in figure 5.4, is applied here. The same four quadrants in the two-by-two table would yield a distribution of environmental factors that would be more or less important and more or less changeable. The policy implication for action on factors in each quadrant would pertain equally to the environmental factors. The only exception might be the greater weight one could give to Quadrant 3, where the environmental factor is apparently changeable but relatively low in objective importance. As Slovic and others have pointed out in their research on risk perception, the subjective importance of an environmental factor for the community is often as important as the objective evidence for its relationship or causal link to the health goal or ecological problem. Risk is not just a scientific construction; it is a social construction (Slovic 1999; 2001). When public health professionals and community stakeholders grapple with problems simultaneously from an objective and subjective perspective, the problems cannot be resolved solely by applying traditional linear, cause-and-effect approaches to problem-solving. Rather, these complex, environmental health problems (sometimes referred to as "wicked problems") are most likely to yield to a combination of the following: (1) the application of effective community health education skills (especially those focusing on stakeholder involvement and participatory research) and systems thinking; (2) a sustained commitment to sound environmental and epidemiological science; and (3) ongoing, transparent communication among all stakeholders and community residents (Kreuter et al. 2004).

Step 5: Stating Environmental Objectives

With the priorities established among environmental factors to be changed, the final step in this phase of the assessment planning process is to state the objectives for environmental change in quantitative terms. Again, we urge planners to follow the same protocol recommended for crafting behavioral objectives, with the exception that it would not be uncommon to see an absence of the "who." For example, in a global warming reduction program with a focus on clean air in the environment, an objective might be focused on air pollution and the built environment (Sallis and Green 2012), not on personal behaviors or the actors who will be responsible for creating the desired change:

The amount of carbon monoxide released into the atmosphere in our community will be reduced by 20% by the year 2025.

In the Roseville case, for example, the planning team might state one of their environmental objectives as follows:

Student access to vaping and tobacco products in Roseville will be reduced by 75% by three years after the launch of the program.

The Roseville group chose to insert a specific "who," as in this version:

Merchants in Roseville gas stations and convenience stores will reduce their sales to minors by 100% by three years after the launch of the program.

If the environmental change objective requires the action of specific groups of people to achieve it, then behavioral objectives might be set for their actions as well. This relationship between environmental and behavioral objectives is reflected in the vertical arrows (between environment and behavior) in the diagram of the PRECEDE-PROCEED model in figure 5.1 at the beginning of this chapter.

EXERCISES

1. Identify behavioral and environmental factors associated with the health problem you chose for chapter 4's exercises.
2. Rate (low, medium, high) each factor according to (a) its relative importance in affecting the health problem, and (b) its potential for change.
3. Discuss the reasons for your ratings.
4. Write an objective for both the highest-priority behavioral factor and the highest-priority environmental factor.

Notes

1. Institute of Medicine of the National Academies Press reports on obesity control have dealt usefully with the genetic, behavioral, and environmental interactions in food supply, marketing, intake, genetic predispositions, physical activity, and the built environment (Green et al. 2013; Koplan et al. 2010; Kumanyika et al. 2010).
2. Access to risk factor data has grown exponentially since the inception of the PRECEDE model in the early 1970s. See, for example, Chronic Disease Interactive Data Applications available from the CDC at https://www.cdc.gov/chronicdisease/data/statistics.htm.

References

Barnoya, J., & Glantz, S.A. (2004). Association of the California tobacco control program with declines in lung cancer incidence. *Cancer Causes and Control, 15*(7), 689–95. https://doi .org/10.1023/B:CACO.0000036187.13805.30

Brownson, R.C., Fielding, J.E., & Green, L.W. (2018). The debate about electronic cigarettes: Harm minimization or the precautionary principle. *Annual Review of Public Health, 39,* 189–92. https://doi.org/10.1146/annurev-publhealth-102417-124810

Crawford, D., & Jeffery, R.W. (2006). *Obesity Prevention and Public Health.* Oxford University Press.

Dannenberg, A.L., Jackson, R.J., Frumkin, H., Schieber, R.A., Pratt, M., Kochtitzky, C., & Tilson, H.H. (2003). The impact of community design and land-use choices on public health: A scientific research agenda. *American Journal of Public Health, 93*(9), 1500–8. https://doi.org/10.2105/ajph.93.9.1500

Farquhar, J. & Green, L.W. (2015). Community intervention trials in high-income countries. In Detels, R., Gulliford, M., Abdool Karim, Q., and Tan, C.C. (Eds.), *Oxford Textbook of Public Health* (6th ed., Vol. 2, pp. 516–27). Oxford University Press. https://doi.org/10.1093 /med/9780199661756.003.0112

Fichtenberg, C.M., & Glantz, S.A. (2000). Association of the California Tobacco Control Program with declines in cigarette consumption and mortality from heart disease. *The New England Journal of Medicine, 343*(24), 1772–7. https://doi.org/10.1056/NEJM200012143 432406

Froguel, P., & Boutin, P. (2001). Genetics of pathways regulating body weight in the development of obesity in humans. *Experimental Biology and Medicine, 226*(11), 991–6. https:// doi.org/10.1177/153537020122601105

Gielen, A.C., & Green, L.W. (2015). The impact of policy, environmental, and educational interventions: A synthesis of the evidence from two public health success stories. *Health Education and Behavior, 42*(Suppl. 1), 20S–34S. https://doi.org/10.1177/1090198115570049

Gielen, A.C., Sleet, D.A., & Green, L.W. (2006). Community models and approaches for interventions. In Gielen, A.C., Sleet, D.A., & DiClemente, R.J. (Eds.), *Injury and Violence Prevention: Behavioural Science Theories, Methods, and Applications* (pp. 65–82). Jossey-Bass.

Glantz, S.A., & Bareham, D.W. (2018). E-cigarettes: Use, effects on smoking, risks, and policy implications. *Annual Review of Public Health, 39,* 215–35. https://doi.org/10.1146/annurev -publhealth-040617-013757

Golden, S.D., McLeroy, K.R., Green, L.W., Earp, J.A., & Lieberman, L.D. (2015). Upending the social ecological model to guide health promotion efforts toward policy and environmental change. *Health Education and Behavior, 42*(Suppl. 1), 8S–14S. https://doi.org /10.1177/1090198115575098

Green, L.W., & Gielen, A.C. (2014). Evidence and ecological theory in two public health successes for health behavior change. In Kahan, S., Gielen, A.C., Fagan, P., & Green, L.W. (Eds.), *Health Behavior Change in Populations* (pp. 26–43). Johns Hopkins University Press.

Green, L.W., Sim, L., & Breiner, H. (Eds.). (2013). *Evaluating Obesity Prevention Efforts: A Plan for Measuring Progress* (p. 489). National Academy Press.

Green, L.W., & Mercer, S.L. (2001). Participatory research: Can public health researchers and agencies reconcile the push from funding bodies and the pull from communities? *American Journal of Public Health, 91*(12), 1926–9. https://doi.org/10.2105/ajph.91.12.1926

Green, L.W., & Ottoson, J.M. (1999). *Community and Population Health* (8th ed.). WCB/ McGraw-Hill.

Green, L.W., & Ottoson, J.M. (2004). From efficacy to effectiveness to community and back: Evidence-based practice vs practice-based evidence. In Green, L., Hiss, R., Glasgow, R., et al. (Eds.), *From Clinical Trials to Community: The Science of Translating Diabetes and Obesity Research* (pp. 15–18). National Institutes of Health.

Green, L.W., Ottoson, J.M., García, C., & Hiatt, R. (2009). Diffusion theory and knowledge dissemination, utilization and integration in public health. *Annual Review of Public Health, 30,* 151–74. https://doi.org/10.1146/annurev.publhealth.031308.100049

Jacobsen, L., Lantz, P.M., Warner, K.E., Wasserman, J., Pollack, H.A., & Ahlstrom, A.A. (2001). *Combating Teen Smoking: Research and Policy Strategies.* University of Michigan Press.

Killingsworth, R., Earp, J., & Moore, R. (2003). Supporting health through design: Challenges and opportunities. *American Journal of Health Promotion, 18*(1), 1–2. https://doi.org/10.4278/0890-1171-18.1.1

Koplan, J., Brownson, R.C., Bullock, A., & Foerster, S.B. (Eds.). (2010). *Progress in Preventing Childhood Obesity: How Do We Measure Up?* National Academies Press.

Kreuter, M.W., De Rosa, C.R., Howze, E., & Baldwin, G. (2004). Understanding wicked problems: A key to environmental health promotion. *Health Education and Behavior, 31*(4), 441–54. https://doi.org/10.1177/1090198104265597

Kumanyika, S.K., Parker, L., & Sim, L.J. (Eds.). (2010). *Bridging the Evidence Gap in Obesity Prevention.* National Academies Press.

Mukherjea, A., & Green, L.W. (2014). Tobacco and behavior change. In Kahan, S., Gielen, A., Fagan, P., & Green, L.W. (Eds.), *Health Behavior Change in Populations* (pp. 153–87). Johns Hopkins University Press.

Richard, L., Potvin, L., Kishchuk, N., Prlic, H., & Green, L.W. (1996). Assessment of the integration of the ecological approach in health promotion programs. *American Journal of Health Promotion, 10*(4), 318–28. https://doi.org/10.4278/0890-1171-10.4.318

Sallis, J.F., & Green, L.W. (2012). Active Living by Design and its evaluation: contributions to science. *American Journal of Preventive Medicine, 43*(5 Suppl. 4), S410–2.

Slovic, P. (1999). Trust, emotion, sex, politics, and science: surveying the risk-assessment battlefield. *Risk Analysis, 19*(4), 689–701.

Slovic, P. (2001). The risk game. *Journal of Hazardous Materials, 86*(1–3), 17–24. https://doi.org/10.1016/S0304-3894(01)00248-5

World Health Organization (WHO). (2000). *Obesity: preventing and managing the global epidemic.* [Report of a WHO Consultation (WHO Technical Report Series 894)]. https://www.who.int/nutrition/publications/obesity/WHO_TRS_894/en/

Educational and Ecological Assessment: Predisposing, Enabling and Reinforcing Factors

•

María E. Fernández, Gerjo Kok, Guy Parcel,
and Lawrence W. Green

Learning Objectives

After completing the chapter, the reader will be able to:

- Describe the definitions and give examples of predisposing, reinforcing, and enabling factors influencing behavior and environmental conditions.
- Explain how to use theory, evidence, and new data to identify predisposing, reinforcing, and enabling factors.
- Describe and provide examples of how factors can interact to influence behavior and environmental conditions.
- Provide examples of how you might engage a community in the identification and prioritization of predisposing, reinforcing, and enabling factors.
- List and describe steps for considering which factors to prioritize in a health promotion planning effort.
- Demonstrate an ability to distinguish and label types of factors influencing behavior and environmental conditions.

INTRODUCTION

The next PRECEDE-PROCEED phase—the educational and ecological diagnosis—identifies factors that are associated with the important behaviors and environmental conditions identified in the previous chapter's social and epidemiologic assessment phase, as seen in figure 6.1. These factors are the immediate targets of an intervention and must be modified to create and sustain desired changes

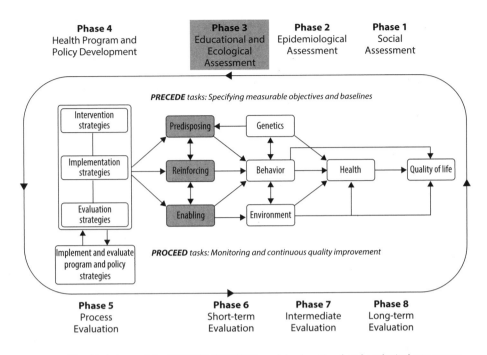

FIGURE 6.1. The third phase of the PRECEDE-PROCEED model, educational and ecological assessment, focuses on the predisposing, enabling, and reinforcing determinants of behavior and the environment.

in behaviors and environments that influence health and quality of life. This assessment phase of PRECEDE helps planners clearly identify and understand the various and multilevel factors influencing health-related behavior and environmental conditions.

We call this phase the educational and ecological diagnosis because it guides the identification of behavioral influences that reside within the individual and will become *educational* targets. It does so using an *ecological* perspective that also considers factors in the environment that influence behavior. The term *educational* refers to the natural social learning process that occurs in everyday living, by which individuals exercise some control over their behavior and environment (Bandura 2001; 2002). "Ecological" refers to the relationships among factors and the idea that a person's behavior influences the social environment and that behavior is, in turn, influenced by multiple levels of the environment (family, peers, organizations) (Bandura 1978; 2001). This phase of PRECEDE underscores this reciprocal relationship and defines three categories of factors affecting individual or collective behavior: predisposing, enabling, and reinforcing factors. Each exerts a different type of influence on behavior, but all three motivate, facilitate, and sustain behavioral and environmental change.

Predisposing factors are antecedents to behavioral change that provide the rationale or *motivation* for the behavior. These include knowledge, attitudes, self-efficacy, perceived social norms, and behavioral intentions. They usually reside within the individual and can be considered the necessary or motivating force behind behavior. For example, for a woman to complete a screening mammogram, she must be aware of the guidelines, believe it is the right thing to do for her health, expect support from her family or friends, and feel confident in her ability to get screened.

Enabling factors are antecedents to behavioral or environmental change that make it easier to change behavior or the environment. Resources, social support, and skills are all examples of enabling factors. An enabling factor that would influence mammography screening may be whether a woman has health insurance, the recommendation she received from her provider, or the encouragement she receives from her friends. In the previous PRECEDE phase, we identified environmental factors—changes needed in the broader community environment to create the required conditions for health. The category of enabling factors includes the skills and personal, family, or community resources necessary to make a behavioral change possible for an individual.

Reinforcing factors follow a behavior and provide the continuing *reward* or incentive for the persistence or repetition of the behavior. The positive feedback or social support she receives from family and peers following the mammogram, or the relief a woman feels after having completed a screening, are examples of reinforcing factors.

These three types of factors typically influence behaviors, but the importance of specific determinants within each category may vary depending on the behavior, setting, or population.

THEORETICAL FOUNDATION

Many theories attempt to explain influences on human behavior at multiple levels; however, no single theoretical model can sufficiently encompass the range of human experience and circumstances. The PRECEDE framework can help understand and organize concepts and constructs from specific theories, observations, and research evidence. A particular behavior or feature of the social or health environment is not caused by just one factor. Instead, each factor increases or decreases the probability the action will be performed or the environment will change. Each potentially affects the influence of other factors (Allegrante 2015; Campbell et al. 2007; Gehlert et al. 2008; Golden et al. 2015; Kawachi and Kennedy 1999; Krieger 2008; Link and Phelan 1995; Marmot 2005; Schölmerich and Kawachi 2015; Stokols 1996; Thoits 2011; Wallerstein and Duran 2006). PRECEDE is based on several common theoretical themes that have proven especially applicable and appropriate to health promotion. PRECEDE helps the planner organize the determinants of behavior and environment into three categories, with the assumption that any behavior or environmental change is caused by the collective influence of these three types of factors (Golden et al. 2015).

How these factors are interdependent and can influence behavior and environment through various pathways is demonstrated in figure 6.2.

The sequence would proceed as follows: (1) A person has an initial reason, impulse, or motivation (predisposing factor) to pursue a given course of action (e.g., reducing fat intake). This first factor (Arrow 1 in figure 6.2)—the desire to lose weight and outcome expectations that reducing fat intake can lead to weight loss—motivates the person to start taking steps toward the behavior, but the person will not engage in the behavior unless they have the resources and skills needed to carry out the behavior. The motivation, then, is followed by (2) the use of skills and resources to enable the action (enabling factor), such as access to lower-fat foods or the ability to prepare foods without added fat. This usually results in at least a tentative enactment of the behavior, followed by (3) a reaction to the behavior that is emotional, physical, or social (reinforcing factor), such as actual weight loss and encouragement from family or friends. Reinforcement strengthens (4) behavior and (5) the search for, mobilization of, or commitment of future resources and motivation. The ready availability of enabling factors provides cues, increases awareness, and activates other factors predisposing the behavior. The social-ecological perspective of health promotion also suggests

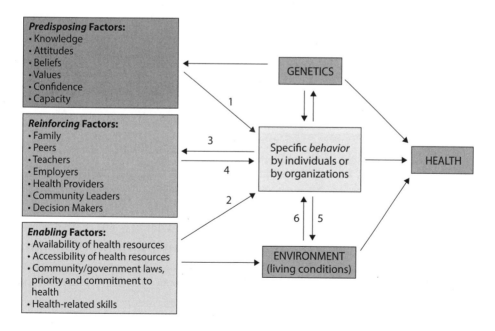

FIGURE 6.2. Examples of predisposing, enabling, and reinforcing factors influencing behavior.

that building up social reinforcement for a behavior through the social environment (social norms) can lead to the *enabling* of behavior in the form of social support and assistance (Arrow 6).

Besides its theoretical value in explaining and predicting behavior, the classification of determinants of behavioral and environmental change into predisposing, reinforcing, and enabling categories makes it possible to select the most effective types of interventions according to what type of factors we are trying to influence. In the next chapter, we describe how identification of these factors helps planners match and map intervention strategies that will most likely influence them. Intervention Mapping (Fernández et al. 2019) describes a similar process of selecting theoretical methods and practical applications of those methods according to specific determinants identified by using a modified PRECEDE diagnostic approach. In both planning frameworks, the assumption is that a careful identification of predisposing, reinforcing, and enabling factors will inform the "mapping," selection, or development of intervention strategies.

PREDISPOSING FACTORS

Certain predisposing factors may be of more immediate concern than others, either because they are prerequisites of other factors or because they are the most important. Predisposing factors relate to the motivation of an individual or group to act. They include cognitive and affective factors. These may include knowledge, attitudes, self-efficacy, beliefs, values, perceived norms, perceived support, and perceived abilities.

Other factors that could predispose a given health-related behavior or condition, through a variety of mechanisms, include personality factors and sociodemographic characteristics such as socioeconomic status, age, gender, ethnic group, genetics, and family size or history. While these types of factors are indeed "determinants" of behaviors and health outcomes, we do not include them in predisposing, reinforcing, or enabling categories because they are not immediately changeable and do not lend themselves readily to health promotion interventions. Nevertheless, they can help identify groups most in need of intervention and whether different interventions should be planned for different groups. This information is critical in the early stages of the planning process in order to identify the specific priority populations and any needs for specific targeting or tailoring or communications with them (Kreuter and Skinner 2000).

Not all health behavior is the result of people processing information to plan and engage in courses of action to improve health (Bartholomew-Eldredge et al. 2016). Some behaviors are automatic, unconscious, impulsive, or have become habitual. Automatic behaviors are often guided by external stimuli or contextual cues with reduced cognitive resources. Determinants of such behaviors are habits, environmental influences, and automatic activation of attitudes. These determinants need interventions other than or in addition to those targeting motivation (Verplanken 2018).

Knowledge

Cognitive learning results over time from exposure to an object, experience with it, and awareness of it. These cumulatively produce recognition knowledge, then recall knowledge, and eventually analytic skills and wisdom pertaining to the object. Positive associations between knowledge and behavior have been found in countless studies over decades of educational research (Blevins and DeGennaro 2018; Fredriksson et al. 2018; Ghisi et al. 2014; Guillaumie et al. 2010). Some studies also show that increased knowledge did not result in behavior change (e.g., Davis et al. 2017; Jerant et al. 2014; Wofford et al. 2007). Nevertheless, health knowledge of some kind is probably necessary before a conscious personal health action will occur—necessary, but not sufficient. For example, knowing the recommendations for preventing COVID-19 infection (mask-wearing, social distancing, vaccination) is important, but after that amount of knowledge is attained, additional information will not necessarily increase behavioral change (Anderson et al. 2009; Burke et al. 2006).

Cognitive learning also accumulates as experience, which produces beliefs, and these combine over time to produce values. Together with social influences, values, in turn, reinforce attitudes. These processes of shaping personal experience and behavior through predisposing factors are shown in figure 6.2.

The specific knowledge requirement for the person or population to carry out an intended behavior can often be inferred through simple logic. Before people will act voluntarily, they need to know *why* they should act, *what* actions are needed, *when* or under what circumstances, *how* to do it, and *where*.

Beliefs, Values, and Attitudes

Beliefs, values, and attitudes are independent **constructs,** yet the differences among them are often fine and complex. Here we describe these factors in a practical way, trusting that those seeking more detail will look further in the theoretical literature (Bartholomew-Eldredge et al. 2016; Glanz et al. 2015). Nevertheless, they are important to consider when identifying determinants of health behaviors.

Beliefs. A *belief* is a conviction that a phenomenon or object is true or real. Health-oriented belief statements include such statements as "I believe it is important to take care of myself so that I can care for my family" or "When your time is up, there's nothing you can do about it." During the planning process, a health promotion plan can consider the following questions: If beliefs such as these are strongly held, to what extent will they influence health behavior? Can they be changed? Will changes facilitate health-promoting or health-protecting behavior?

The **Health Belief Model (HBM)** (Skinner et al. 2015), developed and widely employed over the past 70 years, attempts to explain and predict health-related behavior from certain belief patterns. The model is based on the following assumptions about behavior change:

1. The person must believe that his or her health is in jeopardy of acquiring the condition. This is referred to generally as *belief in susceptibility*. For some conditions, this belief may be expressed as "I may have it and not know it." This "asymptomatic belief" is particularly important when the condition is detected by tests in the absence of felt symptoms.

2. The person must perceive the *potential seriousness* of the condition in terms of pain or discomfort, time lost from work, economic difficulties, and so forth.

3. The person must believe that *benefits* stemming from the recommended behavior outweigh the costs and inconvenience (these are *perceived* benefits and costs).

4. The person must believe in *efficacy*, that the change is possible and within his or her grasp.

5. Another component is "cue to action," a precipitating force that makes the person aware of the need to take action.

The HBM relates largely to the predisposing factors in the PRECEDE-PROCEED model and serves as a useful tool to carry out that part of the educational assessment in PRECEDE. Another construct that is somewhat related to HBM is fear. **Fear** is likely influenced by perceived susceptibility and seriousness. An additional dimension included in fear is anxiety, caused by perceived threat *in combination with* a sense of hopelessness. This combination may lead to denial or rationalization of the threat as unreal. Thus, arousals of fear in health education messages can backfire, unless they are accompanied by an immediate course of action the person can take and messages that improve self-efficacy (Kok et al. 2017).

Values. Values are concepts or ideas upon which we place worth. They are influenced by gender, culture, membership in social groups, religion, and life experience. Values are thus internalized and affect motivations, thoughts, and behavior. They can be seen as standards that become part of a person's identity and can guide behavior. Values tend to cluster within groups (ethnic, political, religious) and across generations of people who share a common history and geography. They form the basis for justifying one's actions in moral or ethical terms. While health promotion programs may not seek to change values, they can help people recognize inconsistencies between their values and their behavior or environment (e.g. values protecting their children, but smokes in their presence), thus serving as a motivation to change the behavior to align better with their values.

Attitudes. In the context of health promotion planning, attitudes are evaluative judgements about a particular behavior or task. Attitudes can range from positive to neutral to negative and typically arise from an inner framework of values and beliefs, developed over time. Kirscht (1974) viewed *attitudes* as a collection of beliefs that always includes an evaluative aspect. Attitudes differ from values in that they are attached to specific objects, persons, or situations and are more amenable to change. Values are more deeply seated and therefore less changeable than are attitudes and beliefs (Fishbein 2008; Montano and Karprzyk 2015; Rokeach 1970). For example, the belief that vaccines are important to protect health is an attitude. The belief that your role as a parent is to protect your children (by having them vaccinated) is a value. In identifying predisposing factors, the following aspects of attitude are important: (1) attitude is a rather *constant* feeling that is *directed toward an object* (be it a person, an action, a situation, or an idea), and (2) inherent in the structure of an attitude is *evaluation*, a good-bad dimension.

Theories that describe beliefs and attitudes such as the HBM, the Social Cognitive Theory (SCT), and the Theory of Reasoned Action (Glanz et al. 2015) can be very helpful to the program planner when identifying predisposing factors.

Self-Efficacy and Social Cognitive Theory. The concept of self-efficacy as a determinant of behavior found early acceptance in health education and health promotion because of its emphasis on learning and on the empowerment of people to have a sense of control or "agency" over their health. Self-efficacy is a central concept in Bandura's original Social Learning Theory (Bandura 1989) to describe a cognitive state of taking control, in which people are not just acted upon by their environments but also feel they can act upon and help influence their environments (Sheeran et al. 2016).

This concept of reciprocal determinism, with its associated concepts of self-management and self-control, is the SCT's major departure from *operant conditioning theories,* which tend to view behavior as a one-way product of rewards and punishment in the environment. Reciprocal determinism makes the SCT ideally suited to the integration of behavioral, environmental, predisposing, enabling, and reinforcing factors and the development of an educational *and* ecological approach to health program planning.

Learning takes place through three processes: (1) direct experience, (2) indirect or vicarious experience from observing others (modeling), and (3) the storing and processing of complex information in cognitive operations. These allow one to anticipate the consequences of actions, represent goals in thought, and weigh evidence from various sources to assess one's own risks and capabilities. Self-efficacy, then, is a perception of one's own capacity for success in organizing and implementing a pattern of behavior. The SCT provides information not only for identifying self-efficacy as a potential predisposing factor, but also for identifying ways to change it (called "theoretical change methods" in Intervention Mapping) (Bartholomew-Eldredge et al. 2016; Glanz et al. 2015). The self-efficacy variable has proved particularly useful in planning health programs using mass media with role models for the vicarious learning and modeling process and for the development of skills.

Behavioral Intention, Perceived Norms, and the Theory of Reasoned Action

The Theory of Reasoned Action (TRA) (Fishbein and Ajzen 2010), reformulated as the Theory of Planned Behavior (TPB) (Ajzen 2015), includes important determinants (motivational factors) of health behaviors that fall into the category of predisposing factors. The TPB postulates that **behavioral intention**, the most important determinant of (planned) behavior, is in turn, influenced by three constructs: attitude, perceived norms, and perceived behavioral control. In the TPB, an attitude is the individual's positive or negative evaluation of performing the particular behavior of interest. **Perceived norms** are the beliefs of people about what important others approve or disapprove, or beliefs about what others like oneself do. Perceived behavioral control is people's perceptions of the degree to which they are capable of, or have control over, performing a given behavior. This is comparable to self-efficacy in the SCT. Fishbein and colleagues later expanded the TPB by adding constructs, calling it the Reasoned Action Approach (RAA) (Fishbein and Ajzen 2010). Later authors expanded the TRA and TPB to include components from other major behavioral theories, including: (1) knowledge and skills to perform the behavior, (2) salience of the behavior, (3) environmental constraints, and (4) habit (Montano and Karprzyk 2015). Applications of these theories in health behavior studies and health program planning can be found in a wide range of health issues (Bartholomew-Eldredge et al. 2016; Glanz et al. 2015). For example, Roncancio et al. (2015) tested the utility of the TPB in predicting cervical cancer screening among Latinas. They found that subjective norms and perceived behavioral control were positively associated with the intention to be screened for cervical cancer, and the intention to be screened predicted actual cervical cancer screening. The study provides support for the use of the TPB in predicting cervical cancer screening among Latinas.

ENABLING FACTORS

Enabling factors are primarily skills or conditions of the environment that *facilitate, allow,* or *permit* the performance of an action by individuals or organizations. Enabling conditions, if present, make the change in behavior or change in the organization more likely, whereas the absence of adequate enabling factors inhibits action. Enabling factors include the availability, accessibility, and affordability of health care and community resources (such as whether free COVID-19 testing is available in one's community). They also include the conditions of living that act as facilitators or barriers to action, such as the availability of transportation or childcare. Enabling factors also include *new* skills that a person, organization, or community needs to implement a behavioral or environmental change.

To plan interventions directed at changing enabling factors, the planner assesses the presence or absence of enabling factors (resources, experience, and organizational structures) in the community of interest. This calls for an organizational or ecological assessment of resources and an educational assessment of required skills.

Enabling factors for health care or medical care behaviors include health care resources (e.g., hospitals, health care providers, availability of personal protective equipment, etc.). Cost, distance, available transportation, hours of operation, available childcare, and so forth are enabling factors that affect the availability and accessibility of the health care services. For each priority behavioral risk factor or capacity identified in the behavioral epidemiology assessment, one can identify environmental enabling factors.

Skills

Skills refer to a person's ability or capacity to perform tasks. Here we are referring to the skills necessary to enact a health-related behavior or skills for creating an organizational or environmental change. Skills relevant to health promotion include the ability to control personal risk factors for a disease (e.g., skills related to choosing healthful snacks, such as the ability to read food labels), skills in the appropriate use of medical care (e.g., the ability to communicate effectively with one's doctor), and skills in changing or controlling exposures to the environment (such as the ability to apply insect repellant to prevent mosquito bites that may carry disease). Skills related to broader community, regional, or national change include the ability to vote and capacities related to coalition-building and community organizing to bring about change in one's neighborhood, community policies, and civic practices and skills (combined with resources) among health personnel to conduct effective mass communications with populations, appropriate to the phase of a health campaign and the beliefs and attitudes of the population.

Health programs working to increase the ability of the people, individually or collectively, to change their environment need to know whether the people possess skills related to influencing their family, their organizations, their environment, or their community (Maclellan-Wright et al. 2007; Shahandeh et al. 2012; Williams and Rhodes 2016).

Assessing the extent to which members of the target population possess enabling skills and resources can give the planner valuable insights into possible program components.

REINFORCING FACTORS

Reinforcing factors are consequences of action that determine whether the actor receives positive or negative feedback, feels rewarded, and is supported socially afterward. They include social support, peer influences, and advice and feedback by health care providers. Reinforcing factors also include the physical consequences of behavior, which may be separate from the social context. For example, the alleviation of respiratory symptoms following the correct use of asthma medication and feelings of well-being or relief from pain caused by physical exercise provide feedback and reinforcement.

Social benefits such as recognition, appreciation, and admiration; physical benefits such as convenience, comfort, and relief of discomfort or pain; tangible rewards such as economic benefits or avoidance of cost; and self-actualizing, imagined, or vicarious rewards such as improved appearance, self-respect, or association with an admired person who demonstrates the behavior—all of these reinforce behavior. That is, they make it more likely that the same behavior will be repeated and even maintained over long periods.

Reinforcing factors also include the adverse consequences of behavior, or "punishments," that can lead to the extinction of a behavior. Rewards also can reinforce behavior that is *not* conducive to health. For individuals, these might include the relief of tension that rewards the smoker, or the masking of emotions that accompanies compulsive eating (Caglar-Nazali et al. 2014). For organizations, these might include the profits that accrue from promoting a harmful product. Tax incentives that support nonpolluting products and penalties or fines that discourage ones that pollute can positively and negatively reinforce changes in organizational behavior, respectively. For each of the priority behaviors from the behavioral diagnosis, the planner can identify important reinforcing factors and build resources and communications into the program plan to address them.

Social reinforcements, as well as social images created by mass media or social media, set up norms of behavior transmitted within social groups and from one generation to another as *culture*. Culture influences personal values; norms influence personal attitudes, and these, in turn, influence behavior. Organizations are often part of an individual's environment. They can affect behavior through enabling and reinforcing factors. For example, a health care clinic's hours of operation may be an enabling factor in seeking medical attention among people who have long workdays and are unable to take time off for routine care.

A person considering performing a behavior can anticipate reinforcement—negative or positive—prior to a behavior, and this can make the behavior more or less likely. Such *anticipated* reinforcement (e.g., social acceptance or disapproval) will influence the subsequent performance of the behavior. Some factors that provide social reinforcement can become enabling ones if they generate ongoing social support, such as financial assistance.

Reinforcement can also be *vicarious*. Vicarious reinforcement is the process of learning behaviors through the observation of reward. For example, a person is more likely to enact a behavior if they have observed someone else model the behavior that is then reinforced. For example, you may begin to exercise after hearing your friend say that she lost weight and feels happier after starting to exercise regularly. Vicarious reinforcement also may contribute to the adoption of unhealthful behaviors. For example, middle-school students who see the "vaping kids" enjoying the activity and being more popular could contribute to increased vaping uptake.

In developing a health program, the source of reinforcement will, of course, vary depending on the objectives and type of program, as well as the setting. In patient care settings, reinforcement may come from nurses, physicians, fellow patients, and, again, family members. Reinforcement for the behavior of staff may come in either of those settings from other staff, from supervisors, or from higher-level administrators who control rewards.

Incremental and easily reversible changes in behavior are more likely to be successful, and thus reinforced by success, compared to drastic or difficult changes. For example, to decrease sodium consumption, people tolerate small steps of a low-salt diet more easily. These are more apt to be reinforced through their successful implementation than are large steps toward the goal.

Behavior that influences environmental or health care conditions also responds to reinforcing factors. Community or social support can reinforce actions to influence these changes, as seen by peer influences on social distancing and mask wearing during the COVID-19 pandemic. Such support can be provided by community residents, health care providers, and health education or health promotion practitioners.

The same considerations influencing health behavior in people whose health is at risk or who seek to improve their health also influence the behavior of health professionals and even organizations to bring about changes to improve health. Knowledge, beliefs, self-efficacy, and other psychological factors influence decisions by those in charge, but other strategic and political considerations must come into play in the implementation of those decisions. The applications of PRECEDE-PROCEED to professional, policy, and implementation decisions and to regulatory and organizational behavior will be addressed in chapters 7 and 8. Those chapters also will address how to use the results of the previous stages of the planning process to produce the final plan for implementation.

The following case study in box 6.1 and figure 6.3 illustrates the use of the PRECEDE framework in understanding HPV vaccination decisions among parents.

BOX 6.1
For Our Children Case Study: An Intervention to Increase Human Papillomavirus (HPV) Vaccination

For Our Children / *Por Nuestros Hijos* is an educational program for parents designed to increase HPV vaccination among Hispanic adolescents between the ages of 11 and 17 who have not had the vaccine. The team at the UTHealth School of Public Health Center for Health Promotion and Prevention Research developed and tested the effectiveness of the program using both PRECEDE-PROCEED (Green and Kreuter 2005) and Intervention Mapping (Bartholomew-Eldredge et al. 2016). HPV vaccination protects against several types of cancer and genital warts and is a recommended vaccine for this age group. Nevertheless, low uptake and completion of the vaccine two- or three-dose series (depending on age of initiation) remains low. The priority population was Hispanic parents recruited from clinical and community sites in Harris County and surrounding areas.

The planning team used PRECEDE-PROCEED (Green and Kreuter 2005) and Intervention Mapping (Bartholomew-Eldredge et al. 2016) to develop the program.

The development of *Por Nuestros Hijos* began with a needs assessment, guided by PRECEDE, to understand the local burden of HPV in low-income Hispanics in the region, as well as factors influencing parental decisions to vaccinate. The team assembled a community advisory committee to guide the needs assessment and conducted a literature review and qualitative research with members of the target population. To ensure identification of all potential factors influencing vaccination, the team conducted a review of the literature using search terms related to HPV vaccination, parent decision-making and vaccinations, parental acceptance of the HPV vaccine, and parental beliefs and attitudes toward the HPV vaccine. This review was supported by ongoing work by one of the team members conducting a systematic literature review of reviews (Rodriguez et al. 2020) which helped identify important factors that were related to HPV vaccination (Rodriguez et al. 2020).

To understand specific factors influencing parent HPV vaccine decision-making, the team conducted focus groups and in-depth interviews with Hispanic parents of adolescents. All focus groups and interviews were recorded and later transcribed for analysis. The results of the literature review and the new data collection identified several factors that were associated with HPV vaccination. Using PRECEDE, the team categorized these factors as predisposing, reinforcing, or enabling, as shown in figure 6.3. Thus, the PRECEDE framework helped both guide the needs assessment by examining various types of factors that could be associated with vaccination and organize identified factors into the three categories, which would subsequently inform the selection of intervention strategies that could influence those factors. The team was able to identify factors that influence parents' decision to vaccinate their children:

- Predisposing factors: HPV and HPV vaccine knowledge (Bastani et al. 2011; Gold et al. 2013; Morales-Campos et al. 2013; Podolsky et al. 2009; Sanderson et al. 2009), perceived safety (Galbraith et al. 2016; Yeganeh et al. 2010), and perceived vaccine effectiveness (Davis et al. 2004; Dempsey et al. 2006; Gerend et al. 2007; Reiter et al. 2009, Trim et al. 2012);

- Reinforcing factors: social support from friends and family (Kepka et al. 2012; Morales-Campos et al. 2013), and advice and feedback from health care provider (Allen et al. 2012);

- Enabling factors: parent (Chao et al. 2009; Dempsey et al. 2009; Perkins et al. 2010; Reiter et al. 2009; Reiter et al. 2013; Rosenthal et al. 2008; Taylor et al. 2014; Yeganeh et al. 2010) and provider behaviors (Chao et al. 2009; Chao et al. 2010; Dempsey et al. 2009; Gerend et al. 2009; Gottlieb et al. 2009; Reiter et al. 2009; Rosenthal et al. 2008; Yeganeh et al. 2010), and HPV vaccine recommendations (Boehner et al. 2003; Davis et al. 2004; Dempsey et al. 2006; Gerend et al. 2007; Kahn et al. 2001; Olshen et al. 2005).

Once identified, they then matched strategies to address these factors using guidance from both PRECEDE and Intervention Mapping (Bartholomew-Eldredge et al. 2016).

The For Our Children/*Por Nuestros Hijos* program consists of a print fotonovela (a booklet illustrated with photos depicting a storyline) and a tailored multimedia intervention (TIMI) delivered on a tablet designed to address parents' questions and concerns about HPV, HPV-related cancers, and the HPV vaccine. The two program components (fotonovela and TIMI) use an entertainment education approach to deliver the messages, including a story about a parent making the decision to vaccinate their child. The program also incorporates theoretical methods such as modeling and persuasion. The TIMI includes videos and interactive educational modules on a tablet, to personalize health messages such that each parent would receive messages focused on the specific questions they might have and determinants identified. There were various themes throughout the program, including the importance of protecting one's child through HPV vaccination. The program also aimed to increase knowledge and self-efficacy as well as parental skills in talking to their provider. It included the modeling of behaviors, featuring a mother making the decision to vaccinate her child against HPV. The program is available in English and Spanish and has been implemented in clinical and community settings (Rodriguez et al. 2018).

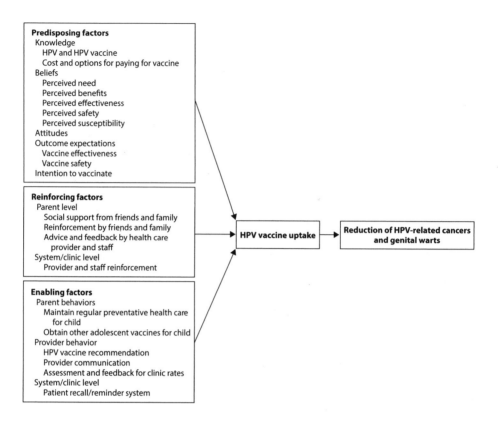

FIGURE 6.3. Predisposing, enabling, and reinforcing factors that influence the behavior of HPV vaccine uptake.

SELECTING DETERMINANTS OF BEHAVIOR AND ENVIRONMENTAL CHANGE

Selecting the predisposing, reinforcing, and enabling factors that, if modified, will help bring about the targeted health-related behavior and environmental change is the core of PRECEDE's educational and ecological phase. The three basic steps in this process are: (1) identifying and sorting factors into the three categories, (2) setting priorities among the categories, and (3) establishing priorities within the categories. In the Intervention Mapping protocol, Bartholomew-Eldredge and colleagues (2016) suggest several *core processes* for making decisions about which determinants to select. Briefly, these include posing questions and brainstorming potential answers to the questions (e.g., what influences the behavioral and environmental conditions identified in the previous phase); reviewing the empirical literature for both theory- and evidence-based "answers" to the questions; addressing needs for new data, particularly practice-based evidence from evaluation of related programs in this or similar populations; and then developing a working list of answers (Bartholomew-Eldredge et al. 2016; Fernández et al. 2019; Ruiter and Crutzen 2018). These processes can be used in each of the steps below.

Step 1: Identifying and Sorting

The list of causal factors initially identified for each behavior and environmental target should be as comprehensive as possible to help the planner avoid overlooking crucial determinants.

Informal Methods. The team designing the intervention plan usually has educated guesses based on personal or organizational experience with similar health issues, and hypotheses about the factors influencing behavior and environmental conditions. Planners should again involve members of the target populations in the planning. Intensive interviews, informal group discussions, nominal groups, focus groups, panels, and questionnaires can provide useful data. Brainstorming sessions with key stakeholders, community members, and planners and nominal group processes are useful techniques for generating data on factors influencing behavioral and environmental change. Focus groups are also a widely applied method for the informal collection of perceived causes of the behavioral and environmental issues. Lists can become long, so a process of ranking or setting priorities among perceived causes, or messages to address them, should be part of the process.

Formal Methods. Searching the literature can help find answers to the question of whether a particular factor is causally related to a health-related behavior or environmental change. Such a search may also yield items that can be used in surveys or other data collection tools that may be useful for understanding whether the identified factors are related to the behaviors or environmental changes of interest. The literature on evaluation and research on the type of program can provide guidance for the quantitative expectation of progress, which can guide the setting of quantitative objectives. They can then also be used for evaluation of the program. Checklists and questionnaires are structured ways of collecting and organizing information from important individuals and groups within the local or "target" population. These can be used to measure knowledge, attitudes, and beliefs as well as perceptions of services. Numerous projects and programs have conducted formal surveys of the predisposing, enabling, and reinforcing factors associated with behavioral and environmental changes required to affect health outcomes. Most of these formal surveys were also used in the follow-up evaluation of the programs and can be used in future assessments with some degree of prior validation.

Community organizations and planning agencies often compile directories of available community resources. These directories are particularly helpful when enabling factors are being examined. Utilization data from health care organizations and attendance records from agencies may be available. Additionally, community organizations may have already conducted needs and assets assessments that may be useful (Springer and Evans 2016).

The predisposing, reinforcing, and enabling categories are meant to help the planner sort the causal factors that are each amenable to the three broad classes of intervention strategies: (1) direct communication to change the predisposing factors, (2) indirect communication and mobilization of support (through family, peers, teachers, employers, and health care providers) to change the reinforcing factors, and (3) organizational, developmental, regulatory, and training strategies to change the enabling factors.

Step 2: Setting Priorities Among Categories

All of the causes for several behavioral and environmental changes cannot be tackled simultaneously. One needs to decide both the relative importance of the factors and the order in which factors need to be addressed by a program. To do this, planning groups must also decide on the most important criteria to use during the prioritization process.

The logical order and development of the three kinds of factors is an important consideration for setting priorities. For example, COVID-19 testing services must have their facility and laboratory in operation before they create a demand for their services. There will be instances, however, when raising public awareness and *demand* is necessary before the political support to fund the necessary services will be forthcoming. In such instances, the use of health education becomes an advocacy tool.

For most health programs, predisposing factors include some of the more immediate targets that must be addressed and preceding changes in other factors that ultimately led to behavior change. People typically will not adopt a set of behaviors to reduce a health risk if they are not aware that there *is* a risk. Belief in the immediacy of the risk and its implications will have to be developed for them to use the *enabling* resources. Finally, reinforcing factors cannot come into play until behaviors have taken place. Thus, for a community program, enabling, then predisposing, then reinforcing factors would be translated into interventions in that order. Nevertheless, the order of needs might vary across a population. Underserved segments of the population will likely need more help with the enabling factors of access to resources, financial support, transportation, and childcare before they can take advantage of services, whereas in the more affluent segments of the population, a little motivation (increase in predisposing factors) will stimulate actions unencumbered by resource barriers.

Step 3: Establishing Priorities Within Categories

Within the three categories of determinants of behavioral and environmental changes, we use the same criteria as those used for selecting high-priority health-related behaviors in the previous chapter: importance and changeability.

Importance. Importance or relevance can be estimated by judging *prevalence*, *immediacy*, and *necessity* according to logic, experience, data, and theory. **Prevalence** asks, "How widespread or frequent is the factor?" If the factor identified is very widespread or prevalent (i.e., high relative to the population size) or occurs often (frequency or "incidence" in epidemiological terms), it should qualify for priority consideration. In addition, importance can be determined by the strength of the association of the selected factor with the health risk or health promoting behavior. Findings from previous research or newly collected data by public health agencies can be used to judge how important a factor may be in the performance of the behavior (Peters 2014).

Immediacy asks, "How compelling or urgent is the factor?" Knowing the symptoms of a heart attack and what is needed to save a victim's life is one example of knowledge that has immediate consequences for people at high risk of heart attacks. Another type of immediacy has to do with how close the connection is between the factor and the group at risk.

Necessity is based on the consideration of factors that must be present (or absent) for the change in behavior or environment to occur. If an outcome cannot be achieved without a certain factor, that factor must be prioritized. Knowledge is often necessary, though insufficient on its own, to bring about an action. It is difficult to envision someone using a mask to avoid contracting COVID-19 without knowing the primary mode of transmission of the virus (which spreads through respiratory droplets when an infected person coughs, sneezes, or talks). Certain beliefs also can be considered necessary. People who wore masks in public consistently likely believed that they were doing the right thing in protecting themselves and others.

Changeability. One can gather evidence of the changeability of a factor by looking at the results of previous programs that have addressed it or the trends in that factor's prevalence in a population over time. Assessments of changeability can also be made using techniques set forth in the literature. One also can analyze changeability and the priority of factors according to a diffusion theory on stages in adoption and diffusion of innovations.

LEARNING AND RESOURCE OBJECTIVES

Writing learning objectives and resource objectives is similar to writing health, behavioral, and other objectives, as presented in other chapters. Learning objectives define the proportion of a population that should possess a predisposing factor or skill by a particular time following the beginning of a program or at the end of a program. Resource objectives define the environmental enabling factors that should be in place at a point in time after the start of a program or by the end of the program.

The predisposing and enabling factors described in figure 6.3 have been restated in terms of learning objectives for parents in table 6.1. Note the variations in the "how much" in these examples. One can usually create a high level of knowledge. A smaller percentage of those who are aware will believe the fact is relevant, important, or useful. Not all of these will develop the requisite skill to carry out recommended actions. Hence, the "leakage" of effect over the sequence of cascading cause-effect linkages provides a rough guide to how to estimate reasonable quantified objectives in the absence of complete baseline data. Results of previous studies can also be used to estimate the expected effect.

One can develop learning objectives not only for the target population but also for those people who will reinforce the target population. In addition, information about environmental enabling factors provides the basis for developing resource objectives.

SUMMARY

This chapter examines the factors affecting behavior and the environment as they relate to health. We call this phase of PRECEDE the educational and ecological assessment because we identify those factors on which health education and community organization can have a direct and immediate influence and thereby an indirect influence on behavior or the social-ecological environment. Three sets of factors are identified: predisposing, reinforcing, and enabling. Each plays an important role in health-related behavior and organization. After identifying the factors, we suggest how to assess their relative importance and changeability. Then, the planning group develops related learning and organizational and resource objectives so that the health promotion program can focus where it will do the most good in facilitating development of or changes in behavior and environment. Formulation of learning objectives follows from the identification of predisposing factors and skills; development of organizational and resource objectives follows from the identification of reinforcing and enabling factors.

TABLE 6.1. Examples of learning objectives and resource objectives based on HPV vaccination example described in box 6.1 and figure 6.3

Problem: Increasing parental acceptance of HPV vaccine
Target group: Parents of Hispanic adolescent 11- to 17-year-old boys and girls

Knowledge: By the end of the program period, 90% of the parents will be able to:

1. Describe the human papillomavirus and its route of transmission;
2. Recognize that there is a safe, effective HPV vaccine that protects their adolescent son/daughter from HPV and HPV-related diseases;
3. Recognize that boys and girls ages 11-17 are eligible for vaccination and the dose schedule for the vaccine;
4. State that their son/daughter can still complete the vaccination schedule even if he/she is late for a subsequent dose;
5. Explain that the HPV vaccine given prior to sexual initiation is more effective;
6. Describe that the HPV vaccine will not increase sexual disinhibition.

Beliefs: By the end of the program, 80% of parents will:

1. Expect that the HPV vaccine can prevent HPV-related diseases and cancer;
2. Believe in the importance of the HPV vaccine for their sons/daughters;
3. Believe that their son/daughter is at risk now or in the future;
4. Believe that the HPV vaccine is safe for their sons/daughters;
5. Believe that HPV infection can have serious consequences;
6. Believe that discussing the HPV vaccine with their son's/daughter's health care provider will address their concerns;
7. Believe that other parents like them are ensuring that their sons/daughters complete the vaccine schedule;
8. Believe that family members and friends would support their decision about vaccinating their sons/daughters against HPV;
9. Believe that it is important to complete the vaccine series.

Skills: By the end of the program, 70% of the parents will be able to:

1. Demonstrate the ability to initiate discussion and ask their son's/daughter's health care provider specific questions about HPV and the HPV vaccine;
2. Demonstrate the ability to make and keep an appointment for their son/daughter;
3. Express confidence and demonstrate the ability to request the HPV vaccine for their son/daughter;
4. Demonstrate the ability to identify a way to pay for the vaccine;
5. Express confidence and demonstrate the ability to make and keep subsequent follow-up appointments.

EXERCISES

1. For one of the high-priority behavioral changes you selected in the previous chapter, list all the predisposing, enabling, and reinforcing factors you can identify. For a priority environmental condition, list the enabling factors.

2. Rate each factor believed to cause the health behavior or environmental condition according to its importance and changeability. Give each factor a rating of low, medium, or high on each criterion.

3. Write learning or resource objectives for the highest-priority predisposing factor, enabling factor, and reinforcing factor.

References

Ajzen, I. (2015). The theory of planned behaviour is alive and well, and not ready to retire: a commentary on Sniehotta, Presseau, and Araújo-Soares. *Health Psychology Review, 9*(2), 131–7. https://doi.org/10.1080/17437199.2014.883474

Allen, J.D., de Jesus, M., Mars, D., Tom, L., Cloutier, L., & Shelton, R.C. (2012). Decision-Making about the HPV Vaccine among Ethnically Diverse Parents: Implications for Health Communications. *Journal of Oncology, 2012*, 401979. https://doi.org/10.1155/2012/401979

Allegrante, J.P. (2015). Policy and Environmental Approaches in Health Promotion: What Is the State of the Evidence? *Health Education & Behavior, 42*(Suppl. 1), 5S–7S. https://doi.org/10.1177/1090198115575097

Anderson, P., de Bruijn, A., Angus, K., Gordon, R., & Hastings, G. (2009). The message and the media: Impact of alcohol advertising and media exposure on adolescent alcohol use: A systematic review of longitudinal studies. *Alcohol and Alcoholism, 44*(3), 229–43. https://doi.org/10.1093/alcalc/agn115

Bandura, A. (1978). The self system in reciprocal determinism. *American Psychologist, 33*(4), 344–58. https://doi.org/10.1037/0003-066X.33.4.344

Bandura, A. (1989). Human agency in social cognitive theory. *American Psychologist, 44*(9), 1175–84. https://doi.org/10.1037/0003-066x.44.9.1175

Bandura, A. (2001). Social cognitive theory: an agentic perspective. *Annual Review of Psychology, 52*, 1–26. https://doi.org/10.1146/annurev.psych.52.1.1

Bandura, A. (2002). Social cognitive theory. In Breslow, L. (Ed.), *Encyclopedia of Public Health* (4th ed., pp. 1121–2). MacMillan.

Bartholomew-Eldredge, L.K., Markham, C., Ruiter, R.A., Fernández, M.E., Kok, G., & Parcel, G. (2016). *Planning Health Promotion Programs: An Intervention Mapping Approach* (4th ed.). Jossey-Bass.

Bastani, R., Glenn, B.A., Tsui, J., Chang, L.C., Marchand, E.J., Taylor, V.M., & Singhal, R. (2011). Understanding suboptimal human papillomavirus vaccine uptake among ethnic minority girls. *Cancer Epidemiology, Biomarkers and Prevention, 20*(7), 1463–72. https://doi.org/10.1158/1055-9965.EPI-11-0267

Blevins, C.S., & DeGennaro, R. (2018). Educational intervention to improve delirium recognition by nurses. *American Journal of Critical Care, 27*(4), 270–8. https://doi.org/10.4037/ajcc2018851

Boehner, C.W., Howe, S.R., Bernstein, D.I., & Rosenthal, S.L. (2003). Viral sexually transmitted disease vaccine acceptability among college students. *Sexually Transmitted Diseases, 30*(10), 774–8. https://doi.org/10.1097/01.OLQ.0000078823.05041.9E

Burke, M.J., Sarpy, S.A., Smith-Crowe, K., Chan-Serafin, S., Salvador, R.O., & Islam, G. (2006). Relative effectiveness of worker safety and health training methods. *American Journal of Public Health, 96*(2), 315–24. https://doi.org/10.2105/AJPH.2004.059840

Caglar-Nazali, H.P., Corfield, F., Cardi, V., Ambwani, S., Leppanen, J., Olabintan, O., Deriziotis, S., Hadjimichalis, A., Scognamiglio, P., Eshkevari, E., Micali, N., & Treasure, J. (2014). A systematic review and meta-analysis of 'Systems for Social Processes' in eating disorders. *Neuroscience and Biobehavioral Reviews, 42*, 55–92. https://doi.org/10.1016/j.neubiorev.2013.12.002

Campbell, M.K., Hudson, M.A., Resnicow, K., Blakeney, N., Paxton, A., & Baskin, M. (2007). Church-based health promotion interventions: Evidence and lessons learned. *Annual Review of Public Health, 28*, 213–34. https://doi.org/10.1146/annurev.publhealth.28.021406.144016

Chao, C., Velicer, C., Slezak, J.M., & Jacobsen, S.J. (2009). Correlates for completion of 3-dose regimen of HPV vaccine in female members of a managed care organization. *Mayo Clinic Proceedings 84*(10), 864–70.

Chao, C., Velicer, C., Slezak, J.M., & Jacobsen, S.J. (2010). Correlates for human papillomavirus vaccination of adolescent girls and young women in a managed care organization. *American Journal of Epidemiology, 171*(3), 357–67. https://doi.org/10.1093/aje/kwp365

Davis, K., Dickman, E.D., Ferris, D., & Dias, J.K. (2004). Human papillomavirus vaccine acceptability among parents of 10- to 15-year-old adolescents. *Journal of Lower Genital Tract Disease, 8*(3), 188–94. https://doi.org/10.1097/00128360-200407000-00005

Davis, S.N., Christy, S.M., Chavarria, E.A., Abdulla, R., Sutton, S.K., Schmidt, A.R., Vadaparampil, S.T., Quinn, G.P., Simmons, V.N., Ufondu, C., Ravindra, C., Schultz, I., Roetzheim, R., Shibata, D., Meade, C.D., & Gwede, C.K. (2017). A randomized controlled trial of a multicomponent, targeted, low-literacy educational intervention compared with a nontargeted intervention to boost colorectal cancer screening with fecal immunochemical testing in community clinics. *Journal of Cancer, 123*(8), 1390–1400. https://doi.org/10.1002/cncr.30481

De Vries, H., Backbier, E., Dijkstra, M., Van Breukelen, G., Parcel, G., & Kok, G. (1994). A Dutch social influence smoking prevention approach for vocational school students. *Health Education Research, 9*(3), 365–74. https://doi.org/10.1093/her/9.3.365

Dempsey, A.F., Abraham, L.M.., Dalton, V., & Ruffin, M. (2009). Understanding the reasons why mothers do or do not have their adolescent daughters vaccinated against human papillomavirus. *Annals of Epidemiology, 19*(8), 531–8. https://doi.org/10.1016/j.annepidem.2009.03.011

Dempsey, A.F., Zimet, G.D., Davis, R.L., & Koutsky, L. (2006). Factors that are associated with parental acceptance of human papillomavirus vaccines: a randomized intervention study of written information about HPV. *Pediatrics, 117*(5), 1486–93. https://doi.org/10.1542/peds.2005-1381

Fernández, M.E., Ruiter, R.A.C., Markham, C.M. & Kok, G. (2019). Intervention Mapping: Theory- and evidence-based health promotion program planning: Perspective and examples. *Frontiers in Public Health, 7*, 209. https://doi.org/10.3389/fpubh.2019.00209

Fishbein, M. (2008). A reasoned action approach to health promotion. *Medical Decision Making, 28*(6), 834–44. https://doi.org/10.1177/0272989X08326092

Fishbein, M., & Ajzen, I. (2010). *Predicting and Changing Behavior: The Reasoned Action Approach* (1st ed.). Psychology Press.

Fredriksson, S.V., Alley, S.J., Rebar, A.L., Hayman, M., Vandelanotte, C., & Schoeppe, S. (2018). How are different levels of knowledge about physical activity associated with physical activity behaviour in Australian adults? *PLoS One, 13*(11), e0207003. https://doi.org/10.1371/journal.pone.0207003

Galbraith, K.V., Lechuga, J., Jenerette, C.M., Moore, L.T.C. Angelo D., Palmer, M.H., & Hamilton, J.B. (2016). Parental acceptance and uptake of the HPV vaccine among African-Americans and Latinos in the United States: A literature review. *Social Science and Medicine, 159*, 116–26. https://doi.org/10.1016/j.socscimed.2016.04.028

Gehlert, S., Sohmer, D., Sacks, T., Mininger, C., McClintock, M., & Olopade, O. (2008). Targeting health disparities: A model linking upstream determinants to downstream interventions. *Health Affairs, 27*(2), 339–49. https://doi.org/10.1377/hlthaff.27.2.339

Gerend, M.A., Lee, S.C., & Shepherd, J.E. (2007). Predictors of human papillomavirus vaccination acceptability among underserved women. *Sexually Transmitted Diseases, 34*(7), 468–71. https://doi.org/10.1097/01.olq.0000245915.38315.bd

Gerend, M.A., Weibley, E., & Bland, H. (2009). Parental response to human papillomavirus vaccine availability: uptake and intentions. *Journal of Adolescent Health, 45*(5), 528–31. https://doi.org/10.1016/j.jadohealth.2009.02.006

Ghisi, G.L., Abdallah, F., Grace, S.L., Thomas, S., & Oh, P. (2014). A systematic review of patient education in cardiac patients: Do they increase knowledge and promote health behavior change? *Patient Education and Counseling, 95*(2), 160–74. https://doi.org/10.1016/j.pec .2014.01.012

Glanz, K., Rimer, B.K., & Viswanath, K. (2015). *Health Behavior: Theory, Research, and Practice* (5th ed.). Jossey-Bass.

Gold, R., Naleway, A., & Riedlinger, K. (2013). Factors predicting completion of the human papillomavirus vaccine series. *Journal of Adolescent Health, 52*(4), 427–32. https://doi.org /10.1016/j.jadohealth.2012.09.009

Golden, S.D., McLeroy, K.R., Green, L.W., Earp, J.A.L., & Lieberman, L.D. (2015). Upending the social ecological model to guide health promotion efforts toward policy and environmental change. *Health Education and Behavior, 42*(Suppl. 1), 8S–14S. https://doi.org/10.1177 /1090198115575098

Gottlieb, S.L., Brewer, N.T., Sternberg, M.R., Smith, J.S., Ziarnowski, K., Liddon, N., & Markowitz, L.E. (2009). Human papillomavirus vaccine initiation in an area with elevated rates of cervical cancer. *Journal of Adolescent Health, 45*(5), 430–7. https://doi.org/10.1016 /j.jadohealth.2009.03.029

Green, L.W., & Kreuter, M.W. (2005). *Health Program Planning: An Educational and Ecological Approach* (Vol. 4). McGraw-Hill Companies, Inc.

Guillaumie, L., Godin, G., & Vézina-Im, L.A. (2010). Psychosocial determinants of fruit and vegetable intake in adult population: A systematic review. *International Journal of Behavioral Nutrition and Physical Activity, 7*, 12. https://doi.org/10.1186/1479-5868-7-12

Jerant, A., Kravitz, R.L., Sohler, N., Fiscella, K., Romero, R.L., Parnes, B., Tancredi, D.J., Aguilar-Gaxiola, S., Slee, C., Dvorak, S., Turner, C., Hudnut, A., Prieto, F., & Franks, P. (2014). Sociopsychological tailoring to address colorectal cancer screening disparities: a randomized controlled trial. *Annals of Family Medicine, 12*(3), 204–14. https://doi.org /10.1370/afm.1623

Kahn, J.A., Emans, S.J., & Goodman, E. (2001). Measurement of young women's attitudes about communication with providers regarding Papanicolaou smears. *Journal of Adolescent Health, 29*(5), 344–51. https://doi.org/10.1016/s1054-139x(01)00254-3

Kawachi, I., & Kennedy, B.P. (1999). Income inequality and health: Pathways and mechanisms. *Health Services Research, 34*(1 Pt. 2), 215–27.

Kepka, D.L., Ulrich, A.K., & Coronado, G.D. (2012). Low knowledge of the three-dose HPV vaccine series among mothers of rural Hispanic adolescents. *Journal of Health Care for the Poor and Underserved, 23*(2), 626–35. https://doi.org/10.1353/hpu.2012.0040

Kirscht, J.P. (1974). The health belief model and illness behavior. *Health Education Monographs, 2*(4), 387–408. https://doi.org/10.1177/109019817400200406

Kok, G., Peters, G.-J.Y., Peters, Kessels L.T.E., ten Hoor, G.A., & Ruiter, R.A.C. (2017). Ignoring theory and misinterpreting evidence: the false belief in fear appeals. *Health Psychology Review, 12*(2), 111–25. https://doi.org/10.1080/17437199.2017.1415767

Krieger, N. (2008). Proximal, distal, and the politics of causation: What's level got to do with it? *American Journal of Public Health, 98*(2), 221–30. https://doi.org/10.2105/AJPH.2007 .111278

Kreuter, M.W., & Skinner, C.S. (2000). Tailoring: what's in a name? *Health Education Research, 15*(1), 1–4. https://doi.org/10.1093/her/15.1.1

Link, B.G., & Phelan, J. (1995). Social conditions as fundamental causes of disease. *Journal of Health and Social Behavior,* 80–94.

Maclellan-Wright, M.F., Anderson, D., Barber, S., Smith, N., Cantin, B., Felix, R., & Raine, K. (2007). The development of measures of community capacity for community-based funding programs in Canada. *Health Promotion International, 22*(4), 299–306. https://doi .org/10.1093/heapro/dam024

Marmot, M. (2005). Social determinants of health inequalities. *The Lancet, 365*(9464), 1099–104. https://doi.org/10.1016/S0140-6736(05)71146-6

Montano, D.E., & Karprzyk, D. (2015). Theory of Reasoned Action, Theory of Planned

Behavior, and the Integrated Behavioral Model. In Glanz, K., Rimer, B.K., & Viswanath, K. (Eds.), *Health Behavior: Theory, Research, and Practice* (5th ed., pp. 95–124). Jossey-Bass.

Morales-Campos, D.Y., Markham, C.M., Peskin, M.F., & Fernandez, M.E. (2013). Hispanic mothers' and high school girls' perceptions of cervical cancer, human papilloma virus, and the human papilloma virus vaccine. *Journal of Adolescent Health, 52*(Suppl. 5), S69–S75. https://doi.org/10.1016/j.jadohealth.2012.09.020

Olshen, E., Woods, E.R., Austin, S.B., Luskin, M., & Bauchner, H. (2005). Parental acceptance of the human papillomavirus vaccine. *Journal of Adolescent Health, 37*(3), 248–51. https://doi.org/10.1016/j.jadohealth.2005.05.016

Perkins, R.B., Pierre-Joseph, N., Marquez, C., Iloka, S., & Clark, J.A. (2010). Why do low-income minority parents choose human papillomavirus vaccination for their daughters? *Journal of Pediatrics, 157*(4), 617–22. https://doi.org/10.1016/j.jpeds.2010.04.013

Peters, G.Y. (2014). A practical guide to effective behavior change: how to identify what to change in the first place. *European Journal of Health Psychology, 16*(5), 142–55.

Podolsky, R., Cremer, M., Atrio, J., Hochman, T., & Arslan, A.A. (2009). HPV vaccine acceptability by Latino parents: a comparison of U.S. and Salvadoran populations. *Journal of Pediatric and Adolescent Gynecology, 22*(4), 205–15. https://doi.org/10.1016/j.jpag.2008.05.010

Reiter, P.L., Brewer, N.T., Gottlieb, S.L., McRee, A.L., & Smith, J.S. (2009). Parents' health beliefs and HPV vaccination of their adolescent daughters. *Social Science and Medicine, 69*(3), 475–80. https://doi.org/10.1016/j.socscimed.2009.05.024

Reiter, P.L., McRee, A.L., Pepper, J.K., Gilkey, M.B., Galbraith, K.V., & Brewer, N.T. (2013). Longitudinal predictors of human papillomavirus vaccination among a national sample of adolescent males. *American Journal of Public Health, 103*(8), 1419–27. https://doi.org/10.2105/AJPH.2012.301189

Rodriguez, S.A., Mullen, P.D., Lopez, D.M., Savas, L.S., & Fernández, M.E. (2020). Factors associated with adolescent HPV vaccination in the U.S.: A systematic review of reviews and multilevel framework to inform intervention development. *Preventive Medicine, 131*, 105968. https://doi.org/10.1016/j.ypmed.2019.105968

Rodriguez, S.A., Roncancio, A.M., Savas, L.S., Lopez, D.M., Vernon, S.W., & Fernandez, M.E. (2018). Using Intervention Mapping to Develop and Adapt Two Educational Interventions for Parents to Increase HPV Vaccination Among Hispanic Adolescents. *Frontiers in Public Health, 6*, 164. https://doi.org/10.3389/fpubh.2018.00164

Rokeach, M. (1970). *Beliefs, attitudes, and values*. Jossey-Bass.

Rosenthal, S.L., Rupp, R., Zimet, G.D., Meza, H.M., Loza, M.L., Short, M.B., & Succop, P.A. (2008). Uptake of HPV vaccine: Demographics, sexual history and values, parenting style, and vaccine attitudes. *Journal of Adolescent Health, 43*(3), 239–45. https://doi.org/10.1016/j.jadohealth.2008.06.009

Ruiter, R.A., Crutzen, R., & Kok, G. (2018). Core Processes for Developing Theory-and Evidence-Based Interventions. https://doi.org/10.31234/osf.io/j4ftz

Sanderson, M., Coker, A.L., Eggleston, K.S., Fernandez, M.E., Arrastia, C.D., & Fadden, M.K. (2009). HPV vaccine acceptance among Latina mothers by HPV status. *Journal of Women's Health (Larchmt), 18*(11), 1793–9. https://doi.org/10.1089/jwh.2008.1266

Schölmerich, V.L.N., & Kawachi, I. (2015). Translating the Social-Ecological Perspective Into Multilevel Interventions for Family Planning: How Far Are We? *Health Education and Behavior, 43*(3), 246–55. https://doi.org/10.1177/1090198116629442

Shahandeh, K.H., Majdzadeh, R., Jamshidi, E., & Loori, N. (2012). Community capacity assessment in preventing substance abuse: A participatory approach. *Iranian Journal of Public Health, 41*(9), 48–55.

Sheeran, P., Maki, A., Montanaro, E., Avishai-Yitshak, A., Bryan, A., Klein, W.M., Miles, E., & Rothman, A.J. (2016). The impact of changing attitudes, norms, and self-efficacy on health-related intentions and behavior: a meta-analysis. *Health Psychology, 35*(11), 1178–88. https://doi.org/10.1037/hea0000387

Skinner, C.S., Tiro, J., & Champion, V.L. (2015). Background on the health belief model. In Glanz, K., Rimer, B.K., & Viswanath, K. (Eds.), *Health Behavior: Theory, Research, and Practice* (5th ed., pp. 75–94). Jossey-Bass.

Springer, A.E., & Evans, A.E. (2016). Assessing environmental assets for health promotion program planning: a practical framework for health promotion practitioners. *Health Promotion Perspectives, 6*(3), 111–8. https://doi.org/10.15171/hpp.2016.19

Stokols, D. (1996). Translating social ecological theory into guidelines for community health promotion. *American Journal of Health Promotion, 10*(4), 282–98. https://doi.org/10.4278/0890-1171-10.4.282

Taylor, J.L., Zimet, G.D., Donahue, K.L., Alexander, A.B., Shew, M.L., & Stupiansky, N.W. (2014). Vaccinating sons against HPV: results from a U.S. national survey of parents. *PLoS One, 9*(12), e115154. https://doi.org/10.1371/journal.pone.0115154

Thoits, P.A. (2011). Mechanisms Linking Social Ties and Support to Physical and Mental Health. *Journal of Health and Social Behavior, 52*(2), 145–61. https://doi.org/10.1177/0022146510395592

Trim, K., Nagji, N., Elit, L., & Roy, K. (2012). Parental Knowledge, Attitudes, and Behaviours towards Human Papillomavirus Vaccination for Their Children: A Systematic Review from 2001 to 2011. *Obstetrics and Gynecology International, 2012*, 921236. https://doi.org/10.1155/2012/921236

Verplanken, B. (2018). *The Psychology of Habit: Theory, Mechanisms, Change, and Contexts* (1st ed.). Springer.

Wallerstein, N.B., & Duran, B. (2006). Using community-based participatory research to address health disparities. *Health Promotion Practice, 7*(3), 312–23. https://doi.org/10.1177/1524839906289376

Williams, D.M., & Rhodes, R.E. (2016). The confounded self-efficacy construct: conceptual analysis and recommendations for future research. *Health Psychology Review, 10*(2), 113–28. https://doi.org/10.1080/17437199.2014.941998

Wofford, T.S., Greenlund, K.J., Croft, J.B., & Labarthe, D.R. (2007). Diet and physical activity of U.S. adults with heart disease following preventive advice. *Preventive Medicine, 45*(4), 295–301. https://doi.org/10.1016/j.ypmed.2007.06.013

Yeganeh, N., Curtis, D., & Kuo, A. (2010). Factors influencing HPV vaccination status in a Latino population; and parental attitudes towards vaccine mandates. *Vaccine, 28*(25), 4186–91. https://doi.org/10.1016/j.vaccine.2010.04.010

CHAPTER 7

Health Program and Policy Development I: Intervention Strategies

•

Michelle C. Kegler and Rodney Lyn

Learning Objectives

After completing the chapter, the reader will be able to:

- Match possible intervention strategies to the various ecological levels for intervention and to specific predisposing, enabling, and reinforcing factors.
- Use "best practices" where available from the research literature and "best experiences" from other programs to address the most important predisposing, enabling, and reinforcing factors.
- Adapt evidence-based strategies with practice-based evidence, observations, and experience of and for the particular population and context.
- Use behavioral and social science theories to design new interventions specific to a population and context.
- Pool and blend interventions into comprehensive programs that address the essential predisposing, enabling, and reinforcing factors identified in the previous chapter.
- Create a logic model or theory of change to ensure a successful transition from planning to the implementation of practical strategies that lead to health improvements and to evaluation of them.

INTRODUCTION

At this point in the PRECEDE-PROCEED program planning process, you have identified your health priorities, selected which behavioral and environment determinants you will target, and identified predisposing, reinforcing, and enabling factors to prioritize based on which are most important and changeable. You also have a set of outcome objectives for your program. You are now going

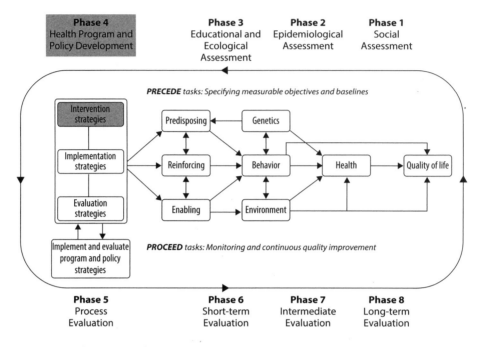

FIGURE 7.1. The fourth phase of the PRECEDE-PROCEED model, health program and policy development, begins with a focus on the identification and formation of, and priorities among, *intervention* strategies to influence determinants of behavioral and environmental change.

to turn the corner from assessment to selecting and aligning intervention strategies with the determinants you identified in the earlier phases of PRECEDE, as shown in figure 7.1. This phase of the planning process will help you describe *how* you will address the determinants of behavioral and environmental change identified during the assessment phases of PRECEDE. A first step in this alignment process is to match potential evidence-based interventions or best practices, when available, to the priority determinants, which includes identifying any adaptations needed to fit your specific context (Alignment 1). This matching process may identify gaps where you will need to develop new interventions or figure out the "how-to" for general best practices based on what you know from theory, systematic reviews of interventions, and prior experience with similar settings and populations.

These efforts lead directly into a second step toward alignment—to *adapt* evidence-based interventions for a better fit in your organizational and community context, in collaboration with your community partners (Alignment 2). Additionally, unless you are working with a very homogeneous population, you may need also to adapt interventions for varied population subgroups. Where evidence-based interventions have been evaluated in settings very different from your program context or they simply do not exist, pilot testing of new theory-based approaches must come into greater play to "patch" the gaps (Alignment 3). "Pilot testing" might range from consultation with experienced professionals in the community, to role-playing or simulating the alternative intervention in a small group. Another step in this pre-implementation alignment of program needs with program components is the strategic *blending* and sequencing of interventions into a cohesive, comprehensive, and affordable program, based on your organizational, personnel, and community context assessment (Alignment 4). Once the plan is fully drafted, the administrative and policy assessment phase of PRECEDE-PROCEED will inform refinement of your comprehensive plan to ensure feasibility and affordability for the implementing organization and partners.

The primary purpose of this chapter is to call your attention to considerations in selecting and aligning intervention strategies with priority determinants of change identified in the previous phase of PRECEDE and adapting intervention strategies in PROCEED to the unique context and reactions of the community. In this phase, you will also identify the specific settings in which health promotion activities must take place, and how each of those settings will have plan modifications that you will require or suggest. The lead or sponsoring organization may itself provide a setting, such as a health department clinic, school or worksite, for implementing the program. Often, the lead or sponsoring organization, such as a public health department, must depend on other organizations (and sometimes multiple organizations) outside of the health sector to share responsibility for implementation. Such planned coordination and collaboration are critical; the setting you are in will dictate many of the specific methods, materials, and other program components. Specific considerations for program planning in settings such as schools, worksites, and primary care are addressed in chapters 10 to 14.

In previous phases of applying PRECEDE, you identified:

1. a population's priority social and health problems;

2. the most important and changeable behavioral and environmental determinants of those problems;

3. the priority predisposing, enabling, and reinforcing factors for the targeted behavioral outcomes; and

4. the enabling factors for the targeted environmental outcomes (noting that some environmental changes will further enable some behavioral changes).

Data from these earlier phases enable you to seek specific intervention strategies that will make up your program and create the changes in predisposing, enabling, and reinforcing factors that you prioritized, within the context of your population, community, and organizational settings. The subsequent chapter will focus more directly on resources needed and available to launch and sustain your program and how to react to or exploit the organizational barriers and facilitators that can affect program implementation.

MATCHING, ADAPTING, PATCHING, AND BLENDING INTERVENTION STRATEGIES INTO A COMPREHENSIVE PROGRAM PLAN

ALIGNMENT 1: Aligning priority determinants with intervention strategies by matching intervention strategies with prioritized predisposing, reinforcing, and enabling factors

An ecological approach calls first for matching intervention strategies with the level at which they can have their effects. We use the term "**matching**" for this level of alignment. The matching process calls for the selection of intervention strategies that correspond to the predisposing, reinforcing, and enabling factors identified in the ecological and educational diagnosis phase of PRECEDE outlined in chapter 6. A complementary approach is to organize the factors and corresponding intervention strategies by the level of the social ecologic framework (Golden et al. 2015; McLeroy et al. 1988) with predisposing factors categorized at the individual level, reinforcing factors categorized at the interpersonal level, and enabling factors categorized at the organizational, community, or policy level. With increased attention to social determinants of health and environmental change, a more nuanced categorization of the enabling factors may aid in more impactful and sustainable interventions (Frieden 2010; Golden and Earp 2012) while acknowledging the need for synergy across levels (Golden et al. 2015; Green and Kreuter 2010). Conceptualizing your program from a social-ecological perspective and targeting a combination of predisposing, reinforcing, and enabling factors acknowledges (1) the complexity of health and social problems, and (2) the reality that relationships across levels and among determinants within levels are multidirectional. We know that organizational, community, and higher governmental levels can influence or moderate the effects of individual and interpersonal factors on individual behavior. We also know that the higher levels of organization—for example, the physical and social environments that they represent or encompass—do not affect health exclusively through behavioral change, but rather can have some direct effects on health independent of the main behavioral effects (e.g., lead in the water can lead directly to negative health effects; violence in the neighborhood can lead directly to stress). We also know that organizational and political action from the bottom up can stimulate change in policies and implementation of policies at higher levels.

Match Priority Determinants with Intervention Strategies

A straightforward way to proceed with matching of interventions with the level at which they can have their effects is to develop a table that lists each determinant and the intervention strategy that you propose for influencing that determinant. This allows you to delineate clearly whether each of the priority determinants is addressed by your developing program plan and which other emerging determinants you still need to find a way to address as they emerge. For example, if you have obesity as your priority health issue and low-income families living in Atlanta, Georgia, as your priority population, you may have prioritized the determinants in table 7.1. At the individual level, you may have prioritized self-efficacy for healthful eating and behavioral capability (knowledge and skills) for healthful food preparation, all constructs from the Social Cognitive Theory (Bandura 1986). At the interpersonal level, you may have prioritized family and church-related social support for healthful eating. At the higher levels of the social-ecological framework, you may have prioritized enabling factors such as limited access to healthful foods in lower-income neighborhoods and within various organizational settings, including homes. But after your program goes to implementation, a local city council initiative to require something new like labeling of calories in certain categories of fresh fruits and vegetables may come to pass. Such policy changes occasionally arise in public debate or legislative initiatives within the environment of your ongoing program, requiring adaptations.

Your next task is to find, adapt, and create intervention strategies that can change self-efficacy, knowledge and skills, family and church-based social support, and household, organizational, and community policies and practices.

TABLE 7.1. Determinants by level of the social-ecological model: healthful eating example

Level	Determinants
Predisposing (individual level)	Self-efficacy for healthful eating Healthy food preparation knowledge and skills Outcome expectations for healthy food preparation
Reinforcing (interpersonal level)	Church-based social support for healthful eating Family-based social support for healthful eating
Enabling (organizational level)	Church policies related to healthful foods Home food environment
Enabling (community level)	Limited access to healthful foods due to high prevalence of fast food, convenience stores and corner stores
Enabling (policy level)	No supermarkets in low-income neighborhoods

Seek Findings from Prior Evidence-Based Intervention Strategies

An important first step is to search for a program that has been well-evaluated and is evidence-based. Seldom will your effort be the first time someone, somewhere, has tried to solve the problem or to address the need that your program plan addresses, nor does your plan start at time zero in this place. Other attempts elsewhere and in your setting should be considered as resources and guides. The intervention **strategy** selection process has two key components: (1) review and pool the best experience of prior attempts to address the problem, and (2) build on effective existing program activities related to the intervention targets.

Evidence-based programs and intervention strategies or "best practices" have become highly valued in recent years, especially by funding agencies seeking to justify their expenditures on programs presumably assured of success. Best practices refer to intervention strategies, and sometimes whole programs consisting of multiple intervention strategies, that have been submitted to rigorous scientific evaluation, ideally in multiple settings and populations, and subjected to critical analysis across multiple studies. Resources are available to support your identification and selection of best practices. The Guide to Community Preventive Services (i.e., The Community Guide) provides a collection of evidence-based findings based on systematic reviews of effectiveness of intervention strategies across a wide range of health topics (https://www.thecommunityguide.org). Beyond the "strength" of evidence based on the rigor of internal validity controls for potential confounding explanations for the outcomes, the Community Guide also has given increased attention in its systematic reviews to the "weight" of the evidence based on the external (practice-based) validity across settings, beyond the "strength" of evidence based on the rigor of internal validity controls for potential confounding explanations for the outcomes (Green 2006; 2008; Vaidya et al. 2017). The National Cancer Institute (NCI)'s Evidence-Based Cancer Control Programs (https://ebccp.cancercontrol.cancer.gov/index.do) provides a searchable database of hundreds of evidence-based cancer control interventions. It is designed to provide program planners and public health practitioners easy and immediate access to research-tested materials (National Cancer Institute 2020). The Cochrane Database of Systematic Reviews (https://www.cochranelibrary.com/cdsr/about-cdsr) includes several thousand systematic reviews of research on health care, health policy, and other health-related interventions (Cochrane n.d.). The Substance Abuse and Mental Health Services Administration's Evidence-Based Practices Resources Center (https://www.samhsa.gov/ebp-resource-center) provides evidence-based programs used to prevent and treat mental and substance use disorders (US Department of Health and Human Services n.d.). Also consider (D'Onofrio 2001):

- Reports of specific interventions in journal articles, which are usually strong on evaluation methods, but skimpy on details regarding the interventions;

- Overview reports or reviews of health programs addressing a particular problem or population, or reviewing specific methods or approaches to a class of problems;

- Meta-analyses of multiple studies of programs addressing the same problem;

- Sections of some professional journals devoted to brief reports from practitioners;

- Books and monographs on specific projects or problems, which often contain much more detail or case study information about the interventions than in the published articles describing the same projects;

- Technical reports containing official guidelines from government agencies or national advisory groups, based usually on consensus among experts, experienced practitioners, and staff reviews of literature;

- Conferences and professional meetings, providing presentations and descriptions of programs before they are published, but also not yet peer-reviewed;

- National clearinghouses and websites for guidelines derived from systematic reviews and the consensus of experts; and

- Funding agencies and their newsletters, websites, or communications directly from their grantees.

Assess Whether Interventions Should Work in Your Setting and the Level of Adaptation Needed

Here is a key question in assessing intervention strategies: when is the pathway toward achieving outcome objectives clear, assuming adequate resources and effective implementation? The answer is: where evidence-based best practices can be matched with the ecological levels and priority determinants for maximum effect, and when evidence is available to suggest it was tested with a population or community similar to yours. Other guiding questions in intervention assessment are shown in box 7.1.

As you go through this planning process, be aware that the ideals of best practices are much easier to achieve in medicine, because they arise from the dozens and sometimes hundreds of randomized, controlled studies on specific medical practices. In some populations and circumstances, the planner will have few, if any, best practices, and most of those will be based on evidence generated in populations and settings fairly different from your context (Brownson et al.

2018; Green 2006; Green 2008). Depending on the scope of the program you are planning, the most likely outcome from identifying best practices that match your determinants is that you will have a couple of evidence-based intervention strategies or best practices that need to be adapted to fit your organizational capacity and community context. Oftentimes, these general best practices do not translate into a clear and detailed set of steps for creating that type of change (e.g., what strategies work to encourage convenience stores to start selling fresh fruits and vegetables?).

Returning to our healthful eating example, perhaps you find a church-based intervention on NCI's Evidence-Based Cancer Control Programs website, such as Body and Soul (Allicock et al. 2012; Campbell et al. 2007; Resnicow et al. 2004), and a home environment intervention in the peer-reviewed literature (Kegler et al. 2016). The church-based intervention may address some of your predisposing determinants (i.e., self-efficacy and knowledge and skills), as well as reinforcing (i.e., church-based social support for healthy eating) and enabling determinants (i.e., policies for healthful foods at church). The Healthy Homes/ Healthy Families intervention may change some aspects of the home food environment (e.g., home food inventory). However, you still need to find a strategy for building family support for healthful eating and a strategy for promoting community policies related to food access. The former may be addressed by adding a component to Healthy Homes/Healthy Families such as a coaching session with the whole family. The latter may require developing some new intervention strategies or learning from other communities doing similar work,

---

BOX 7.1
Questions to Ask When Assessing Evidence-based Interventions for Their Fit with Your Community

When reviewing descriptions and summaries of tested interventions, consider:

- What determinants did the intervention target and how well do these align with your prioritized predisposing, reinforcing, and enabling factors?

- Did the intervention create change in the prioritized determinants? How much change was documented in the prioritized behavioral determinants, environmental conditions, or health problem that was targeted?

- What are the core elements or essential ingredients of the intervention? What can be changed for your context while still maintaining a high probability of achieving desired outcomes?

- Does your organization or your partner organization(s) have the capacity to implement the intervention while maintaining fidelity to the core elements of the original intervention?

such as those working on corner store initiatives or efforts to locate grocery stores in low-income neighborhoods.

Corner store interventions, such as the Healthy Bodegas Initiative, have been shown to improve the community food environment by increasing the availability of fresh fruits and vegetables and other healthful options (Cavanaugh et al. 2014; Dannefer et al. 2012). Such efforts have also shown promise for improving patrons' purchasing intentions (Gittelsohn et al. 2010) and behaviors (Dannefer et al. 2012), especially where healthful products are placed in easy-to-access locations within the store (Wong et al. 2015). Another strategy for improving healthful food access may include policy and advocacy initiatives (intervention strategies) to increase the number of supermarkets in the community (an enabling factor). For example, in Philadelphia, the Food Trust, a nonprofit organization dedicated to increasing access to healthful food, created food access maps and convened a task force. The Supermarket Campaign—a strategic advocacy effort born from their effort—ultimately led to a statewide public-private partnership, the Pennsylvania Fresh Food Financing Initiative, which obtained $120 million in funding that supported an initial group of 74 fresh food outlets (Karpyn et al. 2010). The important takeaway from these examples is that intervention strategies may be needed at the predisposing, reinforcing, and enabling levels and matching determinants to intervention strategies may require consideration of evidence-based and adapted strategies.

ALIGNMENT 2: Adapting Intervention Strategies to "Fit" Organizational and Community Contexts

Most of this discussion has assumed that evidence-based best practices must be supplemented with experience-based and theory-based adaptations and innovations to address some of the predisposing, enabling, and reinforcing factors. Even when the literature offers evidence-based recommendations for a best practice, one is faced in a local situation with the question of whether to adhere strictly to every detail of the intervention or practice, or whether to innovate and adapt to certain local circumstances.

A variety of models for adaptation have been developed in recent years. Escoffery and colleagues (2019; see also the next chapter of this book) conducted a scoping study of adaptation frameworks used in public health. They identified 11 steps common enough across 13 frameworks to warrant routine consideration. These included: conduct community assessment, understand the intervention, select the intervention, consult with experts, consult with stakeholders, decide what needs adaptation, adapt the original program, train staff, test the adapted materials, implement, and evaluate. In describing the typical tasks associated with deciding what needs adaptation, Escoffery and colleagues (2019) highlight identifying differences between the new priority population and setting and the original population and setting in which the program or intervention strategy was tested.

The next task is to systematically reduce "mismatches" between the evidence-based practices and the new situation, while retaining as much fidelity to the core elements of the program or intervention strategy as possible and appropriate. Typical changes to evidence-based programs and intervention strategies include alterations to delivery methods or media, program structure, content, and implementation delivery providers (Carvalho et al. 2013; Escoffery et al. 2019). The most commonly cited adaptation frameworks are the federal Center for Substance Abuse Prevention's guidelines for balancing fidelity and adaptation (Backer 2002), McKleroy's et al. (2006) Map of Adaptation Process, and the APAPT-ITT model (Wingood and DiClemente 2008).

In describing a process for adapting a program or intervention strategy, Highfield and colleagues (2015) identify a series of "fit" considerations. In addition to fit between environmental, behavioral, and more proximal determinants (i.e., predisposing, reinforcing, and enabling factors), they highlight organizational capacity to deliver the program and cultural fit. A number of things to consider in adapting a program or intervention strategy to local circumstances include some that may have been addressed in the situational assessment described in chapters 2 and 3. These include questions about potential organizational collaborators, staff/technical resources, and budget, as demonstrated in box 7.2.

These questions help to assess "fit" and comprise the Intervention Strategies component of the Health Program and Policy Development, Phase 4 of PRECEDE-PROCEED, as seen in figure 7.1. Preliminary assessments of budget, staffing, and organizational mission and priorities can help inform decisions about which intervention strategies are feasible within the local context. For example, an intervention strategy that requires multiple home visits when no home visiting structure is in place may not be feasible, especially when resources are not available for local travel or staff time for delivering an intervention household by household. Concerns about legal liability also may arise from the perspective of the implementing organization. These "mismatches" may necessitate modifying the intervention strategy—in this case, perhaps changing the home visits to telephone-based counseling.

One can also try to improve on previous efforts to change a particular predisposing, enabling, or reinforcing factor by one of two approaches—increasing the intensity or improving the quality of the previous efforts. The evaluation research literature refers to the intensity approach as dose-response, increased exposure time, or increased intensity of the intervention strategies—for example, adding booster sessions. The quality approach seeks to make an intervention strategy or program more effective in changing a predisposing, enabling, or

---

BOX 7.2

Questions to Ask About Organizational Capacity for Intervention Adaptation

- Who are the potential organizational partners, and are they supportive of the potential program?
- Are experienced personnel available for program implementation?
- Will staff require special training for implementation, and is the training available?
- Are the facilities and space necessary for the program available?
- Do the proposed intervention strategies align with the mission of the lead organization or any of its partners?

---

reinforcing factor than in previous efforts by changing some of its features or the mix of strategies in a program—for example, tailoring educational materials rather than providing generic information.

Pretesting, a small-scale trial of an intervention strategy, is critical because it involves potential members of the target audience in assessing the readability, comprehension, feasibility, acceptability, and "fit" of potential strategies within the local context. It does so in real time, before making a commitment to include possible strategies in the program. Program components are tested with samples of typical end users or recipients of the intervention strategies to see whether the presumed feasibility and acceptability actually adhere in the population or program context. Pretesting is seldom, however, a test of efficacy or effectiveness of the program against outcomes specified in the objectives, unless combined with other conditions of controlled trials, including at least a post-test and a comparison group.

Sometimes, clear cultural differences need to be addressed when adapting an intervention. In adapting a smoke-free homes intervention originally developed for a general population for use in Native American families (Kegler et al. 2015; Mullen et al. 2016; Williams et al. 2016), for example, the planners knew that traditional use of tobacco would need to be addressed and that casting all tobacco use in a negative light would be culturally inappropriate. The planners formed a working group of Native American tobacco control experts to advise on initial adaptation to intervention materials. Revised materials were mocked up and then pretested through focus groups in five different tribal communities across the United States (Anderson et al. 2019). Additional determinants were confirmed in the focus groups (e.g., need to address traditional use, respect for elders) and a revised overall theme for the intervention was identified, shifting from "Some Things are Better Outside" to "Respect our Past and Protect our Future." The research team then hired a Native American graphic designer to overhaul the print materials based on focus group findings.

ALIGNMENT 3: Patching the Gaps by Creating Intervention Strategies and Figuring Out "How-to" Steps for General Best Practices

Even after adapting an evidence-based intervention to address some of your assessments of priority determinants, you will often need also to develop new or additional intervention strategies or suggest how to proceed if the guidance for a recommended or "best practice" is vague. Many policy, systems, and environmental change interventions do not include a detailed implementation manual, but instead provide general guidance such as "reduce structural barriers." Behavioral and social science theory can be particularly helpful at this stage in the program planning process. For example, in table 7.2, common predisposing factors are listed, followed by selected relevant theories and a sample of intervention strategies that can be used to address potentially relevant predisposing factors. For a more comprehensive list, see Abraham and Michie (2008), who developed a taxonomy of 26 behavioral change techniques with definitions and their associated theoretical framework.

Behavioral change techniques include providing various types of information (i.e., about behavior-health links, consequences, approval from others), modeling or demonstrating a behavior, prompting specific goal setting, teaching to use prompts or cues, providing contingent rewards, agreeing on a behavioral contract, and motivational interviewing, among many others. An example of how several of these change strategies were used in a smoke-free homes intervention is provided in box 7.3, and figure 7.2 shows some sample material.

Most of the behavior change techniques focus on individual-level determinants. However, when directed toward change agents who control or make decisions regarding organizational, community, and governmental policies (e.g., pastors, school principals, county commissioners), these same techniques also become relevant for targeting enabling factors and higher levels of the social ecologic framework. When the reach to some population segments is limited to mass media, phrasing and illustrating the key messages must depend on consultation, strategic communication, and audience segmentation practices for success.

Bartholomew-Eldredge and colleagues (2016) similarly provide theory-based methods for changing behavior, as shown in chapter 6. They list basic methods such as persuasive communication, active learning, tailoring, modeling, feedback, and reinforcement, among others. For each, they identify supporting theories, provide a definition, describe parameters for use, and give an example.

TABLE 7.2. Common predisposing factors, relevant theories, and related intervention strategies

Dimension	Examples
Factors	Knowledge
	Beliefs
	Attitudes
	Outcome expectations
	Skills
	Self-efficacy
	Stage of change
	Behavioral intention
Relevant theories	Social cognitive theory (Bandura 1986)
	Theory of planned behavior (Fishbein and Ajzen 2010)
	Health belief model (Janz and Becker 1984)
	Transtheoretical model (Prochaska et al. 2015)
	Communication-persuasion matrix (McGuire 1985)
	Elaboration likelihood model (Petty et al. 2009)
Intervention strategies	One-on-one education
	Motivational interviewing
	Persuasive communication
	Small media
	Tailoring
	Role modeling
	Mass media campaigns
	Goal-setting
	Behavioral contracts
	Self-monitoring
	Group education

They also identify theory-based methods to change specific determinants, such as knowledge, awareness and risk perception, habitual, automatic and impulsive behaviors, attitudes, beliefs and outcome expectations, and skills, capability, self-efficacy and overcoming barriers. Once you identify a theory-informed and ideally evaluation-based (at least pretested) intervention, you will have a general blueprint for how to design that particular component of your program. For example, tailoring involves identifying the constructs to target (e.g., beliefs about the benefits of a preventive behavior) and then constructing messages specific to the beliefs held by a program participant (Hawkins et al. 2008). Tailored messages can then be delivered through a variety of means, including print materials, computer or smartphone (i.e., text messages or app-based), via telephone, or in-person contact.

BOX 7.3

Description of Selected Behavioral Change Strategies in the *Smoke-Free Homes: Some Things are Better Outside* Program

Program overview	The purpose of the program is to encourage and support families to create a household smoking ban to reduce secondhand smoke exposure among children and nonsmokers.
Program description	Three mailings of printed materials and a coaching call delivered over a six-week period.
Selected behavioral change strategy	Program component
Information on consequences of behavior	List of reasons to go smoke-free
Modeling creation of a home smoking ban	Photo novella of family creating a home smoking ban
Goal setting	Coach assists participant to set stage-based goal (e.g., make list of reasons to go smoke-free, have family talk about a ban)
Use of prompts or cues	Smoke-free home window cling and stickers

---

Common reinforcing factors, relevant theories, and related intervention strategies are listed in table 7.3. Bartholomew-Eldredge and colleagues (2016) identify strategies for changing social influence, including information about approval from others, resistance to social pressure, mobilizing social support, and providing opportunities for social comparison. They also describe methods for changing social norms, including mass media role modeling, entertainment education, behavioral journalism, mobilizing social networks, enhancing networking linkages, developing new social network linkages, peer education, and use of lay health advisors. For each, they list relevant theories, a definition, parameters for use, and an example.

Attention to enabling factors, which facilitate healthful behaviors by shaping the environmental context, has grown considerably in the last two decades. Historically, researchers and program planners sought to improve health behaviors by developing interventions that focused primarily on modifying individual-level beliefs, attitudes, or preferences (predisposing) and skill-related (enabling) factors. Without adequate focus on broader contextual and enabling factors, such approaches often have limited effectiveness, high cost and poor sustainability (Brownson et al. 2006). A resurgence in focus on the "enabling" role that

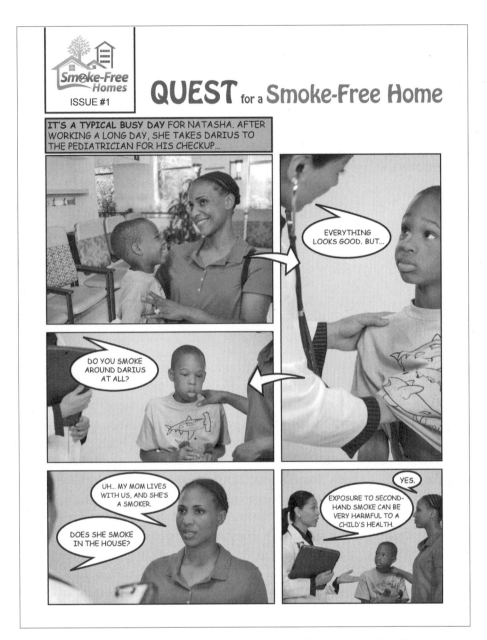

FIGURE 7.2. Sample material from the Smoke-Free Homes: Some Things are Better Outside program.
Source: Emory Prevention Research Center, Rollins School of Public Health, Emory University.

social and environmental factors play in influencing individual health behaviors has resulted in a package of intervention strategies known as policy, systems, and environmental change (PSE) approaches. PSE approaches place emphasis on altering the environmental context to make healthful choices practical for all members of a community (Bunnell et al. 2012). This may be achieved through

TABLE 7.3. Common reinforcing factors, relevant theories, and related intervention strategies

Dimension	Examples
Factors	Social norms
	Social support
	Social networks
Relevant theories and models	Social norms (Lapinski and Rimal 2005)
.	Social support theories (Holt-Lunstad and Uchino 2015)
	Social network theory (Valente 2015)
	Lay health advisor model (Eng et al. 2009)
Intervention strategies	Providing social support (e.g., support groups)
	Mobilizing social networks (e.g., peer education)
	Creating new network linkages
	Entertainment education
	Social norms marketing

changes in policy (e.g., policy, laws, regulations, ordinances, rules, or procedures); changes in systems (e.g., transportation, food, health care, education, social safety net); or changes in the environment (e.g., physical/structural, economic, social). Such approaches warrant particular consideration as you identify strategies with the potential to enable and facilitate desired health behaviors in underserved populations.

Former CDC director Tom Frieden (2010) provided a framework for public health action that supports a focus on enabling factors and is inclusive of PSE approaches. The Health Impact Pyramid included five tiers of interventions aimed at socioeconomic disparities, comprising the base and followed (in ascending order) by interventions that change the context to make individuals' default decisions healthful, clinical interventions that require limited contact but confer long-lasting protection (e.g., vaccination), direct clinical care, and health education and counseling. Interventions focusing on the lower portion of the pyramid tend to be more effective because they reach broader segments of the population and require less individual effort to access direct benefits. Multilevel interventions that target determinants at more than one level may create synergy across levels and aid in sustaining behavior change (Golden et al. 2015). This synergistic impact is likely to be greater than for interventions focused on a single level (Frieden 2010; Golden et al. 2015; for a commentary on Frieden: Green and Kreuter 2010).

As you develop plans to address enabling factors, it will be beneficial to consider using collective action. Collaborative approaches to health promotion and disease prevention, such as the use of coalitions, has been shown to promote PSE changes and modify enabling factors across a wide array of health topics, including obesity, asthma, tobacco, nutrition, and physical activity (Butterfoss et al. 2006; Kreuter et al. 2000; Litt et al. 2013a; Litt et al. 2013b; Lyn et al. 2013; Reinert et al. 2005). The Community Coalition Action Theory (Butterfoss and Kegler 2009) provides guidance on the types of coalitions that can be established and describes steps for the establishment and maintenance of effective coalitions.

Bartholomew-Eldredge and colleagues (2016) provide a useful lens to organize strategies to influence enabling factors into (a) methods to change organizations, (b) methods to change communities, and (c) methods to change policy. For organizations, they list sense-making, organizational diagnosis and feedback, team building and human relations training, structural redesign, and increasing stakeholder influence. For community change, they list problem-posing education, community assessment, community development, social action, forming coalitions, social planning, and framing to shift perspectives. For policy change, they list media advocacy, agenda setting, timing to coincide with policy windows, and creating and enforcing laws and regulations. Since the outset of the PRECEDE-PROCEED model, it has been important to recognize that the focus on organizations, communities, and policy are not mutually exclusive. Organizations may seek to impact community decisions. Communities may leverage collective action to influence public policy. Efforts to impact health determinants and outcomes may involve action at one or preferably (synergistically) more of these levels. Common enabling factors, relevant theories, and related intervention strategies to inform program planning are provided in table 7.4.

ALIGNMENT 4: Pooling and Blending Intervention Strategies into Comprehensive Programs

The next step is to combine all of your intervention strategies, newly developed and adapted, into a comprehensive program plan. Several processes are available to help structure this pooling and blending process. One common tool to aid at this point of the program design is a logic model. A logic model provides a visual representation of the pathways through which intervention strategies, combined into program components, lead to short-term, intermediate, and long-term outcomes (Frechtling 2007; McLaughlin and Jordan 1999). Using the PRECEDE-PROCEED framework, which is among other things, a logic model, predisposing, reinforcing, and enabling factors serve as the short-term outcomes, leading to the intermediate outcomes of behavioral and environmental determinants, which in turn lead to the longer-term outcomes typically defined in terms of health, social, or quality of life outcomes.

TABLE 7.4. Common enabling factors, relevant theories, and related intervention strategies

Dimension	Examples
Factors	Organizational policies and practices
	Community capacity
	Public policies
Relevant theories and models	Organizational development (Shafritz and Ott 2001)
	Community readiness model (Plested et al. 2006)
	Community-based participatory approach (Israel et al. 2008)
	Community coalition action theory (Butterfoss and Kegler 2009)
	Diffusion of innovations (Rogers 2003)
	Multiple streams theory (Kingdon 2003)
	Social-ecological model (McLeroy et al. 1988)
	Social movement theory (De la Porta and Diani 2006)
	Role theory in imitation (Bandura 1997)
Intervention strategies	Facilitation
	Strategic planning
	Stakeholder engagement and education
	Community readiness assessment
	Community coalitions
	Media communication and advocacy
	Photovoice
	Policy advocacy
	Opinion polling
	Health impact assessment

Besides its use as an evaluation tool, drawing a logic model as part of the program planning process can help to establish among planning participants how the various intervention strategies synergistically work together to create the desired change. Logic models can help to identify gaps in logic. For example, one might notice that, despite self-efficacy being identified as a priority short-term outcome, none of the planned intervention strategies focus on increasing self-efficacy. Or perhaps self-efficacy is adequately addressed, but there is a misalignment between self-efficacy and the behavioral determinants that were prioritized. The construction and evolution of a logic model is illustrated sequentially across the earlier chapters of this book as applied generically to the PRECEDE planning process, but planners are strongly encouraged to review examples of specific logic models previously developed in their own or similar organizations when designing—and particularly blending—possible intervention strategies into a comprehensive program plan. A logic model representing the healthful eating example discussed in this chapter is displayed in figure 7.3.

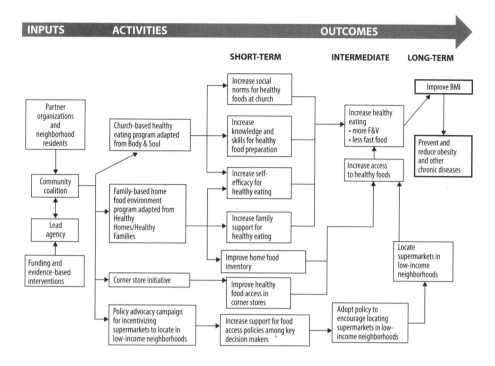

FIGURE 7.3. Logic Model for Multi-Level Healthy Eating and Obesity Prevention Program

Details on how to operationalize your plan into a detailed work plan with time-lines and sequencing of various program components are provided in chapters 9 and 10 on implementation and evaluation.

REFINING THE FULL PROGRAM PLAN TO ENSURE ORGANIZATIONAL AND COMMUNITY FIT

We turn now to the process of fine-tuning your program plan to your organizational and community context based on an administrative and policy assessment of the implementation setting. This includes the capacity of your organization to implement the full complement of intervention strategies you are proposing, such as resources (i.e., funding and staff) required and available to mobilize and deploy the proposed interventions. At this stage, begin by budgeting the time and material resources needed to implement the methods and strategies chosen in the preceding steps. Budgeting and staffing are described in detail in chapter 8. When sufficient resources are not available, the fallback position, of course, is to trim the sails on your program plan and propose more modest objectives. Logically, such action will indeed reduce the potential impact of a proposed intervention program. Because this course represents a compromise of the plan, you should undertake it only with due consideration of the consequences for the integrity of the plan, the commitments made during the participatory planning process, and the program's scope, reach, and impact. Specific questions you should ask before giving up too many parts of the plan or levels of intervention due to budget cuts include the following:

1. *The threshold level:* Will the reduced level of resources still allow enough intervention to reach a threshold of impact that will achieve subsequent objectives? The notion of a threshold level of resources suggests that there is a minimum level of investment below which the program will be too weak to achieve a useful result.

2. *The point of diminishing returns:* Is there a point of diminishing returns beyond which additional resources do not necessarily achieve commensurate gains in impact or outcome? If so, fewer resources might not hinder the achievement of at least some benefits.

3. *Critical elements:* Does the program plan have a critical element without which the objectives cannot be achieved? If so, will the budget cut or shortage of resources preclude achieving that one objective or element?

4. *Critical expectations:* Can the target levels of the objectives be lowered without jeopardizing the integrity of the program or the expectations of the constituents or sponsors of the program? If the behavioral change target of immunization can be reduced from 94% to 92% for schoolchildren without risking a major outbreak of measles, the savings in outreach resources could be considerable. This is because, as seen in Diffusion theory (Green et al. 2009; Rogers 2003), the late adopters are harder for a program to reach than the late majority. An equivalent reduction in the target levels during the early phases of a program—say, from 14% to 10%—would not yield a commensurate cost savings because early adopters are easier to reach and often less likely to be exposed to the disease (e.g., COVID-19) than late adopters.

5. *Critical timing and cash flow:* Can the target dates for the objectives be set back to spread the program effort over a longer period? By itself, this will not save resources in the long run, but it will reduce costs in the initial year by shifting them to later periods. The initial costs could be the major budgetary barrier because of temporary fiscal circumstances. By slowing the pace of the program implementation, some outlays could be delayed in anticipation of better budgetary times. This amounts to an adjustment of cash flow.

In addition to budget considerations, one needs to know how a proposed program fits with existing organizational mission, policies, and regulations. How do political forces influence the planning or implementation of a health promotion program? In any situation where finite resources have to be allocated among several programs but the decision makers do not agree on the distribution of those finite resources, politics will likely influence the ultimate decision. Specifically, decisions will be influenced by what the decision makers do or do not know about the goals and content of the competing programs and also by how their peers or constituents value the proposed program. For example, a program that plans to test community or school garden soil for heavy metal contamination may encounter political concerns related to liability if the soil is found to contain lead (Hunter et al. 2019). Time and resources should be invested as early as possible to engage and educate stakeholders and to build support among decision makers for proposed programs and policies. Where politics shape decisions, it is vital to have laid the foundation for favorable perceptions among the public and stakeholders of the proposed work.

Be aware that most organizations operate under a blend of formal and informal mandates—most of which are not set in stone. The first question one can ask about any policy that appears to be inconsistent with a program plan is: how flexible is that policy? Most good policies are flexible or worded broadly rather than specifically because it is impossible to know in advance all the problems and opportunities an implementing organization or program will face, especially from a distance, where many policies are made. The best test of flexibility is to find a previous program implemented under the policy and to examine its deviations, if any, from the policy. This will provide one with both an indicator of flexibility and a precedent to cite in defending one's request for an exception to, or waiver of, policy. If the previous implementation experience was uniformly or mostly positive, one may have a reason to invoke the policy in support of the program, but flexibility might still be the reason other programs flourished under the policy.

The political milieu can be analyzed at both the intra-organizational and the inter-organizational level. If one attempts to bring about change in another organization as an outsider, one has a greater need and justification for employing political methods, because organizations resist change from without. In health promotion, the inter-organizational level of analysis is particularly important, because many of the programs and policies needed to alter lifestyles and environments that are controlled by multiple organizations, some of them entirely outside the health sector. Anticipating challenges and being flexible are helpful for navigating intra-organizational and inter-organizational political forces. Health promotion programs are often implemented in partnership with other organizations. Conflicts might arise also with the policies of a collaborating organization or group. In the face of such incompatibilities, one has three choices: (1) to adapt the proposed plan to be consistent with the organizational mission and policies, (2) to seek to change the policy or organizational mandate, or (3) some of both.

A plan can be in alignment with the organization's mission but inconsistent or at odds with a policy or position held by stakeholders or an influential organization or unit within the host organization. Health practitioners concerned with violence prevention, comprehensive school health, HIV/AIDS education, and tobacco control have learned the value of anticipating the reactions of these groups early in the planning process. Failure to address the concerns of groups with conflicting policy perspectives can have serious negative consequences, such as budget cuts or conflicts with key decision makers or legislators. Addressing such a situation after the fact is inevitably an uphill battle. By anticipating a potential conflict, planners can rely on their negotiation and communication skills, their political acumen, and the scientific and theoretical soundness of their plan to achieve support for the proposed outcome.

Additional considerations for selecting, developing, and implementing the methods and strategies will be addressed in the setting-specific chapters (chapters 10 to 14), because it is the setting or channel through which one will reach the population that dictates which intervention strategies are most appropriate. A comprehensive program may involve several settings. Representatives of those settings would ideally have been included in the planning processes leading up to this point; however, at times it only becomes clear at this point that a setting not previously involved needs to be a channel for the program. Involvement in this phase of planning can help ensure that developers will address the resource requirements of such a setting.

SUMMARY

To summarize, the foregoing steps in crafting a comprehensive program include reviewing the coverage of intervention strategies across essential targets. The first step was the matching of possible intervention strategies to the various ecological levels for intervention and to specific predisposing, enabling, and reinforcing factors, using "best practices" where available from the research literature and "best experiences" from previous and concurrent programs to address the most important predisposing, enabling, and reinforcing factors. Intervention strategies may involve the adaptation of evidence-based strategies for your particular population and context, or may involve using behavioral and social science theories to design new interventions specific to your context. This process sets up the final step of pooling, adapting, and blending these interventions into comprehensive programs that address the essential predisposing, enabling, and reinforcing factors identified in the previous chapter. Pooling the various intervention strategies together into a cohesive whole by creating a logic model or theory of change helps to ensure a successful and practical transition from planning to the implementation of practical strategies that lead to health improvements.

References

Abraham, C., & Mitchie, S. (2008). A taxonomy of behavior change techniques used in interventions. *Health Psychology, 27*(3), 379–81. https://doi.org/10.1037/0278-6133.27.3.379

Allicock, M., Campbell, M.K., Valle, C.G., Carr, C., Resnicow, K., & Gizlice, Z. (2012). Evaluating the dissemination of Body & Soul, an evidence-based fruit and vegetable intake intervention: challenges for dissemination and implementation research. *Journal of Nutrition Education and Behavior, 44*(6), 530–8. https://doi.org/10.1016/j.jneb.2011.09.002

Anderson, K., Kegler, M., Bundy, Ł., Henderson, P., Halfacre, J., & Escoffery, C. (2019). Adaptation of a brief smoke-free homes intervention for American Indian and Alaska Native families. *BMC Public Health, 19*(1), 981. https://doi.org/10.1186/s12889-019-7301-4

Backer, T. (2002). *Finding the balance: Program fidelity and adaptation in substance abuse prevention: A state-of-the-art review.* Substance Abuse and Mental Health Services Administration.

Bandura, A. (1977). *Social Learning Theory.* Prentice Hall.

Bandura, A. (1986). *Social Foundations of Thought and Action: A Social Cognitive Theory.* Prentice Hall.

Bartholomew-Eldredge, L., Markham, C., Ruiter, R., Fernández, M., Kok, G., & Parcel, G. (2016). *Planning Health Promotion Programs: An Intervention Mapping Approach* (4th ed.). Jossey-Bass.

Brownson, R., Fielding, J.E., & Green, L.W. (2018). Building capacity for evidence-based public health: Reconciling the pulls of practice and the push of research. *Annual Review of Public Health, 39*, 27–53. https://doi.org/10.1146/annurev-publhealth-040617-014746

Brownson, R., Haire-Joshu, D., & Luke, D. (2006). Shaping the context of health: a review of environmental and policy approaches in the prevention of chronic disease. *Annual Review of Public Health, 27*, 341–70. https://doi.org/10.1146/annurev.publhealth.27.021405.102137

Bunnell, R., O'Neil, D., Soler, R., Payne, R., Giles, W., Collins, J., Bauer, U., & Communities Putting Prevention to Work Program Group. (2012). Fifty communities putting prevention to work: accelerating chronic disease prevention through policy, systems and environmental change. *Journal of Community Health, 37*(5), 1081–90. https://doi.org/10.1007/s10900-012-9542-3

Butterfoss, F., Gilmore, L., Krieger, J., Lachance, L., Lara, M., Meurer, J., Orians, C., Peterson, J., Rose, S., & Rosenthal, M. (2006). From formation to action: how Allies Against Asthma Coalitions are getting the job done. *Health Promotion Practice, 7*(Suppl. 2), 34S–43S. https://doi.org/10.1177/1524839906287063

Butterfoss, F., & Kegler, M. (2009). The Community Coalition Action Theory. In DiClemente, R., Crosby, R., & Kegler, M. (Eds.), *Emerging Theories in Health Promotion and Practice.* Jossey-Bass.

Campbell, M.K., Resnicow, K., Carr, C., Wang, T., & Williams, A. (2007). Process evaluation of an effective church-based diet intervention: Body & Soul. *Health Education and Behavior, 34*(6), 864–80. https://doi.org/10.1177/1090198106292020

Carvalho, M.L., Honeycutt, S., Escoffery, C., Glanz, K., Sabbs, D., & Kegler, M.C. (2013). Balancing fidelity and adaptation: implementing evidence-based chronic disease prevention.

Journal of Public Health Management and Practice, 19(4), 848–56. https://doi.org/10.1097/PHH.0b013e31826d80eb

Cavanaugh, E., Green, S., Mallya, G., Tierney, A., Brensinger, C., & Glanz, K. (2014). Changes in food and beverage environments after an urban corner store intervention. *Preventive Medicine, 65*, 7–12. https://doi.org/10.1016/j.ypmed.2014.04.009

Cochrane. (n.d.) *Cochrane Library*. Retrieved February 13, 2019, from https://www.cochrane library.com/

Dannefer, R., Williams, D., Baronberg, S., & Silver, L. (2012). Healthy bodegas: Increasing and promoting healthy foods at corner stores in New York City. *American Journal of Public Health, 102*(10), e27–e31. https://doi.org/10.2105/AJPH.2011.300615

De la Porta, D., & Diani, M. (2006). *Social Movements: An Introduction* (2nd ed.). Blackwell Publishing.

D'Onofrio, C. (2001). Pooling information about prior interventions: A new program planning tool. In Sussman, S. (Ed.), *Handbook of Program Development for Health Behavior Research and Practice* (p. 158–203). SAGE Publishing.

Eng, E., Rhodes, S., & Parker, E. (2009). Natural helper models to enhance a community's health and competence. In DiClemente, R., Crosby, R., & Kegler, M. (Eds.), *Emerging Theories in Health Promotion and Practice*. Jossey-Bass.

Escoffery, C., Lebow-Skelley, E., Udelson, H., Böing, E., Wood, R., Fernandez, M.E., & Mullen, P. (2019). A scoping study of frameworks for adapting public health evidence-based interventions. *Translational Behavioral Medicine, 9*(1), 1–10. https://doi.org/10.1093/tbm/ibx067

Fishbein, M., & Ajzen, I. (2010). *Predicting and Changing Behavior: The Reasoned Action Approach*. Psychology Press.

Frechtling, J. (2007). *Logic Modeling Methods in Program Evaluation*. Jossey-Bass.

Frieden, T. (2010). A framework for public health action: the health impact pyramid. *American Journal of Public Health, 100*(4), 590–5. https://doi.org/10.2105/AJPH.2009.185652

Gittelsohn, J., Song, H., Suratkar, S., Kumar, M., Henry, E., Sharma, S., Mattingly, M., & Anliker, J. (2010). An urban food store intervention positively affects food-related psychosocial variable and food behaviors. *Health Education and Behavior, 37*(3), 390–401. https://doi.org/10.1177/1090198109343886

Golden, S., McLeroy, K., Green, L.W., Earp, J.A., & Lieberman, L.D. (2015). Upending the social ecological model to guide health promotion efforts toward policy and environmental change. *Health Education and Behavior, 42*(Suppl. 1), 8S–14S. https://doi.org/10.1177/1090198115575098

Golden, S.D., & Earp, J. (2012). Social ecological approaches to individuals and their contexts: Twenty years of *Health Education & Behavior* health promotion interventions. *Health Education and Behavior, 39*(3), 364–72. https://doi.org/10.1177/1090198111418634

Green, L.W., & Kreuter, M.W. (2010). Evidence hierarchies versus synergistic interventions. *American Journal of Public Health, 100*(10), 1824–5. https://doi.org/10.2105/AJPH.2010.197798

Green, L.W. (2006). Public health asks of systems science: to advance our evidence-based practice, can you help us get more practice-based evidence? *American Journal of Public Health, 96*(3), 406–9. https://doi.org/10.2105/AJPH.2005.066035

Green, L.W. (2008). Making research relevant: if it is an evidence-based practice, where's the practice-based evidence? *Family Practice, 25*(Suppl. 1), i20–4. https://doi.org/10.1093/fampra/cmn055

Green, L.W., Ottoson, J.M., García, C., & Hiatt, R. (2009). Diffusion theory and knowledge dissemination, utilization and integration in public health. *Annual Review of Public Health, 30*, 151–74. https://doi.org/10.1146/annurev.publhealth.031308.100049

Hawkins, R., Kreuter, M., Resnicow, K., Fishbein, M., & Dijkstra, A. (2008). Understanding tailoring in communicating about health. *Health Education Research, 23*(3), 454–66. https://doi.org/10.1093/her/cyn004

Highfield, L., Hartman, M., Mullen, P., Rodriguez, S., Fernandez, M., & Bartholomew, L. (2015). Intervention mapping to adapt evidence-based interventions for use in practice: Increasing mammography among African American women. *BioMed Research International, 2015*, 160103. https://doi.org/10.1155/2015/160103

Holt-Lunstad, J., & Uchino, B. (2015). Social support and health. In Glanz, K., Rimer, B., & Viswanath, K. (Eds.), *Health Behavior: Theory, Research, and Practice.* Jossey-Bass.

Hunter, C., Williamson, D., Gribble, M., Bradshaw, H., Pearson, M., Saikawa, E., Ryan, P., & Kegler, M. (2019). Perspectives on heavy metal soil testing among community gardeners in the United States: A mixed methods approach. *International Journal of Environmental Research and Public Health, 16*(13), E2350. https://doi.org/10.3390/ijerph16132350

Israel, B.A., Schulz, A., Parker, E., Becker, A., Allen, A., & Guzman, J. (2008). Critical issues in developing and following CBPR principles. In Minkler, M., and Wallerstein, N. (Eds.), *Community-Based Participatory Research for Health: From Process to Outcomes* (2nd ed., pp. 47–66). Jossey-Bass.

Janz, N., & Becker, M. (1984). The Health Belief Model: A decade later. *Health Education Quarterly, 11*(1), 1–47. https://doi.org/10.1177/109019818401100101

Karpyn, A., Manon, M., Treuhaft, S., Giang, T., Harries, C., & McCoubrey, K. (2010). Policy solutions to the 'grocery gap'. *Health Affairs, 29*(3), 473–80. https://doi.org/10.1377/hlthaff.2009.0740

Kegler, M., Bundy, Ł., Haardörfer, R., Escoffery, C., Berg, C., Yembra, D., Kreuter, M., Hovell, M., Williams, R., Mullen, P., Ribisl, K., & Burnham, D. (2015). A minimal intervention to promote smoke-free homes among 2-1-1 callers: A randomized controlled trial. *American Journal of Public Health, 105*(3), 530–7. https://doi.org/10.2105/AJPH.2014.302260

Kegler, M., Haardörfer, R., Alcantara, I., Gazmararian, J., Veluswamy, J., Hodge, T., Addison, A., & Hotz, H. (2016). Impact of improving home environments on energy intake and physical activity: A randomized controlled trial. *American Journal of Public Health, 106*(1), 143–52. https://doi.org/10.2105/AJPH.2015.302942

Kingdon, J.W. (2003). *Agendas, Alternatives, and Public Policies* (2nd ed.). Longman.

Kreuter, M., Lezin, N., & Young, L. (2000). Evaluating community based collaborative mechanisms: implications for practitioners. *Health Promotion Practice, 1*(1), 49–63. https://doi.org/10.1177/152483990000100109

Lapinski, M., & Rimal, R. (2005). An explication of social norms. *Communication Theory, 15*(2), 127–47. https://doi.org/10.1111/j.1468-2885.2005.tb00329.x

Litt, J., Reed, H., Zieff, S., Tabak, R., Eyler, A., Tompkins, N., Lyn, R., Gustat, J., Goins, K.V., & Bornstein, D. (2013a). Advancing environmental and policy change through active living collaboratives: Exploring compositional, organizational, and community engagement as correlates of group effectiveness. *Journal of Public Health Management and Practice, 19*(3 Suppl. 1), S49–S57. https://doi.org/10.1097/PHH.0b013e3182848056

Litt, J., Reed, H., Tabak, R., Zieff, S., Eyler, A., Lyn, R., Goins, K.V., Gustat, J., & Tompkins, N. (2013b). Active living collaboratives in the United States: understanding characteristics, activities, and achievement of environmental and policy change. *Preventing Chronic Disease, 10*, 120162. https://doi.org/10.5888/pcd10.120162

Lyn, R., Davis, T., Aytur, S., Eyler, A., Chriqui, J., Cradock, A., Evenson, K., & Brownson, R. (2013). Policy, systems, and environmental change for obesity prevention, a framework to inform local and state action. *Journal of Public Health Management and Practice, 19*(3, Suppl. 1), S23–S33. https://doi.org/10.1097/PHH.0b013e3182841709

McGuire, W. (1985). Attitudes and attitude change. In Lindzey, G., & Aronson, E. (Eds.), *Handbook of social psychology: Special fields and applications* (Vol. 2, 3rd ed.). Random House.

McLeroy, K., Bibeau, D., Steckler, A., & Glanz, K. (1988). An ecological perspective on health promotion programs. *Health Education Quarterly, 15*(4), 351–77. https://doi.org/10.1177/109019818801500401

McKleroy, V.S., Galbraith, J.S., Cummings, B., Jones, P., Harshbarger, C., Collins, C., Gelaude, D., Carey, J.W., & ADAPT Team. (2006). Adapting evidence-based behavioral interventions for new settings and target populations. *AIDS Education and Prevention, 18*(Suppl. A), 59–73. https://doi.org/10.1521/aeap.2006.18.supp.59

McLaughlin, J., & Jordan, G. (1999). Logic models: a tool for telling your program's performance story. *Evaluation and Program Planning, 22*(1), 65–72. https://doi.org/10.1016/S0149-7189 (98)00042-1

Mullen, P., Savas, L., Bundy, Ł., Haardörfer, R., Hovell, M., Fernández, M., Monroy, J., Williams, R., Kreuter, M., Jobe, D., & Kegler, M. (2016). Minimal intervention delivered by 2-1-1 information and referral specialists promotes smoke-free homes among 2-1-1 callers: A Texas generalization trial. *Tobacco Control, 25*(Suppl. 1), i10–i18. https://doi.org/10.1136 /tobaccocontrol-2016-053045

National Cancer Institute. (2020, October 2). *Evidence-Based Cancer Control Programs (EBCCP).* Retrieved February 13, 2019, from https://rtips.cancer.gov/rtips/index.do

Petty, R., Barden, .J, & Wheeler, S. (2009). The Elaboration Likelihood Model of persuasion: Health promotions that yield sustained behavioral change. In DiClemente, R., Crosby, R., & Kegler, M. (Eds.), *Emerging Theories in Health Promotion Practice and Research* (pp. 185–214). Jossey-Bass.

Plested, B., Edwards, R., & Jumper-Thurman, P. (2006). *Community readiness: A handbook for successful change.* Tri-Ethnic Center for Prevention Research.

Prochaska, J., Redding, C., & Evers, K. (2015). The Transtheoretical Model of Stages of Change. In Glanz, K., Rimer, B., & Viswanath, K. (Eds.), *Health Behavior: Theory, Research, and Practice* (5th ed., pp. 168–222). Jossey-Bass.

Reinert, B., Carver, V., & Range, L. (2005). Evaluating community tobacco use prevention coalitions. *Evaluation and Program Planning, 28*(2), 201–8. https://doi.org/10.1016 /j.evalprogplan.2004.09.003

Resnicow, K., Campbell, M., Carr, C., McCarty, F., Wang, T., Periasamy, S., Rahotep, S., Doyle, C., Williams, A., & Stables, G. (2004). Body and soul. A dietary intervention conducted through African-American churches. *American Journal of Preventive Medicine, 27*(2), 97–105. https://doi.org/10.1016/j.amepre.2004.04.009

Rogers, E. (2003). *Diffusion of Innovations* (5th ed.). Simon and Schuster.

Shafritz, J., & Ott, J.S. (2001). *Classics of Organization Theory* (5th ed.). Wadsworth Publishing.

US Department of Health and Human Services, Substance Abuse and Mental Health Services Administration (SAMHSA). (n.d.) *Evidence-Based Practices Resource Center.* Retrieved February 13, 2019, from https://www.samhsa.gov/ebp-web-guide

Vaidya, N., Thota, A.B., Proia, K.K., Jamieson, S., Mercer, S.L., Elder, R.W., Yoon, P., Kaufmann, R., & Zaza, S. (2017). Practice-based evidence in community guide systematic reviews. *American Journal of Public Health, 107*(3), 413–20. https://doi.org/10.2105/AJPH.2016 .303583

Valente, T. (2015). Social networks and health behavior. In Glanz, K., Rimer, B., & Viswanath, K. (Eds.), *Health Behavior: Theory, Research, and Practice.* Jossey-Bass.

Williams, R., Stollings, J., Bundy, Ł., Haardörfer, R., Kreuter, M., Mullen, P., Hovell, M., Morris, M., & Kegler, M. (2016). A minimal intervention to promote smoke-free homes among 2-1-1 callers: North Carolina randomized effectiveness trial. *PLoS One, 11*(11), e0165086. https://doi.org/10.1371/journal.pone.0165086

Wingood, G.M., & DiClemente, R.J. (2008). The ADAPT-ITT model: a novel method of adapting evidence-based HIV interventions. *Journal of Acquired Immune Deficiency Syndromes, 1*(47 Suppl. 1), S40–6. https://doi.org/10.1097/QAI.0b013e3181605df1

Wong, M., Nau, C., Kharmats, A., Vedovato, G., Cheskin, L., Gittelsohn, J., & Lee, B. (2015). Using a computational model to quantify the potential impact of changing the placement of healthy beverages in stores as an intervention to "Nudge" adolescent behavior choice. *BMC Public Health, 15*, 1284. https://doi.org/10.1186/s12889-015-2626-0

Health Program and Policy Development II: Implementation Strategies

•

Cam Escoffery and Lawrence W. Green

Learning Objectives
After completing the chapter, the reader will be able to:
- Understand the concept of implementation.
- Discuss how implementation tools can assist with program delivery.
- Describe factors relating implementation to planning and evaluation.
- Describe phases of implementation.

INTRODUCTION

At this point in the PRECEDE-PROCEED program planning process, you have developed your program, with intervention strategies, through systematic diagnoses of the quality of life and health problems in a population, the behavioral and environmental determinants of those problems, and the predisposing, enabling, and reinforcing determinants of behavior and environmental change. You also have formed theoretical or evidence-based strategies (including the use of diagnostic evidence from the previous steps) for *how*, through *what channels*, and *to whom* to deliver the interventions. Now, we will focus on program implementation, as shown in figure 8.1. This is where we turn the corner in the model from the planning of PRECEDE to the actions of PROCEED.

This chapter describes **implementation readiness** based on administrative assessments of available resources relative to needed resources. It covers the development of an implementation plan and **implementation phases**, **implementation tools**, and **program monitoring**. Tracking your program progress and being cognizant of factors related (positively or negatively) to implementation ensures that your program staff puts into practice strategies that can ensure implementation quality. Finally, a consideration of implementation research and practice-based research will inform your program's early considerations for the program's evaluation (Shillinger 2010).

IMPLEMENTATION

We focus now on planning for program implementation. Implementation is the act of converting program objectives into actions through policy and organization changes, regulation, and interventions. Fundamentally, implementation challenges the notion that having a good idea or plan is enough. It asks, how will that idea or plan express itself as action in the *real world?* It is important that you consider the stages of implementation, necessary steps and the key actors (or implementers), and supporting structures needed for implementation. Often, in the real word, implementation is complex and challenging. Greenhalgh and colleagues (2004) proposed that you have to make implementation happen by actively using strategies to support program adoption and delivery and capitalize on supports for the operations of the program. Reviews of implementation studies (Green 2014; Ottoson et al. 2013; Ottoson and Green 1987; Yano et al.

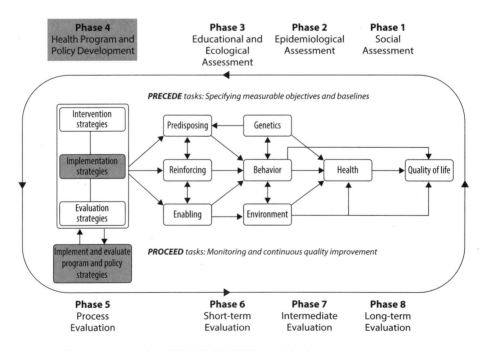

FIGURE 8.1. The fourth phase of the PRECEDE-PROCEED model, health program and policy development, continues with the identification, formation, and initiation of priorities among *implementation* strategies to influence determinants of behavioral and environmental change.

2012) have found numerous ways that implementation alters program outcomes in the range of people reached and influenced, the intensity or duration of the influence, and the diffusion of the influence across secondary intended populations (Calonge et al. 2013).

IMPLEMENTATION PHASES

The delivery of a program is a process, not just a single event. As you create program work plans, you can categorize key tasks for program administrators, staff, and stakeholders into key steps to ensure that you are making progress toward the desired program goals and objectives.

A program work plan often divides activities into program phases. Fixsen and colleagues (2005) describe six stages of program implementation, as shown in figure 8.2. Note that all of these phases are important to consider so that you have resources and people in place at the start of the program and, if it is successful in achieving its outcomes, steps to ensure sustainability.

Exploration and Adoption. This stage spans program planning and program or intervention selection. You would have identified the need for an intervention through prior phases of needs assessment, assessed some of the readiness of your organization to implement the program, and now have created

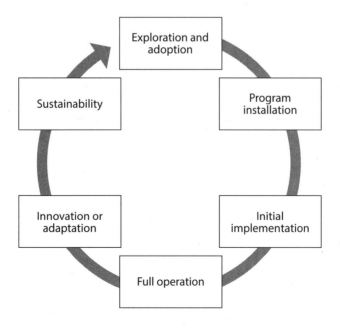

FIGURE 8.2. Stages of Program Implementation (Following Program Planning)

implementation tools such as a budget, work plan, and timeline to put the program into action (e.g., hiring staff, seeking funds, training, etc.). Now we turn to the additional implementation phases and tasks.

Program Installation. This stage involves securing *structural supports* to initiate the program. These supports include locating funding, hiring staff, training implementers, securing space and creating intervention materials. Your detailed program work plan and budget will assist in listing the needed personnel, materials, and resources to implement the program.

Initial Implementation. The first delivery of the program to and with the intended audience in the setting occurs in this stage. This allows for full implementation of the planning activities, the protocol outlined in the implementation manual, and evaluation. You can learn collaboratively with representatives of the community, program sponsors, and the program's recipients from this initial experience, documenting challenges and lessons learned as program monitoring and process evaluation proceed. These lessons can help you make corrections, adjust program components collaboratively, or build supports for future program implementation.

Full Operation. Here the program operates with the full support of program sponsors, participation from the intended audience, and staffing. You begin to offer the program routinely. Over time, especially with continuing evaluation and adaptation, it becomes regarded as a usual practice within the organization or community. In addition, ongoing training and coaching of implementers is critical to making implementation go smoothly. Research on capacity building suggests a variety of strategies that you can use, including training, manuals, technical assistance, and assessment and feedback (Leeman et al. 2015).

Innovation or Adaptation. These processes occur over time with each attempted implementation of the program. Each implementation could lead to changes in the original program—**adaptations**, for example, or shifts in fidelity[2] to the core elements and implementation protocols. **Fidelity** is the adherence to procedures as specified by the original program when delivering it as a new program (Aarons et al. 2009). It is important to innovate, but also to document changes to the original program in relation to a recipient population's composition, context, content, delivery, training, resources, and evaluation (Escoffery et al. 2018; Green 2008; Stirman et al. 2013) and to note the program process and effects.

An example of such adaptation is the Chronic Disease Self-Management Program (CDSMP) developed in English to educate adults with chronic illnesses about strategies for self-management, as shown in box 8.1. To meet the needs of other populations, Lorig and colleagues implemented the program in Texas and New Mexico with English-speaking Latinos who had chronic diseases (mostly diabetes) and created an adapted version, called Tomando Control de su Salud (Taking

Control of Your Health), for Spanish-speaking adults in Chihuahua, Mexico (Lorig et al. 2005). The adapted version was not just a literal translation; they performed cultural adaptations of the contents, changed some activities (e.g., from pair to group discussions), and translated the evaluation survey as well.

Lorig and colleagues found similar effects to the original program, with both groups of participants showing improvements in health behaviors, health status, and self-efficacy at both four months and one year post-intervention (Lorig et al. 2005). The Spanish-speaking group also had significant increases in health care utilization. The work of Lorig and her colleagues show how you can plan to innovate programs by potentially making adaptations and taking systematic steps to perform the modifications and evaluation (Escoffery et al. 2019). In chapter 10, Ramirez and Chelela provide additional examples of translating and implementing PRECEDE-PROCEED to chronic disease prevention strategies in Latinx communities.

Sustainability. Scheirer and Dearing (2011) define **sustainability** as "the continued use of program components and activities for the continued achievement of desirable program and population outcomes" (206). This concept is important because funders often want evidence for the likelihood that your program will continue beyond initial implementation and external funding and that it is having the intended effects. This is why implementation and evaluation need to be linked processes. The timeframe for sustainability varies, but it is often delineated as two or more years after implementation (Glasgow et al. 1999; Stirman et al. 2012).

BOX 8.1

Improving Self-efficacy to Manage Symptoms and Health Behaviors: Chronic Disease Self-Management Program (CDSMP)

The CDSMP is a self-management education program for people with a chronic disease such as diabetes and arthritis. Kate Lorig and colleagues developed it in 1993, and it continues to be adopted at other sites internationally. It is a peer-led intervention consisting of six highly participative classes held for 2.5 hours each, once a week, for six consecutive weeks. It covers topics such as techniques to deal with problems associated with arthritis, appropriate exercise, appropriate use of medications, communicating effectively with family, friends, and health professionals; nutrition, and how to evaluate new treatments (further information can be found at https://www.selfman agementresource.com/programs/small-group/chronic-disease-self-management). The program has been delivered in senior centers, faith-based organizations and other community settings. Evaluations of the program found participant improvements in exercise and ability to do social and household activities, with less depression, fear, and frustration or worry about their health and increased confidence in their ability to manage their condition (Lorig et al. 2001a; 2001b).

Schell and colleagues (2013) defined sustainability capacity as "the existence of structures and processes that allow a program to leverage resources to implement and maintain evidence-based policies and activities." They found nine areas of importance for their "capacity for sustainability framework" from literature reviews, expert panels, and concept mapping research. The domains include political support, funding stability, partnerships, organizational capacity, program evaluation, program adaptation, communications, public health impacts, and strategic planning (Schell et al. 2013). Furthermore, these factors can be divided into intervention characteristics, organizational supports, and environmental supports.

The existence of national policies that sustain program priorities are key to the survival of local programs (Green and Fielding 2011). In your program planning, consider if and how you have these elements in place or how to prepare for them to help sustain the program in the long-term. The Program Sustainability Assessment Tool[3] is a detailed resource on factors important to sustainability, offering an assessment of your program's capacity for sustainability and sample work plans for sustainability (Luke et al. 2014). It can serve as a useful tool for sustainability planning for your program.

As discussed above, key activities identified by Fixsen and colleagues may be helpful to consider and plan for at certain times in the six stages of implementation. You may also find other implementation frameworks can help to guide the identification of challenges and strengths for evidence-based practice implementation (Nilsen 2015; Ottoson and Hawe 2009). The EPIS (Exploration, Preparation, Implementation, and Sustainment) model describes implementation as a process influenced by multilevel factors over time (Aarons et al. 2011). It has the four phases of EPIS in its title and some critical steps to achieve within them. Another model is the Stages of Implementation Completion (SIC), an eight-stage tool of implementation processes and milestones. The stages span three implementation phases of pre-implementation, implementation, and sustainability. Items delineate the date that a site completes implementation activities, yielding measures of duration (time to complete a stage), proportion (of stage activities completed), and progression (how far an organization moved in the implementation process) (Saldana et al. 2014). These process models can specify steps in stages or phases and the needed supports for program delivery.[4]

ADMINISTRATIVE ASSESSMENT

We now turn to the process of accessing the resources required and available to mobilize and deploy the intervention strategies identified. You begin at this stage by considering the time and material resources needed to implement the methods and strategies chosen in the preceding steps. This administrative assessment includes three assessments: (1) resources needed, (2) resources available, and (3) other prevailing factors expected to impede or facilitate implementation. This assessment helps determine how ready you, your agency, and your community are to deliver the proposed intervention strategies.

Step 1: Assess the Resources Needed

As with earlier objective-setting, where the mantra was "who will accomplish how much of what change, and by when," time, personnel, and other cost-bearing and time-consuming factors must be considered. The first step in an administrative assessment is to review the resources required to implement the proposed program methods and strategies. This will entail an examination of the time frames for accomplishing the objectives, the types and numbers of people needed to carry out the program, and the material resources they will need.

Time. Because it is nonrenewable, the first and most critical resource is time. It is inflexible in its supply and it affects the availability and cost of all other resources. Time required is estimated at several levels of PRECEDE with the formulation of realistic objectives. Each **SMART objective**, as seen in the next chapter on evaluation, states the time (date) by which that objective needs to be accomplished for the next higher-level objective to be accomplished. Thus, certain short-term predisposing, enabling, and reinforcing objectives must be accomplished before intermediate behavioral and environmental objectives can be expected to materialize. These, in turn, should be expected to precede any palpable change in long-term health or quality of life outcomes. For example, suppose you have established the following short-term predisposing educational objectives:

> Within the first four months of a measles immunization program, parents in the target population will show:
> - 60% increase in a percentage of parents having a threshold of adequate knowledge that a measles vaccine is available; and
> - 50% increase in those who believe that their children are susceptible to measles.

Your enabling objectives might include a four-month target of dispatching 60 mobile immunization stations, one for each school and shopping center in the community, and a three-month target of obtaining commitments from 50 school principals and 10 shopping-center managers. All these objectives must be accomplished within the time frames stated to achieve a behavioral objective of a four percentage-point increase in schoolchildren receiving measles immunization (from 90% previously immunized to 94%) at the end of six months. These objectives clearly would limit your time frame for implementing specific aspects of the program plan.

Personnel. Staffing requirements take precedence over other budgetary considerations in the resource analysis because the personnel category generally constitutes the largest and most restricted line item in most budgets. In most health promotion programs, you may find a common assumption: existing personnel will suffice throughout the implementation of the program. If the preceding assessments, however, have produced a program design that requires more personnel than the sponsoring organization or unit has at its disposal or can afford to hire, then you may need to consider the following options:

1. Identify and seek part-time commitments from personnel from other departments or units within your organization. If they are not authorized to allocate their own time, you will need commitments from their supervisors as well. Temporary arrangements of this kind are common when separate departments share common goals, which is often the case if the other department has the kind of personnel you need.

2. Retrain personnel within your department to take on tasks outside their usual scope.

3. Explore the potential for recruitment of volunteers from the community. Short-term programs, in particular, can tap the underutilized pool of talent and energy available for volunteer effort for a worthy cause. But don't assume that volunteers don't incur costs and burdens of their own (Institute of Medicine [IOM, now National Academies Press] 2012).

4. Explore the potential for cooperative agreements with other agencies or organizations in the community to fill in the gaps in your personnel. Be sure your organization can reciprocate in the future.

5. Develop a grant proposal for funding, partial funding, or matched funding of your program by a government agency, philanthropic foundation, or corporate donor. With the program plan and addition of your evaluation plan (shown in chapter 9) and a final budget request, you will have a grant application in hand that could attract grant funding from another agency or foundation.

6. Appeal directly to the public for donations or seek a sponsor.

7. Price the service at a cost-recovery level of fees that you will charge some or all users of the service. Diversity and equity considerations come very much into play in many of these options, but especially where the financial affordability of services is concerned.

8. If none of the previous options seem appropriate, feasible, or sufficient and if the program represents a permanent or long-term priority and commitment of the organization, then you may justifiably pursue policy changes in the organization such that a more fundamental reorganization or redistribution of resources to your department or unit would be established before embarking on the program.

Budget. From your planning, you will need to determine your overall budget, including the personnel, equipment, travel, and other expenses required to implement your program. You can retrieve ideas from your logic model (under inputs), timeline, and work plan for people to understand what is required from them. Start with knowing the allocation from your organization for program costs or the grant budget amount that you are seeking for your program.

Step 2: Assess the Resources Available

You will need to create and negotiate a budget to ensure that you have the needed resources to implement the program. A budget details the costs associated with implementing program activities and interventions. However, budgets assist in planning for program delivery and ensure that you have the monetary resources to implement all parts of a program from the start through to the evaluation. Budgets are divided typically into direct costs (explicit project expenses) and indirect costs (organizational overhead charges). To create budgets, computer spreadsheets such as those created in Excel enable you to enter and manipulate costs, and recalculate if you have changes. They also allow you to have tables to budget future years for a program using the same major budget line items. The major sections of a representative program budget, as illustrated for the delivery of four courses over a year of the Chronic Disease Self-Management Program, are shown in table 8.1 (and revisited in box 8.1).

Personnel. Projects need key individuals who are critical to the program. This could include the director, health educators, implementers such as peer educators, and an evaluator. You would convert each person's time into cost estimates by multiplying an average hourly wage or salary estimate by time contributed or by estimating or negotiating a flat consulting fee.

Travel. Travel may include costs for travel related to program development, delivery or dissemination (sharing of results). This would include staff travel to delivery sites (e.g., schools, worksites), training, and conference travel for dissemination of program results. You should use your organization's *per diem* rates for travel (i.e., hotel, meals) and mileage, or the federal rate.

Equipment. If you will be offering PowerPoint slide presentations as part of community education for staff training, then you might include the cost of a laptop computer and projector. You may also need tablets for a technology-based program. Remember to read your funder's guidelines, since some equipment costs are not allowed without a strong justification and some will depend on existing inventory.

TABLE 8.1. Budget for delivery of the Chronic Disease Self-Management Program (CDSMP)

Budget item	Hours/salary	Rate/percentage time	Total
Personnel			
Project coordinator	$65,000	30%	$19,500
Health educator	$45,000	50%	$22,500
Evaluator	$55,000	15%	$8,250
Two people with chronic diseases	44 hours = (12 sessions + 2 meetings + 8 training × 2 people)	$150/hr	$6,600
Fringe benefits		25%	$12,563
Total personnel			$69,413
Travel			
Sessions	120 miles × 4 people × .55		$264
Training	60 miles × 4 people × .55		$132
Area on aging meeting	$600 airfare; $150 per diem; $125 hotel × 2 people		$1,750
Total travel			$2,146
Supplies			
Participant books	$25 × 12		$300
Printing fliers			$120
Office supplies			$500
Total supplies			$920
Other			
Photocopying			$500
CDSMP training	$450 web training × 4		$1,800
Consultant—graphics	16 hours × $40		$640
Total other			$2,940
Total direct costs			$75,419
Indirect costs		25%	$18,855
Total budget			**$94,274**

Other costs. This is a residual category that covers usually smaller costs. These should be separated by major categories to cover participant materials or monetary incentives, food or refreshments for sessions, etc. The term *in kind*, or *gratis*, is often used to highlight the capability of your organization or partners to supply some of these needs.

Indirect costs. These costs, often referred to as *overhead*, are necessary for the general operation of an organization and the conduct of program operations. This is an average maintenance rate that organizations add to any direct cost estimate to provide for the administrative services of the front office, the rental and upkeep of the building and offices, the cost of utilities, and sometimes local telephone or other fixed costs of the offices in which special projects will be housed. These costs may be a proportion of a total budget to cover building maintenance, telephone and internet expenses, general supplies, and so forth. Often, the indirect cost rate is set by either your organization or a funding agency's limit; it can vary from 10% to 50%. For example, if the direct cost of a program is estimated at $10,000 in personnel time and materials, the budget might be $12,000 to cover the usual 20% overhead the agency has established as necessary from experience.

Budget narrative or justification. Most program plans will include a budget justification. This is a narrative that describes major line items in the budget and provides the rationale for why that cost is needed for program delivery. You should always be prepared to back up every line item in the budget with a more detailed version and narrative justification, even if one does not submit the detailed budgets. For example, if travel costs are listed as a lump sum on a summary project budget, that sum should be derived from estimates for the number of staff involved and component parts, such as air travel, meals, ground transportation, hotel costs, and the mileage between project sites to justify the cost of ground travel.

For the personnel section, you would usually describe the title and role of each person, the amount of effort or time in dollars that each key person is contributing to the project, and any special qualifications they have. This justification is usually essential if you need to ask for funds to deliver a program from internal administrators or external funders. An alternative to increasing paid professional personnel, one that has proved itself sometimes even more effective, is the support of mutual self-help groups.

Step 3: Assess the Factors Influencing Implementation

Besides the availability of resources, a host of other considerations may enhance or hinder the smooth implementation of your program plan. Durlak and DuPre (2008) and others have cataloged factors related to implementation. We have identified the classically recognized factors influencing implementation in a multilevel, ecological perspective in table 8.2. The table groups these factors according to five categories: the program or policy, the implementing organization, the implementers, the political milieu, and the community context or environment. Notice that each variable, depending upon the circumstances, can be a positive, facilitating force or a negative, hindering one. We have highlighted and elaborated some of these factors below.

TABLE 8.2. Factors affecting implementation

Program

- Compatibility or fit of the program to an organization's mission and priorities[c,d]
- Adaptability, i.e., extent a program can be adapted or modified[a,c]
- Theory and evidence[a]
- Resources[a]
- Impact[a]

Implementing organization

General organizational factors

- Positive work climate[b,c,d]
- Organizational norms regarding change[c]
- Integration of new programming[c,d]
- Shared vision (shared mission, consensus, commitment, staff buy-in)[c]
- Leadership[b,c,d]
- Program champion (internal advocate)[b,c,d]
- Managerial/supervisory/administrative support[b,d]

Specific practices and processes

- Shared decision-making (local input, community participation)[b,c,d]
- Coordination with other agencies (partnerships, networking, intersector collaboration)[b,c,d]
- Communication[c,d]
- Formulation of tasks (i.e., teams, internal functioning, effective human resource management)[b,c,d]

Implementers

- Perceived need for innovation[c,d]
- Perceived benefits of innovation[c]
- Skill proficiency[b,c]

Political milieu

- Politics[b,c]
- Power—strength[a]
- Power—support[a]

Community

- Intended beneficiaries/populations[a,d]
- Funding[b,c,d]
- Other organizations[a,d]

---

[a] Ottoson and Green (1987); [b] Fixsen et al. (2005); [c] Greenhalgh et al. (2004); [d] Damschroder (2009)

During program planning, especially in the formative stages, it is important to discuss these factors with the participatory planning team and decide how to address them in program delivery. For example, you may need to train implementers with specific competency-building exercises related to their specific skills in delivering the program. Beyond your organization, factors such as community shared decision-making and roles (e.g., participation, partnerships) can enhance program implementation (Durlak and DuPre 2008; Balagna et al. 2020).

Organizational Factors. The presence of a positive work climate, norms of openness to change and innovative programming, and strong leadership are important. Other organizational factors to consider are listed below, from a program's goals to its complexity.

Program Goal(s). Plans that require changes in standard operating procedures call the goals and objectives of the new plans into question. If these conflict with previously accepted goals and objectives, you must resolve the conflict by clarifying priorities. Sometimes the justification for the changes in goals and objectives must be found in the documentation of changing circumstances, new technologies, new personnel, or sometimes changes in the community.

Rate of Change. Incremental change is easier to implement than radical, ambitious changes, or changes that challenge the status quo (Rogers 2003). Break your program plan's implementation steps down into small, manageable steps.

Space. One of the most precious commodities in many organizations is office space. If your program plan proposes to use existing office space for another purpose or to move staff members from one space to another, you will likely step on someone's toes. Space should be treated as a resource to be allocated according to rules or procedures similar to those suggested earlier for personnel and other budgetary items. Parking space is another precious commodity to be arranged at specified hours for potential collaborators.

Staffing. When organizational staff or the implementation team perceive the need for a new program or innovation, attitudes about the program and skills in the conduct of their role within the program delivery need to be accommodated. Meetings help build the priorities for the program during the early phases of its implementation.

Commitment and Attitudes. Before a program work plan is complete, it needs to make the rounds of comments and suggestions from those who will have a role in implementing it, especially if they have not yet been directly involved in formulating the plan. They should be cautioned that decisions already sealed by those who signed off on plans in which they participated as co-planners cannot be radically or easily changed at this stage. Staff members of the implementing agencies will be in the best position to anticipate barriers in their various roles and will welcome the opportunity to point out some of the pitfalls in your plan before you ask them to implement it.

Familiarity. Are the procedures and methods to be employed familiar to staff members who must implement them? Do they depart radically from standard operating procedures? Even if skills are not lacking, unfamiliar methods and procedures require careful introduction and orientation to avoid being rejected, ignored, or poorly implemented (MacDonald and Green 2001).

Complexity. A change requiring multiple transactions or complex relationships and coordination will be more difficult to implement than will single-action or single-person procedures (Rogers 2003).

Political Factors. These could include political will or support at the national to local levels related to the context in which you are delivering your program. They also can entail leadership support related to your programming or the health issue. For example, if you are delivering your program focused on nutrition and physical activity in the context of a county-wide obesity prevention coalition, it will likely be supported in its implementation if it enhances rather than competes for the resources of their broader program.

Community Factors. Beyond your own organization, the community will respond to your proposed program at several levels. The principle of participation, emphasized throughout our previous chapters, should alert one to the need to weigh the community's perceived and measured assets and barriers as one moves through the planning process. Inevitably, even among those who have participated in the planning process, some will express misgivings about how the new program will affect them and their other programs. Some of these misgivings will translate into passive resistance, and some into subtle efforts to minimize, discredit, or even sabotage the program. The best protection against these defensive maneuvers in the community, besides education and earlier involvement in the planning, is to invite those organizations most threatened by the program to be co-sponsors or collaborators. If, for whatever reason, early engagement and involvement did not occur, it is never too late to invite others to share in the credit and the public visibility of the program in exchange for their support.

Even the most thoughtful strategic plan will fail to take every asset, potential barrier, and source of opposition into account. What then? The remaining barriers and sources of support to be assessed, such as broader political and structural barriers, must be discovered in the evaluation phase. Some of them can only be changed through external political processes because they lie beyond the direct control of one's agency.

DEVELOPMENT OF IMPLEMENTATION TOOLS

Once you have conducted your administrative assessment described earlier in this chapter, the next critical step is to assemble the necessary tools to execute the program. The most important steps for this are those identified above as steps for a detailed and feasible implementation plan. The plan describes the program (logic model), its timeline for implementation, and key detailed activities or tasks in a work plan. You may have developed these as part of your program plan in seeking funding for the program. If not, it is critical to create these tools prior to the implementation of your program. Each of these tools is described below.

Logic model. The logic model is a depiction of all parts of a program (i.e., activities and their relationship to outcomes, also discussed in chapters 7 and 9). It offers a global view, usually with boxes and arrows similar to graphics of the PRECEDE-PROCEED model in previous chapters and in the chapter to follow. Elements of a program's **logic model** might include specific agencies, organizations, and staff in place of general categories of stakeholders and resources (inputs); key program activities; immediate objectives or deliverables (outputs) of the components; and the short-term to long-term outcomes that could be measured or assessed in evaluation. It is a valuable communication tool to share the program overview with the entire implementation team in early meetings of the program planning process and during training on the program. Logic models are described further in chapter 9, which includes a table that outlines the general differences between the PRECEDE-PROCEED model and generic program logic models.

Implementation manual. An implementation manual details the essential steps and actors who play a role in them for the program. Ideally, it includes all protocols for procedures or steps for each implementer or program component, curriculum, program core elements, checklists for activities, reporting, and evaluation. These represent "knowledge-to-action" products that are fundamental intervention components in having a program translated to other settings or communities (Wilson et al. 2011). You or a designated staff committee should describe all procedures in sufficient detail such that the implementers will know what tasks to perform. In the future, others will be able to replicate your program if it is designated as an evidence-based intervention and the manual is published in a program registry for sharing. If you are creating a program *de novo*, then you should develop a manual with descriptions of key specific steps that are sufficiently detailed enough to enable the evaluation of the program to include consistent measures of the quality and performance.[1]

Timeline. A timeline or **Gantt chart** can be laid out as in figure 8.3. It shows graphically the start and finish dates for each major activity related to program implementation. It also shows the sequence and overlap of activities in time, as well as the different activities that will be proceeding simultaneously during each period.

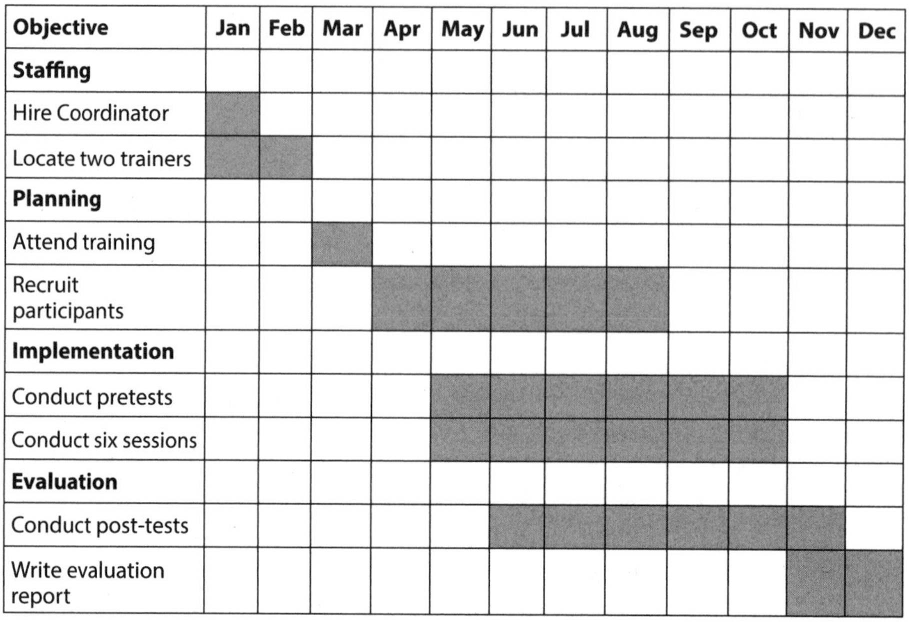

Objective	Jan	Feb	Mar	Apr	May	Jun	Jul	Aug	Sep	Oct	Nov	Dec
Staffing												
Hire Coordinator	▓											
Locate two trainers	▓	▓										
Planning												
Attend training			▓									
Recruit participants				▓	▓	▓	▓	▓				
Implementation												
Conduct pretests					▓	▓	▓	▓	▓	▓		
Conduct six sessions					▓	▓	▓	▓	▓	▓		
Evaluation												
Conduct post-tests						▓	▓	▓	▓	▓		
Write evaluation report											▓	▓

FIGURE 8.3. Chronic Disease Self-Management Program GANTT Chart

Work plan. A work plan is a program planning tool, sometimes required for program grant applications. Detailed, systematic planning can lead to successful interventions if the work plan (or action plan) includes the *what, how much, who,* and *when* for each program objective. Completing a work plan requires:

- Identifying overall goal and objectives for the program;
- Developing a list of activities to support accomplishing the objectives;
- Determining the key steps needed to achieve each objective, including an appropriate sequence and priority;
- Drawing up a timeline for achieving each work plan activity and objective(s).

The work plan also summarizes the key staff or person responsible and resources needed for completing the activity. Once the plan is drafted, share it with staff and other identified departments for their input and revisions. Once it is reviewed and finalized, you are ready for program execution. Just remember to revisit it at least every quarter and revise it as needed as part of the process evaluation described in chapter 9. A sample work plan for delivery of the Chronic Disease Self-Management Program (Lorig et al. 2001a) in urban Atlanta is presented in table 8.3 (revisit box 8.1).

TABLE 8.3. Annual workplan for annual delivery of the Chronic Disease Self-Management Program (CDSMP)

Project period goal (3-year): Increase self-efficacy for chronic disease management by 30% for program participants by the end of the program.

Annual Objective (Year 1): Deliver four entire courses of the CDSMP to adults with chronic illnesses in metro Atlanta by December 2019.

Annual activity description	Evaluation indicator/ outcome	Date to begin	Completion date	Staff/party responsible
Hire for health education	Health educator hired	1/5/19	2/5/19	Project coordinator
Locate two trainers who have chronic disease	Two trainers selected	2/5/19	2/28/19	Project coordinator, health educator
Attend CDSMP web-based training	Attendance of training date and # of participants	3/1/19	3/5/19	Health educator, two trainers
Identify site for program and referral sources for participants	Number of program sites Number of partners who are referring participants	3/6/19	3/31/19	Health educator
Recruit participants	Number of participants recruited	3/6/19	7/31/19	Health educator
Create evaluation plan and surveys	A pretest and post-test survey	3/6/19	3/31/19	Evaluator, health educator
Implement six sessions Conduct pretest	Number of rounds of CDSMP Number of sessions delivered per round Number of pretests completed	4/1/19 5/19/19 6/30/19 8/18/19	5/11/19 6/28/19 8/9/19 9/27/19	Trainers, health educator
Conduct post-test evaluation	Number of post-tests completed	5/11/19 6/28/19 8/9/19 9/27/19	5/18/19 7/5/19 8/16/19 10/4/19	Trainers, health educator
Conduct three-month follow-up evaluation	Number of three-month follow-up surveys completed	8/11/19 9/27/19 11/9/19 12/27/19	9/18/19 10/4/19 11/16/19 1/3/19	Evaluator, health educator
Conduct data analysis	Number of tables and graphs with data	1/6/20	1/31/20	Evaluator, health educator
Write evaluation report	An evaluation report	2/3/20	2/28/20	Evaluator, health educator, coordinator
Share evaluation results	Number of evaluation summaries An infographic created Number of presentations	3/2/20	5/29/20	Health educator, coordinator, trainers

Resources needed: training materials, workplan, GANTT chart, participant materials

QUALITY ASSURANCE, TRAINING, AND SUPERVISION

Effective implementation, addressing each factor of a health promotion program, requires competence and skill on the part of those delivering the program. Durlak and DuPre's (2008) review of implementation factors, such as those in table 8.2, found that few studies have attained levels greater than 80% implementation with **fidelity** (meaning the implementation is conducted with close if not exact replication of the methods and resources used in the main experimental study that led to the program's status as an evidence-based practice).

Some adaptation is justifiable—indeed, sometimes essential—in place of elements that do not fit the local community or population circumstances. Studies have shown that adaptation is common in practice (Carvalho et al. 2013; Moore et al. 2013; Stirman et al. 2013) and often essential if the studies identifying best practices and insisting on fidelity of implementation were conducted without external validity—for example, in very different populations, settings or circumstances than those in which your program will be implemented (Green 2008; Green and Nasser 2018). The Durlak and DuPre findings suggest the need for monitoring the implementation process as the first step in process evaluation, as will be seen in chapter 9. Deviations from fidelity to the original research should be applied cautiously and documented assiduously, but policies and programs must provide for professional discretion and options so that they can be adapted to local situations and changing circumstances (Card et al. 2011).

Training and supervision of personnel provide the best assurance of implementation. Each training program is an educational program in itself and deserves a similar planning process to the one described by the behavioral, environmental, and educational assessments in the PRECEDE framework. Supervision also can be approached as an educational process. Behavior change goals can be set mutually by the supervisor and supervisee. Factors predisposing, enabling, and reinforcing the intended behavior of staff can be analyzed periodically, and corresponding interventions can be planned to predispose, enable, and reinforce implementation through staff meetings, training, written materials, and rewards for high performance.

PROGRAM MONITORING

Program monitoring is the routine collection of information about most, or selected, program activities. It is essential to offering information on what a program is doing, how well it is performing, and whether it is achieving its aims and objectives. It is an ongoing activity that should be incorporated into the daily/weekly administration of the program. The program coordinator should collect, analyze, and document information on the program activities outlined in the work plan, documentation of program components (e.g., logs, satisfaction surveys, etc.), implementation facilitators and barriers, timeline delays or shifts, use of resources, and budget. Regular meetings with the implementation team should facilitate the timely reporting of these data. If challenges or delays in program implementation arise, then the coordinator can identify issues and work to resolve the challenges quickly. The coordinator also needs to keep track of this information to describe the program's progress in achieving major objectives and activities in annual progress reports or final reports to program administrators or funding agencies, and possibly in articles or other publications. In addition, this information about the program can be incorporated as implementation data for process evaluation, and can highlight the contributions of individuals and cooperating or contributing agencies.

IMPLEMENTATION OUTCOMES

Measuring outcomes related to implementation is another tier of evaluation. Often this is called process evaluation or implementation research (defined below). Proctor and colleagues (2011) have identified implementation outcomes in addition to service (i.e., effectiveness, efficiency, safety) and patient or community health-related outcomes such as behavior change, functioning, and disease status, as illustrated in figure 8.4. The implementation outcomes of programs include adoption (uptake by the organization), penetration (reach within the community), acceptability, appropriateness, feasibility of implementation, and costs. Each of the eight implementation outcomes is presented in table 8.4 with a short definition and examples of sources for each. In the design of your evaluation, articulate the key implementation outcomes of interest to you and your stakeholders. For example, if the program is a pilot, then collecting data about its acceptability and feasibility would be important for program revisions. The time required to complete phases of the program implementation would be another indicator to document. Then you can build data collection to capture those outcomes as part of your process evaluation, as seen in chapter 9.

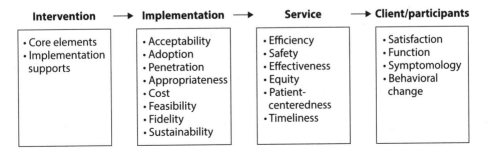

FIGURE 8.4. Types of implementation outcomes. *Source:* Adapted from Proctor et al. (2011).

TABLE 8.4. Implementation outcome definitions and examples of sources

Implementation outcome	Definition	Example of sources include . . .
Acceptability	The degree that an intervention is agreeable and satisfactory among program stakeholders.	A satisfaction survey of the content, delivery, comfort, and user-friendliness of the program.
Adoption	The initial use or uptake of a program.	Administrative data on what settings were adopted and who (and how many) adopted the program.
Appropriateness	The perception of the relevance and fit of a program for a given population or setting.	Qualitative interviews of implementers and program participants about the relevance of the program.
Costs	The actual or incremental expenses for program delivery.	A resource audit of personnel, travel, program materials, indirect costs, and other budgeted items.
Feasibility	The extent to which a program can be successfully conducted within an organization or setting.	An administrative survey of program staff and implementers.
Fidelity	The degree to which a program is delivered as prescribed by the developer.	A checklist of completion of each core element of a program.
Penetration	The integration of a program within a setting; the notion of the number of service users over all people who are eligible for the program.	Program records of participants over eligible participants served by the clinic in the past year.
Sustainability	The degree to which a program is maintained.	Scores on the Program Sustainability Assessment Tool (Luke et al. 2014).

Source: Proctor, E., Silmere, H., Raghavan, R., Hovmand, P., Aarons, G., Bunger, A., Griffey, R., & Hensley, M. (2011). Outcomes for implementation research: conceptual distinctions, measurement challenges, and research agenda. *Administration and Policy in Mental Health, 38*(2), 65–76. https://doi.org/10.1007/s10488-010-0319-7

IMPLEMENTATION SCIENCE

To this point, chapter 8 has focused on the practicalities of implementation. Here we dig deeper into an understanding of the **implementation science** that has informed our recommendations for practice. Implementation science has been defined as the study of methods to promote the systematic uptake of evidence-based interventions into practice and policy and hence improve health (Foy et al. 2015). We have added to that definition that it is "the strategic combination of evidence-based strategies from the cumulative research literature with practice-based evidence from the local population and circumstances that would require adaptations of the scientific evidence" (Green and Ottoson 2004, 16). The purpose of implementation science is to improve the adoption or adaptation, delivery, and sustainment of effective programs in clinical, organizational, or community settings. It also can help your organization learn from each program delivery to enhance its operations and to build capacity within the organization and community for health promotion (WHO 2013).

Implementation science research questions can cover varied topics related to your program (Peters et al. 2013; Tabak et al. 2012). From these questions, you can determine the best methods to collect data to answer your questions. Some examples of research questions are:

- What factors and implementers (key actors) can enhance the delivery of a program?
- What factors influence implementation in a particular type of setting or population?
- How does implementation vary across settings in strategies/activities and implementers?
- How does program delivery lead to changes in implementation outcomes (e.g., feasibility and acceptability) and health or other outcomes (i.e., changes in behavior, environment, policies)?
- What are appropriate networks of organizations or channels for disseminating a program?
- What can assist with scaling up an effective program?

THE "PIPELINE" FROM EVIDENCE-BASED PRACTICE TO PRACTICE-BASED EVIDENCE

The references to a *pipeline* from research to guidelines for evidence-based medicine or evidence-based practice have grown out of traditions in modern medicine and public health that have been institutionalized by international organizations such as the World Health Organization (2013) and federal agencies such as the National Institutes of Health, National Cancer Institute, and Centers for Disease Control and Prevention in their funding and shepherding of research into practice. Central to implementation science is an understanding that the translation pipeline of research to practice, illustrated in figure 8.5 (Green 2008), gets squeezed repeatedly by critical peer review of the science at the stages of its odyssey from grant applications, to publication, to systematic reviews of evidence, to guidelines for evidence-based practice. It encounters the frustrations of the real world where patient or population circumstances and practice conditions or resources don't match the requirements of the evidence-based practice. As noted in the figure 8.5 pipeline, it has been estimated that this odyssey (as of the turn of the century) takes an average of some 17 years for research evidence to be widely implemented in medical practice (Balas and Boren 2000).

The Institute of Medicine (Institute of Medicine [IOM, now National Academies Press] 2009) adapted the pipeline metaphor to apply to implementation studies. From **efficacy** studies, which involve the testing of programs in ideally rigorous, usually experimental conditions, **effectiveness** studies then involve the testing of programs in less controlled, real-world conditions with a more heterogeneous group of participants (Brown et al. 2017), as seen in figure 8.6. For example, efficacy refers to results of an intervention that is tested under close-to-ideal experimental methods of research. Effectiveness refers to the results of a quasi-experimental study within real, contemporary communities where a random assignment of people and other experimental controls might be overly burdensome or impossible.

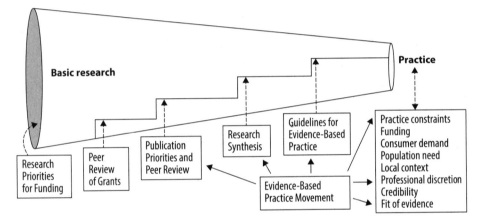

FIGURE 8.5. Pipeline to evidence-based practice. *Source:* Adapted from Green (2008).

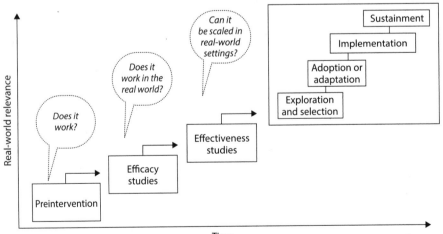

FIGURE 8.6. Translation pipeline. *Source:* Adapted from IOM (2009).

From online repositories of evidence-based programs such as Evidence-based Cancer Control Programs (EBCCP) (formerly known as Research-Tested Intervention Programs or RTIPs) or HIV Effective Interventions that Work (CDC 2021; NCI 2018), health professionals engaging in program planning will then explore relevant programs to their missions and communities and select an intervention with the best fit. They will then implement the program. If the program proves successful, they can justify maintaining its delivery to their organization. But if these best practice interventions do not work, it may be because they were often tested under ideal research circumstances that do not match the different circumstances of the community where the program is implemented and evaluated (Green 2008).

BENEFITS OF IMPLEMENTATION RESEARCH

There are many benefits to implementation research (IR). First, it can identify factors in the clogged evidence-to-practice pipeline that could limit program adoption, implementation, and sustainment. Green et al. (2009a; 2009b) have documented that implementation of evidence-based guidelines or practices depends on a pipeline in which evidence is produced by researchers, then evaluated and only some of it disseminated to policy makers and practitioners. As observed by Balas and Boren, however, obstructions in that translation pipeline could take an average of nearly two decades (~17 years) from discovery to local implementation, as noted in figure 8.5.

Secondly, IR emphasizes an understanding of the factors associated with quality implementation, or putting a program into practice in a manner that meets the standards to accomplish its outcomes (Meyers et al. 2012) and overcome barriers and facilitators to implementation. These findings can inform future program delivery and allow for program revisions. Therefore, IR helps describe implementation delivery and does not solely focus on studying program outcomes. In addition, even if an intervention or practice has been demonstrated in previous research to be effective, if it is not implemented properly or without sufficient fidelity, then it will be more likely to fail (Carroll et al. 2007; Elliott and Mihalic 2004). Therefore, IR can assess factors related to poor quality implementation, such as the program did not truly fit the community, the program was too difficult to implement (e.g., staff burden, program complexity), or the implementers did not have all the skills necessary to perform their roles (Durlak and DuPre 2008; Granja et al. 2018; Pearson et al. 2015).

Thirdly, implementing programs is complex and involves multiple delivery staff and structures that have to work together optimally as systems. IR assesses an array of factors that includes the innovative program, delivery team, cultural sensitivity, inner setting or organizational context, and outer setting, or factors external to the organization (Damschroder et al. 2009; Greenhalgh et al. 2004). Finally, IR is rooted in stakeholder and community engagement. Its methods often require data collection from all aspects of implementation (i.e., leadership, implementers, and partners) as participants in the program or its implementation (Palinkas et al. 2015).

Program Dissemination and Strategies. Once a program is effective, program planners and researchers will want to disseminate the intervention so that others know that it is evidence-based. Dissemination is actively spreading an effective intervention to a target audience with planned strategies and specified channels (Lomas 1993; Rabin and Brownson 2017). In a review of dissemination studies related to cancer prevention, active and multimodal strategies for dissemination (including training, technical assistance or support, print materials, media channels, and financial resources) were most effective (Rabin et al. 2010).

Program Scale-up. Scale-up is defined as the "process by which health interventions shown to be efficacious on a small scale or under controlled conditions are expanded under real-world conditions into broader populations, policy or practice" (Milat et al. 2015, 2). Milat and colleagues (2016) conducted a systematic review of the literature of factors and barriers to scaling up public health interventions. The top five facilitators to scale-up were establishing a monitoring and evaluation system, costing of the intervention, active engagement of the implementers and the target community, tailoring scale-up approaches to the local context, and the presence of a well-defined scale-up strategy. Conversely, the top five barriers were no adaptations to the local context, not measuring intervention costs, lack of human resources, resistance to the creation of new practices due to resource constraints, and insufficient investment in the implementation infrastructure.

As you consider the possibility of the scale-up of your program, it is important to address these barriers and foster the facilitators' continual engagement with the target community and having a developed plan for scaling up. In addition, health professionals should inventory their costs associated with the full program delivery and publish or share these data to encourage an understanding of resources needed for future replication or scale-up.

An example of a program that has been successfully taken to scale is the Chronic Disease Self-Management Program (CDSMP, the case study described earlier; revisit box 8.1). The purpose of this program was to offer self-management education to people who have a variety of health conditions such as diabetes, asthma, heart disease, and arthritis, and it was offered in community settings (Lorig et al. 2001a; 2001b). The program developers horizontally scaled the program over 20-plus years by implementing it in a variety of settings. In a study of its dissemination, Smith and colleagues (2014) examined the characteristics of the first 100,000 program participants and detailed the range of delivery sites of the program, from health care organizations to casinos, with the most common settings being senior centers/agencies on aging (29%), health care settings (21%), residential facilities (18%), other community facilities (10%), and faith-based organizations (8%). Such diversity in program settings calls for additional attention at the level of central planning and monitoring to variations in the program plan to accommodate local environmental conditions (Green 2008; 2014; Green et al. 2009a; Green and Nasser 2018).

PRACTICE-BASED EVIDENCE

Part of implementation research is to determine optimal methods to implement and expand programs to alternative settings. This information is important in determining whether interventions found to be effective in efficacy trials are appropriate and feasible for implementation in a new setting. This view is supported by growing calls for funding and reporting of intervention trials that address contextual issues and external validity to promote translation of evidence-based programs and strategies (Glasgow and Emmons 2007; Green and Nasser 2018; Rychetnik et al. 2012). **External validity** is defined as the extent to which program effects can be generalized to different populations, settings, program variables, and outcome variables (Shadish et al. 2001). It answers the question for health practitioners of whether an intervention (and its causal effects) is relevant to their setting, community, or local circumstances (Steckler and McLeroy 2008). Practitioners should replicate evidence-based interventions to see whether they are effective in local settings or adapt interventions to practitioners' local situations and evaluate them to generate practice-based evidence (Green 2008; Green and Nasser 2018; Green and Ottoson 2004; Green et al. 2009b). At its heart, practice-based evidence is learning from real-world practice and experience.

To elevate practice-based evidence, the field can learn from your program's implementation and evaluations, adaptations, and implementation research. Guidelines have been developed to guide practitioners in describing key elements of their programs so others can learn from your implementation failures and successes. Transparent Reporting of Evaluations with Nonrandomized Designs (TREND) is a guideline to assist in the reporting standards of nonrandomized evaluations of behavioral and public health interventions; it offers a checklist of 22 areas for reporting about the program (Des Jarlais et al. 2004). It is located at the EQUATOR (Enhancing Quality and Transparency Of health Research) website with other reporting guidelines (Equator Network 2018). Elements that you would want to describe in more detail about your intervention in reports or published articles to advance the field, addressing both internal and external validity issues, are found in table 8.5 (Des Jarlais et al. 2004; Green and Nasser 2018).

TABLE 8.5. Reporting elements for programs

Elements[a]	Reporting elements to expand external validity[b]
Participants • Eligibility criteria • Recruitment methods • Recruit setting • Settings and location of data collection	**Setting and populations participation** • Target audience • Representativeness of setting • Representativeness of the program participants
Intervention details • Content • Delivery method • Unit of delivery • Deliverer • Setting • Exposure quantity and duration • Time span • Activities to increase compliance/adherence (i.e., incentives)	**Program or policy implementation and adaptation** • Consistent implementation • Staff expertise • Program adaptation • Mechanisms of change
Outcome • Primary and secondary outcomes • Methods to collect data • Information on validated instruments	**Outcomes and decision-making** • Significance • Adverse consequences • Moderators • Sensitivity • Costs
	Time maintenance and institutionalization • Long-term effects of program • Institutionalization • Attrition

Source: Adopted from the Trend Statement, Des Jarlais et al. (2004)[a] and Green and Nasser (2018)[b].

SUMMARY

This chapter makes the turn from PRECEDE to PROCEED, as shown in the *Implementation Strategies* of Phase 4, figure 8.1. It consists of some of the final steps in diagnostic planning (administrative assessment) and initial steps in implementation and process evaluation. Implementation is a specified set of activities designed to put a program or policy into practice. A first step in implementation is the administrative assessment, which entails the analysis of resources required by a given program, the resources available in the organization or community, and the barriers to implementation of the program. These steps take you from the PRECEDE assessment to the actual program implementation—ideas to action—and then evaluation that occurs throughout PROCEED, as shown in the Implement and Evaluate Program and Policy Strategies in Phase 5, figure 8.1.

Planning and policy in health education, health promotion, and related programs can provide a clear purpose, resources, and protection for sustainability for the programs they produce. It is important to consider and plan for implementation barriers and facilitators at multiple levels. Addressing factors related to implementation in early planning meetings of a program is strategic and potentially will reduce pitfalls or roadblocks in implementation. Plans and policies must leave room to adapt to changing local circumstances, personalities, opportunities, and feedback from evaluation.

PRECEDE assures that a program will be *appropriate* to a person's or population's needs and *feasible* in relation to its circumstances. PROCEED assures that the program will be *available*, *accessible*, *acceptable*, and *accountable*. Only an appropriate program is worth implementing, but even the most appropriate program will fail to reach those who need it if the program is unavailable, inaccessible, or unacceptable to them. PROCEED assesses the resources required to assure a program's *availability*, organizational changes required to assure its *accessibility*, and political and regulatory changes required to assure its *acceptability*. Finally, program monitoring and quality assurance through evaluation and training assures that the program will be *accountable* to the policy makers, administrators, consumers, clients, and any other stakeholders who need to know whether the program met their standards of acceptability.

Implementation relies on a well-thought-out program logic model, work plan, adequate budget, solid organizational and policy support, constructive training and supervision of staff, and careful monitoring in the process evaluation stage. Planning for implementation may require outlining key tasks into phases of implementation. The description of the program phases and key activities can ensure quality implementation. Beyond this, successful implementation depends on experience, sensitivity to people's needs, flexibility in the face of changing circumstances, maintaining a long-term perspective, and having a sense of humor.

Implementation research focuses on the transfer of effective programs, policies and practices into the real world. Conducting implementation research can answer many questions about the adoption, delivery, and sustaining of programs in local settings. We encourage you to advance practice-based evidence by disseminating information about your program's implementation, adoption of evidence-based practices, and adaptations of them to produce practice-based evidence of their fit with the population, resources, and environment (Green 2008; Green and Nasser 2018; Green and Ottoson 2004). To that end, the last table presented offers guidelines for reporting about your program for reports and publications.

————————— **EXERCISES** —————————

1. Identify the resources required for your program and develop a program budget.

2. Analyze what factors may affect the implementation of your program as facilitators and barriers. Develop potential solutions to the implementations barriers.

3. Develop a detailed work plan for a specific program that you are about to implement.

4. Describe the approaches your program might take to ensure its sustainability beyond the initial funding cycle.

5. Describe some implementation outcomes, in addition to health outcomes, that will be important to measure for your program.

Notes

The authors are indebted to Chris Lovato, PhD, Judith M. Ottoson, MPH, EdD, and American and Canadian experts on implementation for their review and contributions to this chapter; and to Virginia Young, MPH candidate, University of British Columbia.

You can find some examples of these manuals on websites that store packaged "evidence-based programs" such as the evidence-based cancer control programs websites at https://ebccp.cancercontrol.cancer.gov/index.do and *The Community Guide* from the CDC-sponsored Task Force on Community Health Services at https://www.thecommunityguide.org.

Note that the "innovation or adaptation" stage is where care should be taken to document adaptations in the protocol needed to make the "evidence-based intervention" fit appropriately in the local population, culture, resources and circumstances, as seen in Green et al. (2009a).

Center for Public Health System Science. (n.d.) *Program Sustainability Assessment Tool.* https://sustaintool.org/

Examples of steps of the phases are described in more detail in Fixsen et al. (2005).

References

Aarons, G.A., Hurlburt, M., & Horwitz, S.M. (2011). Advancing a conceptual model of evidence-based practice implementation in public service sectors. *Administration and Policy in Mental Health, 38*(1), 4–23. https://doi.org/10.1007/s10488-010-0327-7

Aarons, G.A., Sommerfeld, D.H., Hecht, D.B., Silovsky, J.F., & Chaffin, M.J. (2009). The impact of evidence-based practice implementation and fidelity monitoring on staff turnover: evidence for a protective effect. *Journal of Consulting and Clinical Psychology, 77*(2), 270–80. https://doi.org/10.1037/a0013223

Balagna, J., Williams, C.R., Wang, J., Burch, S., Dalton, E., Kirchick, J., & Sosa, P. (2020). Consensus-driven approach for decision-making in diverse groups. *American Journal of Public Health, 110*(1), 5. https://doi.org/10.2105/AJPH.2019.305427

Balas, E.A., & Boren, S.A. (2000). Managing clinical knowledge for health care improvement. In Bemmel, J., & McCray, A. (Eds.), *Yearbook of medical informatics: patient-centered systems* (pp. 65–70). Schattauer.

Brown, C.H., Curran, G., Palinkas, L.A., Aarons, G.A., Wells, K.B., Jones, L., Collins, L.M., Duan, N., Mittman, B.S., Wallace, A., Tabak, R.G., Ducharme, L., Chambers, D.A., Neta, G., Wiley, T., Landsverk, J., Cheung, K., & Cruden, G. (2017). An overview of research and evaluation designs for dissemination and implementation. *Annual Review of Public Health, 38,* 1–22. https://doi.org/10.1146/annurev-publhealth-031816-044215

Card, J.J., Solomon, J., & Cunningham, S.D. (2011). How to adapt effective programs for use in new contexts. *Health Promotion Practice, 12*(1), 25–35. https://doi.org/10.1177/15248399 09348592

Carroll, C., Patterson, M., Wood, S., Booth, A., Rick, J., & Balain, S. (2007). A conceptual framework for implementation fidelity. *Implementation Science, 2,* 40. https://doi.org/10.1186 /1748-5908-2-40

Carvalho, M.L., Honeycutt, S., Escoffery, C., Glanz, K., Sabbs, D., & Kegler, M.C. (2013). Balancing fidelity and adaptation: implementing evidence-based chronic disease prevention programs. *Journal of Public Health Management and Practice, 19*(4), 348–56. https://doi.org /10.1097/PHH.0b013e31826d80eb

Centers for Disease Control and Prevention. (2021). *HIV Effective Interventions that Work.* https://effectiveinterventions.cdc.gov/home/hiv-prevention-that-works

Calonge, N., Chin, M., Clymer, J., Fielding, J., Glanz, K., Goetzel, R., Green, L.W., Grossman, D., Johnson, R., Kumanyika, S., Orleans, T., Pronk, N., Ramirez, G., Remington, P., & Rimer, B. (2013). Notes from the field: Planting, nurturing, and watching things grow. *American Journal of Preventive Medicine, 45*(6), 687–702. https://doi.org/10.1016/J.AMEPRE.2013.09 .006

Damschroder, L.J., Aron, D.C., Keith, R.E., Kirsh, S.R., Alexander, J.A., & Lowery, J.C. (2009). Fostering implementation of health services research findings into practice: a consolidated framework for advancing implementation science. *Implementation Science, 4*(1), 50. https://doi.org/10.1186/1748-5908-4-50

Des Jarlais, D.C., Lyles, C., Crepaz, N., & TREND Group. (2004). Improving the reporting quality of nonrandomized evaluations of behavioral and public health interventions: the TREND statement. *American Journal of Public Health, 94*(3), 361–6. https://doi.org/10.2105/ajph .94.3.361

Durlak, J.A, & DuPre, E.P. (2008). Implementation matters: a review of research on the influence of implementation on program outcomes and the factors affecting implementation. *American Journal of Community Psychology, 41*(3–4), 327–50. https://doi.org/10.1007 /s10464-008-9165-0

Elliott, D.S., & Mihalic, S. (2004). Issues in disseminating and replicating effective prevention programs. *Prevention Science, 5*(1), 47–53. https://doi.org/10.1023/b:prev.0000013981 .28071.52

Equator Network. (2018). *Enhancing the QUAlity and Transparency of Health Research.* Retrieved May 16, 2021, from https://www.equator-network.org/

Escoffery, C., Lebow-Skelley, E., Haardoerfer, R., Boing, E., Udelson, H., Wood, R., Hartman, M., Fernandez, M.E., & Mullen, P.D. (2018). A systematic review of adaptations of evidence-based public health interventions globally. *Implementation Science, 13*(1), 125. https://doi .org/10.1186/s13012-018-0815-9

Escoffery, C., Lebow-Skelley, E., Udelson, H., Böing, E.A., Wood, R., Fernandez, M.E., & Mullen, P.D. (2019). A scoping study of frameworks for adapting public health evidence-based interventions. *Translational Behavioral Medicine, 9*(1), 1–10. https://doi.org/10.1093 /tbm/ibx067

Fixsen, D.L., Naoom, S.F., Blase, K.A., Friedman, R.M., & Wallace, F. (2005). *Implementation Research: A Synthesis of the Literature.* University of South Florida, Louis de la Parte Florida Mental Health Institute.

Foy, R., Sales, A., Wensing, M., Aarons, G.A., Flottorp, S., Kent, B., Michie, S., O'Connor, D., Rogers, A., Sevdalis, N., Straus, S., & Wilson, P.J. (2015). Implementation science:

a reappraisal of our journal mission and scope. *Implementation Science, 10*(1), 51. https://doi.org/10.1186/s13012-015-0240-2

Glasgow, R.E., & Emmons, K.M. (2007). How can we increase translation of research into practice? Types of evidence needed. *Annual Review of Public Health, 28*, 413–33. https://doi.org/10.1146/annurev.publhealth.28.021406.144145

Glasgow, R.E., Vogt, T.M., & Boles, S.M. (1999). Evaluating the public health impact of health promotion interventions: the RE-AIM framework. *American Journal of Public Health, 89*(9), 1322–7. https://doi.org/10.2105/ajph.89.9.1322

Granja, C., Janssen, W., & Johansen, M.A. (2018). Factors Determining the Success and Failure of eHealth Interventions: Systematic Review of the Literature. *Journal of Medical Internet Research, 20*(5), e10235. https://doi.org/10.2196/10235

Green, L.W. (2008). Making research relevant: if it is an evidence-based practice, where's the practice-based evidence? *Family Practice, 25*(Suppl. 1), i20–i24. https://doi.org/10.1093/fampra/cmn055

Green, L.W. (2014). Closing the chasm between research and practice—evidence of and for change. *Health Promotion Journal of Australia, 25*(1), 25–9. https://doi.org/10.1071/HE13101

Green, L.W., & Fielding, J. (2011). The U.S. Healthy People initiative: its genesis and its sustainability. *Annual Review of Public Health, 32*, 451–70. https://doi.org/10.1146/annurev-publhealth-031210-101148

Green, L.W., Glasgow, R.E., Atkins, D., & Stange, K. (2009a). Making evidence from research more relevant, useful, and actionable in policy, program planning, and practice: slips "twixt cup and lip". *American Journal of Preventive Medicine, 37*(6 Suppl. 1), S187–91. https://doi.org/10.1016/j.amepre.2009.08.017

Green, L., & Nasser, M. (2018). Furthering dissemination and implementation research: The need for more attention to external validity. In Brownson, R., Colditz, G., & Proctor, E. (Eds.), *Dissemination and Implementation Research in Health: Translating Science to Practice* (2nd ed., pp. 301–16). Oxford University Press.

Green, L.W., & Ottoson, J.M. (2004). From efficacy to effectiveness to community and back: Evidence-based practice vs practice-based evidence. In Green, L., Hiss, R., Glasgow, R., et al. (Eds.), *From Clinical Trials to Community: The Science of Translating Diabetes and Obesity Research* (pp. 15–18). National Institutes of Health.

Green, L.W., Ottoson, J.M., García, C., & Hiatt, R.A. (2009b). Diffusion theory and knowledge dissemination, utilization, and integration in public health. *Annual Review of Public Health, 30*, 151–74. https://doi.org/10.1146/annurev.publhealth.031308.100049

Greenhalgh, T., Robert, G., Macfarlane, F., Bate, P., & Kyriakidou, O. (2004). Diffusion of innovations in service organizations: systematic review and recommendations. *Milbank Quarterly, 82*(4), 581–629. https://doi.org/10.1111/j.0887-378X.2004.00325.x

Institute of Medicine. (2009). *Preventing Mental, Emotional, and Behavioral Disorders Among Young People: Progress and Possibilities*. National Academies Press.

Institute of Medicine. (2012). *An Integrated Framework for Assessing the Value of Community-Based Prevention*. National Academies Press.

Leeman, J., Calancie, L., Hartman, M.A., Escoffery, C.T., Herrmann, A.K., Tague, L.E., Moore, A.A., Wilson, K.M., Schreiner, M., & Samuel-Hodge, C. (2015). What strategies are used to build practitioners' capacity to implement community-based interventions and are they effective?: a systematic review. *Implementation Science, 10*, 80. https://doi.org/10.1186/s13012-015-0272-7

Lomas, J. (1993). Diffusion, dissemination, and implementation: who should do what? *Annals of the New York Academy of Sciences, 703*(1), 226–37. https://doi.org/10.1111/j.1749-6632.1993.tb26351.x

Lorig, K.R., Ritter, P., Stewart, A.L., Sobel, D.S., Brown, B.W. Jr., Bandura, A., Gonzalez, V.M., Laurent, D.D., & Holman, H.R. (2001a). Chronic disease self-management program:

2-year health status and health care utilization outcomes. *Medical Care, 39*(11), 1217–23. https://doi.org/10.1097/00005650-200111000-00008

Lorig, K.R., Sobel, D.S., Ritter, P.L., Laurent, D., & Hobbs, M. (2001b). Effect of a self-management program on patients with chronic disease. *Effective Clinical Practice, 4*(6), 256–62.

Lorig, K.R., Ritter, P.L., & Jacquez, A. (2005). Outcomes of border health Spanish/English chronic disease self-management programs. *Science of Diabetes Self-Management and Care, 31*(3), 401–9. https://doi.org/10.1177/0145721705276574

Luke, D.A., Calhoun, A., Robichaux, C.B., Elliott, M.B., & Moreland-Russell S. (2014). The Program Sustainability Assessment Tool: a new instrument for public health programs. *Preventing Chronic Disease, 11*, 130184. https://doi.org/10.5888/pcd11.130184

MacDonald, M.A., & Green, L.W. (2001). Reconciling concept and context: The dilemma of implementation in school-based health promotion. *Health Education and Behavior, 28*(6), 749–68. https://doi.org/10.1177/109019810102800607

Meyers, D.C., Durlak, J.A., & Wandersman, A. (2012). The quality implementation framework: a synthesis of critical steps in the implementation process. *American Journal of Community Psychology, 50*(3–4), 462–80. https://doi.org/10.1007/s10464-012-9522-x

Milat, A.J., Bauman, A., & Redman, S. (2015). Narrative review of models and success factors for scaling up public health interventions. *Implementation Science, 10*, 113. https://doi.org/10.1186/s13012-015-0301-6

Milat, A.J., Newson, R., King, L., Rissel, C., Wolfenden, L., Bauman, A., Redman, S., & Giffin, M. (2016). A guide to scaling up population health interventions. *Public Health Research and Practice, 26*(1), e2611604. https://doi.org/10.17061/phrp2611604

Moore, J.E., Bumbarger, B.K., & Cooper, B.R. (2013). Examining adaptations of evidence-based programs in natural contexts. *Journal of Primary Prevention, 34*(3), 147–61. https://doi.org/10.1007/s10935-013-0303-6

National Cancer Institute. (2018). *Evidence-Based Cancer Control Programs (EBCCP)*. Retrieved May 16, 2021, from https://ebccp.cancercontrol.cancer.gov/index.do

Nilsen, P. (2015). Making sense of implementation theories, models and frameworks. *Implementation Science, 10*(1), 53. https://doi.org/10.1186/s13012-015-0242-0

Ottoson, J.M,, & Green, L.W. (1987). Reconciling concept and context: Theory of implementation. In Ward, W.B., & Becker, M.H. (Eds.), *Advances in Health Education and Promotion* (pp. 353–82). JAI Press.

Ottoson, J.M. & Hawe, P. (Eds.) (2009). *Knowledge Utilization, Diffusion, Implementation, Transfer, and Translation: New Directions for Evaluation* (No. 124). Jossey-Bass.

Ottoson, J.M., Ramirez, A.G., Green, L.W., & Gallion, K.J. (2013). Exploring potential research contributions to policy: The *Salud America!* experience. *American Journal of Preventive Medicine, 44*(3 Suppl. 3), S282–9. https://doi.org/10.1016/j.amepre.2012.11.025

Palinkas, L.A., Horwitz, S.M., Green, C.A., Wisdom, J.P., Duan, N., & Hoagwood, K. (2015). Purposeful Sampling for Qualitative Data Collection and Analysis in Mixed Method Implementation Research. *Administration and Policy in Mental Health, 42*(5), 533–44. https://doi.org/10.1007/s10488-013-0528-y

Pearson, M., Chilton, R., Wyatt, K., Abraham, C., Ford, T., Woods, H.B., & Anderson, R. (2015). Implementing health promotion programmes in schools: a realist systematic review of research and experience in the United Kingdom. *Implementation Science, 10*, 149. https://doi.org/10.1186/s13012-015-0338-6

Peters, D.H., Adam, T., Alonge, O., Agyepong, I.A., & Tran, N. (2013). Implementation research: what it is and how to do it. *The BMJ, 347*, f6753. https://doi.org/10.1136/bmj.f6753

Proctor, E., Silmere, H., Raghavan, R., Hovmand, P., Aarons, G., Bunger, A., Griffey, R., & Hensley, M. (2011). Outcomes for implementation research: conceptual distinctions, measurement challenges, and research agenda. *Administration and Policy in Mental Health, 38*(2), 65–76. https://doi.org/10.1007/s10488-010-0319-7

Rabin, B.A., Glasgow, R.E., Kerner, J.F., Klump, M.P., & Brownson, R.C. (2010). Dissemination and implementation research on community-based cancer prevention: a systematic review. *American Journal of Preventive Medicine, 38*(4), 443–56. https://doi.org/10.1016/j.amepre.2009.12.035

Rabin, B.A., & Brownson, R.C. (2017). Developing the terminology for dissemination and implementation research. In Brownson, R.C., Colditz, G.A., & Proctor, E.K. (Eds.), *Dissemination and Implementation Research in Health: Translating Science to Practice* (pp. 19–45). Oxford University Press.

Rogers, E.M. (2003). *Diffusion of Innovations* (5th ed.). Free Press.

Rychetnik, L., Bauman, A., Laws, R., King, L., Rissel, C., Nutbeam, D., Colagiuri, S., & Caterson, I. (2012). Translating research for evidence-based public health: key concepts and future directions. *Journal of Epidemiology and Community Health, 66*(12), 1187–92. https://doi.org/10.1136/jech-2011-200038

Saldana, L., Chamberlain, P., Bradford, W.D., Campbell, M., & Landsverk, J. (2014). The cost of implementing new strategies (COINS): A method for mapping implementation resources using the stages of implementation completion. *Children and Youth Services Review, 39*, 177–82. https://doi.org/10.1016/j.childyouth.2013.10.006

Scheirer, M.A., & Dearing, J.W. (2011). An agenda for research on the sustainability of public health programs. *American Journal of Public Health, 101*(11), 2059–67. https://doi.org/10.2105/AJPH.2011.300193

Schell, S.F., Luke, D.A., Schooley, M.W., Elliott, M.B., Herbers, S.H., Mueller, N.B., & Bunger, A.C. (2013). Public health program capacity for sustainability: a new framework. *Implementation Science, 8*, 15. https://doi.org/10.1186/1748-5908-8-15

Shadish, W.R., Cook, T.D., & Campbell, D.T. (2001). *Experimental and Quasi-Experimental Designs for Generalized Causal Inference.* Houghton Mifflin.

Shillinger, D. (2010). *An Introduction to Effectiveness, Dissemination and Implementation Research: A Resource Manual for Community-Engaged Research.* Clinical and Translational Science Institute at the University of California San Francisco.

Smith, M., Ory, M.G., Ahn, S., Kulinski, K.P., Jiang, L., Horel, S., & Lorig, K. (2014). National dissemination of chronic disease self-management education programs: an incremental examination of delivery characteristics. *Frontiers in Public Health, 2*, 227. https://doi.org/10.3389/fpubh.2014.00227

Steckler, A., & McLeroy, K.R. (2008). The importance of external validity. *American Journal of Public Health, 98*(1), 9–10. https://doi.org/10.2105/AJPH.2007.126847

Stirman, S.W., Miller, C.J., Toder, K., & Calloway, A. (2013). Development of a framework and coding system for modifications and adaptations of evidence-based interventions. *Implementation Science, 8*, 65. https://doi.org/10.1186/1748-5908-8-65

Stirman, S.W., Kimberly, J., Cook, N., Calloway, A., Castro, F., & Charns, M. (2012). The sustainability of new programs and innovations: a review of the empirical literature and recommendations for future research. *Implementation Science, 7*, 17. https://doi.org/10.1186/1748-5908-7-17

Tabak, R.G., Khoong, E.C., Chambers, D.A., & Brownson, R.C. (2012). Bridging research and practice, models for dissemination and implementation research. *American Journal of Preventive Medicine, 43*(3), 337–50. https://doi.org/10.1016/j.amepre.2012.05.024

Wilson, K.M., Brady, T.J., Lesesne, C., & NCCDPHP Work Group on Translation. (2011). An organizing framework for translation in public health: the Knowledge to Action Framework. *Preventing Chronic Disease, 8*(2), A46.

World Health Organization. (2013). *Implementation Research in Health: A Practical Guide.* Alliance for Health Policy and Systems Research.

Yano, E.M., Green, L.W., Glanz, K., Ayanian, J.Z., Mittman, B.S., Chollette, V., & Rubenstein, L.V. (2012). Implementation and spread of interventions into the multilevel context of routine practice and policy: implications for the cancer care continuum. *Journal of the National Cancer Institute, 2012*(44), 86–99. https://doi.org/10.1093/jncimonographs/lgs004

CHAPTER 9

Health Program and Policy Development III: Evaluation Strategies

•

Chris Y. Lovato and Judith M. Ottoson

Learning Objectives

After completing the chapter, the reader will be able to:

- Define program evaluation, including the different types of evaluation and how they are used.
- Explain how the PRECEDE-PROCEED model integrates with the US Centers for Disease Control and Prevention (CDC)'s *Framework for Program Evaluation in Public Health*.
- Describe the steps involved in conducting an evaluation and how the widely adopted "Evaluation Standards" are applied to each step of the process.
- Identify key resources that you can use to support program evaluation.

INTRODUCTION

How will you know if the program developed and implemented achieves the objectives identified in earlier phases of PRECEDE-PROCEED? One of the priorities in Phase 4 is to develop an evaluation plan with strategies that addresses this question and will be used to guide evaluation work in Phases 5–8, as seen in figure 9.1. You will be reassured to see that you have already built, in previous phases, the foundational pieces for an evaluation. This chapter offers a public health framework for evaluation that is conceptually compatible with the PRECEDE-PROCEED model. It addresses key principles and methods to consider in planning, implementing, and using evaluation results for practice-based evidence and evidence-informed public health practice.

It is not feasible to learn everything you need to know about evaluation in a single chapter. There are many formal training programs, courses, books, journals, and websites that focus on the topic, some of which are highlighted or referenced in this chapter. Here we focus on the essential principles of planning an evaluation within the context of PRECEDE-PROCEED, beginning with the earliest planning steps when quantitative program objectives are being developed. Our goal is to provide a practical framework to support planning and implementing an evaluation and to alert you to some key questions and processes to consider as you move forward.

Program planning and evaluation are very closely related; the best planning builds evaluation into a program from the very beginning. The best evaluation will be designed so that results will be used continuously to improve program performance and inform ongoing planning and implementation. The planning activities in early PRECEDE-PROCEED phases result in SMART objectives[1] related to social conditions and quality of life (Phase 1); health, behavior, and the environment (Phase 2); and predisposing, enabling, and reinforcing factors (Phase 3). In Phase 4, the practitioner gathers the objectives identified from each previous phase and begins to develop specific intervention, implementation, and evaluation strategies. The evaluation plan developed in Phase 4 will outline a systematic process to assess implementation of the program and the

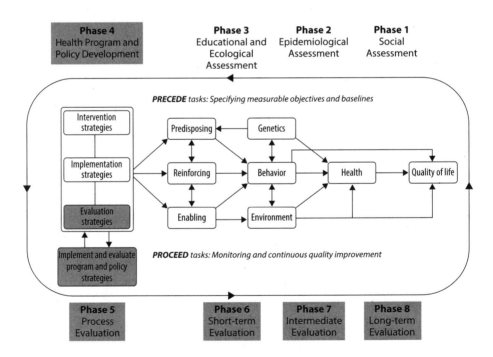

FIGURE 9.1. The fourth phase of PRECEDE-PROCEED model, health program and policy development, continues with the identification, formation, and initiation of priorities among *evaluation* strategies. Evaluation continues in Phases 5–8 to assess whether and how program or policy interventions were implemented as intended and set in motion changes that ultimately affect health and quality of life.

attainment of objectives over time, while at the same time considering the context, resources available, and priorities set by sponsors and stakeholders.

In addition to providing evidence for decision-making, program evaluation supports practice by rendering information that is specific to the context and is informed by stakeholders. Over time, information from evaluation supports the pathway to evidence-informed practice by providing **practice-based evidence** (Green 2008; Green and Ottoson 2004; Institute of Medicine 2012).

WHAT IS PROGRAM EVALUATION?

At the most basic level, program evaluation asks: Did the program we planned work the way we thought it would? Did the program make the intended difference, or even any difference? What did we learn that is useful to practice? The focus of program evaluation—a program, policy, intervention, product, process, component, or whole system (but not a person)—is referred to as the **evaluand**. In this chapter, we use the word "program" interchangeably with "evaluand."

While varying definitions of evaluation populate the literature, we offer the following definition:

> **Evaluation** *is the systematic comparison of an object of interest with a standard of acceptability to provide evidence that is useful to inform decision-making and to demonstrate accountability to social values or policies.*

This definition reflects common understandings of program evaluation, including: (1) questions about the program (*object of interest*); (2) statements of what will be valued or counted as "good" (*standards of acceptability*); (3) design and methodology to answer evaluative questions (*systematic comparison*); (4) a plan for use of the evaluation process and outcomes by stakeholders (*informed decision-making*); and (5) standards for an evaluation practice that is ethical, useful, feasible, accurate, and accountable (*social values*) (Green and Lewis 1986; Patton 2008; Rossi et al. 2019; Shadish et al. 1991; Weiss 1998; Yarbrough et al. 2011).

Many comparisons have been made between research and evaluation, and not everyone agrees on what distinguishes one from the other. Although both use the same designs and methods of systematic investigation, e-*valu*-ation makes value judgements regarding the worth or merit of the evaluand. Key differences between evaluation and research are the involvement of stakeholders in identifying and prioritizing questions, a focus on valuing a program, and the intent that findings will be used for decision-making.

Among the different types of evaluation, it is important to select the type that best suits the evaluation purpose and questions being asked. A description of common evaluation types is provided in table 9.1.

PROGRAM EVALUATION STANDARDS

How will you know if the evaluation itself is well-designed and operating at its full potential? To address these questions and support all types of evaluation, there are five primary standards for program evaluation, as shown in table 9.2. While the evaluation plan enables value judgments about a program, these standards enable judgment about the quality and value of the evaluation itself.[2]

TABLE 9.1. Types and uses of evaluation

Evaluation type	When should this type of evaluation be used?	The evaluation demonstrates . . .	The evaluation is useful because it . . .
Formative evaluation ensures that a program or program activity is feasible, appropriate, and acceptable before it is fully implemented.	• During the development of a new program. • When there are changes in the structure, population, or context of an existing program.	• Whether program elements are needed, understood, and accepted by the population. • The feasibility of evaluation.	• Allows for modifications before full implementation. • Maximizes the likelihood of program success.
Process evaluation, program monitoring or **implementation evaluation** determine whether program inputs, activities, and outputs have been implemented as intended.	• Before (inputs), during (activities), and after (outputs) the program is implemented.	• The extent to which the program is being implemented as designed. • Whether the program is accessible and acceptable to the intended population.	• Can provide early warning signs that the implementation is not proceeding as planned. • Monitors whether and how well the program plans and activities are implemented. • Helps explain the influences on program outcomes.
Outcome evaluation (short-term and intermediate) assesses program "near-term" effects in the intended population.	• After the program has had contact with its intended recipients.	• The extent to which the program is having an effect on the target population and their attitudes, knowledge and behaviors.	• Can tell whether the program is being effective in meeting its short-term and intermediate objectives.

TABLE 9.1. (*continued*)

Evaluation type	When should this type of evaluation be used?	The evaluation demonstrates . . .	The evaluation is useful because it . . .
Outcome evaluation (long-term and social impact) assesses program effects in the intended population by assessing ultimate program objectives and goals.	• During the operation of an existing program, at appropriate intervals. • At the end of a program.	• The degree to which the program meets its ultimate health and quality of life objectives.	• Provides evidence for use in strategic planning, policy and funding decisions. • Provides evidence that behavioral and/or health status changes resulted in population health improvements or social change.
Economic evaluation assesses the costs or consequences of one or more alternative programs or interventions.	• At the beginning of a program. • During the operation of an existing program. • At the end of a program.	• Direct and indirect resource use compared to the program's outcomes.	• Provides program managers and funders data about return on investment.

Sources: Adapted from Centers for Disease Control and Prevention. (n.d.) *Types of Evaluation.* Retrieved April 10, 2021, from https://www.cdc.gov/std/Program/pupestd/Types%20of%20Evaluation.pdf; and Task Force on Community Preventive Services. (2005). Understanding and using the economic evidence. In Zaza, S., Briss, S., Briss, P.A., & Harris, K.W. (Eds.), *The Guide to Community Preventive Services: What Works to Promote Health* (pp. 449–63). Oxford University Press.

TABLE 9.2. Program evaluation standards

Standard	Definition
Utility	Ensure an evaluation will serve the information needs of intended users.
Feasibility	Ensure an evaluation will be realistic, prudent, diplomatic, and frugal.
Propriety	Ensure an evaluation will be conducted legally, ethically and with due regard for the welfare of those involved in the evaluation, as well as those affected by its results.
Accuracy	Ensure an evaluation will reveal and convey technically adequate and useful information about the features that determine worth or merit of the program being evaluated.
Evaluation accountability	Ensure responsible use of resources to produce value.

Source: Adapted from Yarbrough, D.B., Shulha, L.M., Hopson, R.K., & Caruthers, F.A. (2011). *The Program Evaluation Standards: A Guide for Evaluators and Evaluation Users* (3rd ed.). SAGE Publishing.

WHY CONDUCT PROGRAM EVALUATION?

The overarching purpose of evaluation is to contribute to evidence-informed decision-making about programs and policies intended to influence the community's quality of life. Rather than deciding a program's fate by whim, assumptions, bias, or hopes, data from an evaluation bring evidence to bear on whether and how a program works (or not). Evaluation also helps to confirm whether evidence-based practices from the experimentally-controlled research literature are consistent with the practice-based evidence from the actual setting in which you are working (Green 2008; Green and Glasgow 2006). For example, there may be research evidence from a randomized controlled trial that a program to reduce vaping is successful, but there may not be evidence that it is successful in a low-income, bilingual Asian population of males between 13 and 17 years of age (Green and Ottoson 2004).

Some may argue that resources are better invested in program delivery than evaluation. Yet despite comprehensive planning, there is no guarantee a program will work as intended or as demonstrated in a controlled research trial (Green and Ottoson 2004). Real-world contexts are messy and can be filled with competing expectations, power differentials, limited resources, and morphing plans (Bechar and Mero-Jaffe 2014; Cashman et al. 2008; Donaldson et al. 2002; Flicker 2008; Ottoson and Hawe 2009). Evaluation seeks evidence about programs that is gathered systematically. It doesn't take it on faith that programs unfold as planned or achieve intended or unintended outcomes, or any outcomes at all.

Misunderstandings about the purpose of an evaluation can lead to seemingly opposite expectations for evaluation. For example, some stakeholders warmly welcome evaluation as a way to market only the positive aspects of their programs to funders or intended recipients, while leaving out areas needing improvement. Other stakeholders may find evaluation so threatening to their work, their constituents, or their livelihood that they want nothing to do with it and might actively resist it. They may grudgingly work with the evaluation or even obstruct it or deny its veracity. For some, the mere mention of the word "evaluation" may trumpet the possible detection of something gone awry or sound a warning that scarce program resources may be diverted (Green and Kreuter 1999).

Whatever triggers misunderstanding and anxiety about evaluation can be considerably diminished by attending to a systematic and participatory planning process that precedes the implementation and evaluation of the program, as seen in chapter 2. In the context of PRECEDE-PROCEED, program evaluation does *not* start with the assumption that the program is "good" or "bad"; rather, the evaluation is designed to assess elements of the program useful to decision-making and help to manage, improve, and adapt the program to its context. Sound decisions and credible evaluation cannot be based on evaluation findings that only highlight positive aspects of the program or ignore negative aspects (or vice versa). Quality evaluations meet all the program evaluation standards as laid out in table 9.2.

INTEGRATING PRECEDE-PROCEED WITH THE US CDC EVALUATION FRAMEWORK

The widely applied CDC *Framework for Program Evaluation in Public Health* provides a step-by-step guide to support evaluation planning (Centers for Disease Control and Prevention, 1999; 2017). The framework sets out a series of six actions or steps that are centered around five evaluation standards, as shown in figure 9.2. All five standards are applied within each of the six steps of the evaluation process. A checklist that aligns the evaluation standards with each of the evaluation steps is provided in Appendix C.

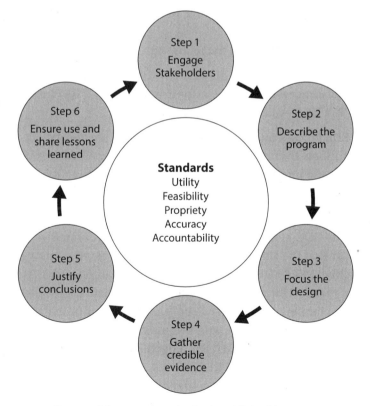

FIGURE 9.2. Framework for program evaluation in public health. *Source:* Adapted from Centers for Disease Control and Prevention (2017).

Like PRECEDE-PROCEED, the CDC framework emphasizes an in-depth understanding of context and engagement of program stakeholders to develop and implement an evaluation plan. Both PRECEDE-PROCEED and the CDC framework encourage a systematic process to address questions about "what works" and provide practical information to support evidence-informed decision-making. We emphasize that although these frameworks describe the planning and evaluation processes in phases or steps, these actions are iterative and usually overlap in practice.

While we introduce the CDC framework to highlight the evaluation process, please note that it is consistent with and complementary to PRECEDE-PROCEED, which we have aligned in figure 9.3. Keep in mind that PRECEDE phases (i.e., Phases 1–3 and the intervention and implementation strategies in Phase 4) are critical to the early steps of an evaluation plan. If the planner has not continuously linked with stakeholders, or has not described and set priorities among needs, or understood the context, or described the proposed intervention, there is no foundation for an evaluation plan. It is in such circumstances, "the sins of the planner are often visited on the evaluation" (Weiss 1977, 122). If the early steps in the process have been completed, these elements will have been addressed and constructing an evaluation plan will be feasible and productive.

As you study figure 9.3, note the following:

- The eight planning phases of PRECEDE-PROCEED are aligned with their corresponding evaluation steps; for example, PRECEDE Phase 1 aligns with PROCEED evaluation step 1.

- PRECEDE Phase 4 and evaluation steps 2 and 3 are fleshed out in more detail to show the constituent components of a comprehensive plan, including the intervention, implementation, and evaluation strategies.

- Evaluation steps 4, 5, and 6 are reiterated in PROCEED Phases 5–8.

Linking the CDC evaluation framework to the PRECEDE-PROCEED model makes it clear that the key aspects of the evaluation planning process are situated throughout PRECEDE Phases 1–4; evaluation planning doesn't just happen at one point in time. Unfortunately, evaluation is sometimes the last thing considered when planning a program, which leads to various problems. Remember that planning, implementation, and evaluation are not silos, but interactive with each other and the context.[3] For a detailed description of the alignment between evaluation steps and PRECEDE-PROCEED phases, see Appendix D. We turn now to a more in-depth understanding of each of the steps in the evaluation process.

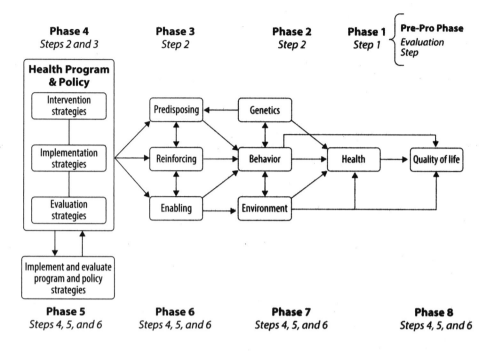

Phase 4   **Phase 3**   **Phase 2**   **Phase 1**   **Pre-Pro Phase**
Steps 2 and 3   *Step 2*   *Step 2*   *Step 1*   *Evaluation Step*

Phase 5   **Phase 6**   **Phase 7**   **Phase 8**
Steps 4, 5, and 6   *Steps 4, 5, and 6*   *Steps 4, 5, and 6*   *Steps 4, 5, and 6*

FIGURE 9.3. PRECEDE-PROCEED Phases aligned with Evaluation Steps

EVALUATION STEP 1: ENGAGE THE STAKEHOLDERS

Sage advice to anyone considering an evaluation is to ask: "Who wants the evaluation, and why?" (Weiss 1998). Multiple stakeholders are likely to be interested in the evaluation of program process and outcomes, including social impact (Institute of Medicine 2012).[4] The CDC framework suggests three broad categories of stakeholders (Centers for Disease Control and Prevention 2018):

1. *Managers and practitioners.* Those involved in program planning, or operation: management, program staff, partners, funding agencies, and coalition members.

2. *Recipients and intended beneficiaries.* Those served or affected by the program: patients or clients, advocacy groups, community members, employers, and elected officials.

3. *Policy decision makers.* Those who are the intended users of evaluation findings: persons in a position to make decisions about the program, such as partners, funding agencies, coalition members, and the general public or taxpayers.

The first two groups will have been engaged in the planning process (see Community Engagement in chapter 2). At this stage, you may also be recruiting additional stakeholders who will be evaluation users (the third group) and are critical to meeting the utility standard, as seen in table 9.2. Engaging stakeholders helps planners and practitioners identify the purposes of evaluation, likely uses, what might count as program success or failure, possible resources, and contextual dynamics. Those who need to make decisions about the program, such as whether to renew funding or to adopt or continue the program, need a say in what will be useful and accurate bases for such decisions. Those who need to implement the program and the evaluation need a say in what is operationally feasible. Those affected by the program need a say in the evaluation's **propriety** or appropriateness.

Engaging stakeholders involves not only talking to them, but listening, studying their materials, determining priorities, understanding their questions about the program, and uncovering power differentials. Such discovery includes understanding not only the overt or legitimate purposes of the evaluation, such as program improvement, but possible covert or nefarious purposes for the evaluation, such as the elimination of a program or the grudge removal of program personnel (Weiss 1998). Understanding all such reasons for evaluation helps to align the evaluation with the program evaluation standards.

When working with stakeholders, it is important to observe who has been included, excluded, or minimized from engagement. Funders, for example, have a lot at stake in program planning and evaluation outcomes and will sometimes be deferred to as the key stakeholder voice. Intended beneficiaries may be difficult to access for their views on program valuing. Program operations may enable or facilitate some stakeholders' or staff viewpoints, but not others. When engaging stakeholders, be aware of who is at the evaluation table and who is not. Maintain cultural sensitivity to the context and circumstances of the evaluation. Through the kind of participatory planning that is a hallmark of PRECEDE-PROCEED, the planner will already have a good sense of the stakeholders, what is important to them, and their interest in the program. For questions that will guide you in engaging stakeholders and achieving the evaluations standards, see the Step 1 checklist in Appendix C.

EVALUATION STEP 2: DESCRIBE THE PROGRAM

In earlier phases of PRECEDE-PROCEED, you will have compiled the situational evidence necessary to describe the program and develop a logic model that addresses Step 2 of the CDC evaluation framework. Step 2 tasks the evaluation planner with confirming that there is an accurate description of the program or evaluand, including its purpose, inputs/resources, activities, outputs (i.e., the products delivered), and outcomes over time, as well as graphically portraying this understanding in an evaluation logic model. Remember, you cannot plan *how* to evaluate if you do not know *what* you are evaluating. To apply the evaluation standards to Step 2 of the evaluation framework, use the checklist in Appendix C.

Why are logic models useful? The PRECEDE-PROCEED model and the evaluation logic model provide a visual representation of the program and its intended effects. These complementary models serve as communication tools for stakeholders to work out how they think or theorize programs work.[5] An evaluation logic model sharpens the evaluation perspective on the program by revealing the intended causal chain and details of program inputs, activities, outputs, and levels of outcomes. As such, it is a roadmap of the planned program; it is *not* a roadmap for how we will conduct an evaluation (e.g., survey a population or analyze data). Characteristics of the PRECEDE-PROCEED model and an evaluation logic model are compared in table 9.3.

TABLE 9.3. Comparison between PRECEDE-PROCEED and an evaluation logic model

The PRECEDE-PROCEED model . . .	An evaluation logic model . . .
Focuses on the full program cycle (planning, implementation, and evaluation).	Focuses only on the evaluation and outlines the program's expected or theoretical cause-and-effect chain.
Outlines a broad program rationale, showing connections between quality of life, health issues and their associated factors, mechanisms for change, the intervention, and the results when it is implemented.	Outlines the intended causal link among inputs, activities, outputs, and outcomes that will be addressed in the evaluation.
Is prescriptive in nature because it sets out a systematic process using theory and evidence to plan, implement, and evaluate a program.	Is descriptive in nature because it focuses on the chain of causes and effects leading to short-term, intermediate, and ultimate outcomes of interest.

Numerous open-access resources are available to guide the development of an evaluation logic model.[6] These resources exemplify different visual representations of logic models. Although logic models are often drawn in a unidimensional, linear fashion using boxes and arrows, they can be drawn as circles, three-dimensional diagrams, and any number of figures, such as a tree, rainbow, or a wheel.

The generic evaluation logic model shown in figure 9.4 has much in common with the PRECEDE-PROCEED model:

- Long-term, intermediate, and short-term outcomes of the generic evaluation logic model are products of PRECEDE Phases 1–3 and are used for development of the evaluation plan in Phase 4. Further, the outcomes assessed over time in this generic logic model correspond with PROCEED Phases 5, 6, 7, and 8.

- Inputs, activities, and outputs of the generic logic model are the products of intervention and implementation planning that occur in PRECEDE Phase 4. These products are expanded in the generic model (figure 9.4) to show the process and intended casual chain to be evaluated. Also, note that the process evaluation components of the generic model align with PROCEED Phase 5.

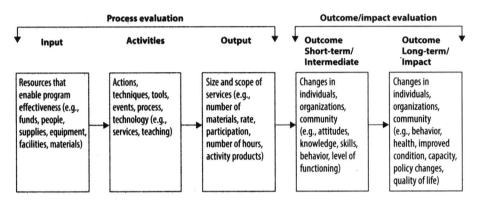

FIGURE 9.4. Generic logic model. *Source:* Adapted from W.F. Kellogg Foundation. (2004). *Logic Model Development Guide.* https://www.wkkf.org/resource-directory/resources/2004/01/logic-model-development-guide

EVALUATION STEP 3: FOCUS THE DESIGN

This evaluation step begins with an understanding of stakeholder questions about the program or intervention. It moves on to specify standards and criteria, choose an appropriate evaluation design, determine who will be sampled, and identify methods needed to collect the relevant data on activities (inputs) and effects (outcomes). As you work through the various components involved in focusing the evaluation design, use the checklist in Appendix C to ensure you are addressing the evaluation standards.

Evaluation Questions

Once you have a good understanding of the program to be evaluated, the next step is to understand what questions stakeholders have about the program. Evaluation questions are derived from the program and its stakeholders. Some stakeholders may be outsiders, such as funding agencies, donors, or policy makers upstream in regional, state, national, or multinational organizations. Some of them may set conditions on the evaluation and sharing of data.

In PRECEDE, evaluation questions are inherent in the goals and SMART objectives that have already been identified and prioritized in Phases 1, 2 and 3. Compare the objective and its inherent question below:

- SMART Objective: There will be a 15% reduction in unplanned pregnancies in the Lindwood School District within three years.

- Evaluation question: Was there a 15% reduction in unplanned pregnancies in the Lindwood School District within three years?

Note that both the objective and the corresponding question identify the criterion or object of interest (unplanned pregnancies) and both contain two standards of acceptability (15% reduction and "within three years"). Much of the work you have done so far to identity and prioritize program objectives can lead seamlessly to evaluation questions. With such similarity, why bother to frame the objective as a question? Answer: Communication!

Questions about the program are much more inviting to stakeholders than the technical precision required for objectives. Getting stakeholders to specify "objects of interest" is often hard enough. Getting them to specify "standards of acceptability" can be even harder. By approaching this task with the familiarity of questions, stakeholders are welcomed into the evaluation process. Also, consider that stakeholders may have evaluative questions about the program that are different from the objectives identified during the planning process. These questions need to be considered for their potential priority, usefulness, and relevance. It may be necessary to convert those questions into objectives. Differences of opinions, the usefulness and feasibility of results, and design possibilities arise when stakeholders understand the relevance of key questions. The bottom line is that good objectives and clear questions go hand in hand. Which will be most engaging to stakeholders? An expanded generic logic model is shown in figure 9.5 (building on figure 9.4) that identifies three layers of generic evaluation questions: (Layer 1) process and outcome questions; (Layer 2) input, activity, output, and outcome questions; and (Layer 3) more program-specific questions.

Effective evaluation questions have several key characteristics. They (1) are derived from the program plan (not the evaluator's agenda); (2) reflect various stakeholder priorities, needs, and interests; (3) fit the stage of the program (developing, new, or existing); (4) consider valuing (what will count as success or not); (5) are useful for decision-making; and (6) are answerable within available resources and constraints. Setting priorities among all the possible questions from a wide range of stakeholders is necessary to ensure and gain support for the wise use of resources and the provision of information useful to key decision makers. Work from previous PRECEDE-PROCEED phases in setting priorities

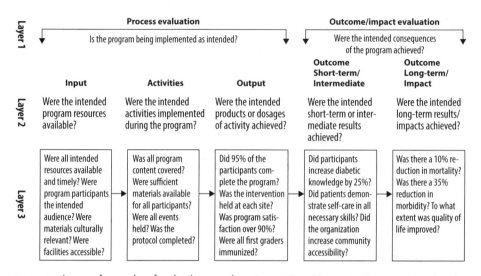

FIGURE 9.5. Layers of examples of evaluation questions. *Source:* Adapted from W.F. Kellogg Foundation. (2004). *Logic Model Development Guide.* https://www.wkkf.org/resource-directory/resources/2004/01/logic-model-development -guide   .

among objectives will also be helpful in setting priorities among evaluation questions. As you do this work, keep in mind that over time these objectives may evolve with the further understanding that comes with program development and implementation.

Valuing: Objects of Interest and Standards of Acceptability

E-*valu*-ation is fundamentally about placing value on something. This is the heart of the evaluation process and one of its most challenging steps. Determining value involves answering the overarching question: What will count as "success" or "goodness"? A case in which evaluators worked with stakeholders to determine what would count as evidence of program success is described in box 9.1.

In keeping with the definition of evaluation offered earlier in this chapter, there are two key components of the valuing process: (1) object(s) of interest; and (2) standard(s) of acceptability. An object of interest is "what" component(s) or process(es) will be used to "value" the program. Many such objects of interest, such as resources (input), tools or processes (activities), size and scope of services (output), knowledge and skills (from short- to intermediate-range outcomes), and behavior or capacity changes (long-term outcomes), are shown in figure 9.5. The work already done to identify objectives will have these objects of interest clearly identified if they are SMART objectives. From a planning perspective, these are the objects of interest that the program will implement or work towards; from an evaluation perspective, the success of the program will be based on these priority objects of interest.

BOX 9.1
Policy Evaluation: What Will Count as "Success?"

The Robert Wood Johnson Foundation requested a utilization-focused evaluation of its Active Living Research (ALR) program. The intent of the ALR program is to translate and disseminate evidence to advocates, policy makers, and practitioners aimed at preventing childhood obesity and promoting active communities. A key evaluation question was: To what extent did ALR contribute to policy?

An early task for the evaluators and stakeholders was to determine "what" would count as evidence of successful policy contribution. The evaluators conducted key informant interviews, with 136 representatives of first-line potential users of ALR research products such as state physical activity and nutrition program coordinators, policy makers, scientists, and funders. Literature and document reviews supplemented a deeper understanding of the ALR contexts.

Results of the evaluation showed ALR contributions to policy discussions were found across a spectrum of policy development phases that included describing the problem, raising awareness of alternative strategies, convening partners, and evaluating policy implementation (as seen in the figure).

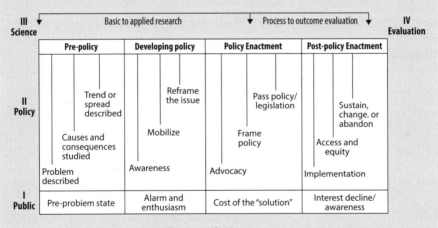

Policy contribution spectra

These various phases and criteria are the "objectives of interest" needed in evaluation to determine "success." Working through the early phases of the PRECEDE-PROCEED model, by engaging the stakeholders, these objects of interest can emerge. Without them, "what" are you evaluating?

Source: Ottoson, J.M., Green. L.W., Beery, W.L., Senter, S.K., Cahill, C.L., Pearson, D.C., Greenwald, H.P., Hamre, R., & Leviton, L. (2009). Policy-contribution assessment and field-building analysis of the Robert Wood Johnson Foundation's Active Living Research Program. *American Journal of Preventive Medicine, 36*(2 Suppl. 1), S34–S43. https://doi.org/10.1016/j.amepre.2008.10.010

If the object of interest changes during or after the program in an intended direction—increases, decreases, stabilizes—then the program is "successful" or "good." Standard(s) of acceptability set "how much" or "by when" the object of interest has to change enough to be considered successful or good. An example of standards of acceptability applied to a school program is shown in table 9.4.

Standards of acceptability can be set in several ways (Green and Kreuter 1999). They may be *scientific standards* based on best practices or best processes derived from systematic literature reviews. *Historical standards* may be used by administrators based on past performance of the program. *Normative standards* are those based on performance by comparable organizations, jurisdictions, or programs. *Compromise standards* result from negotiation and consensus by multiple stakeholders. Perhaps the most problematic are *arbitrary standards*. Without any rationale, such standards can easily be set unrealistically high and doom the program to fail, or too low to assure the program will be viewed as successful no matter what. In all cases, those involved in evaluation should establish standards that are realistic and attainable given local resources and circumstances.

TABLE 9.4. Standards of acceptability, illustrated with a school program example

Standard of acceptability	Example of an evaluation question
Extent, amount, duration	Have at least 95% of kindergarteners completed all required vaccinations?
Accurate, efficient, effective	Did the instructor cover the five program components?
Speed, timing	Were all program supplies delivered before the fall semester commenced?
Useful, enlightening	Did the school principal fully implement one of the report's recommendations?
Costs	Was the program completed within the given budget?
Inclusive, fair, just	Were program participants proportional to the diversity of the school?

Evaluation Designs

Having worked with stakeholders to clarify the purposes, questions, values, resources, and intended uses of the evaluation, you are ready to decide upon a design for the evaluation. An evaluation design, like a research design, clarifies when data are collected (timing), from whom (sampling), and how (methods). Design provides a systematic basis for comparing each "object of interest" with a "standard of acceptability" (Green and Kreuter 1999). The strength of the evaluation design contributes to the credibility of the methods and analyses used to evaluate.

Design is an important consideration for both process and outcome evaluation and is relevant to the different standards of acceptability previously described. This section provides an overview of commonly used quantitative and qualitative designs that are often applied in multiple- or mixed-method evaluations. For some, this material may be a review; for others, it will be new territory and consultants or academic partners may be helpful in constructing a credible design. Many additional resources are available that address evaluation design and may also be helpful.[7]

Quantitative Designs

A *quantitative evaluation design* is appropriate when your evaluation question includes an object of interest and standard of acceptability that both require numerical measurement. For example, the quantitative measure might be whether there has been a change in vaccination rates. To evaluate numerical outcomes, there are four categories of design: (1) experimental, (2) quasi-experimental, (3) natural experiments, and (4) non-experimental (Shadish et al. 2002). The following types of designs are commonly used to assess the intended program effect:

- *Experimental designs* are considered the most rigorous approach because they involve the random assignment of participants (either as individuals, or as large numbers of neighborhoods, census tracts, organizations, or other aggregates of people) to treatment and control groups so that differences found between the groups can be attributed to the intervention and not something else distinguishing the groups. In evaluation, they can be used to assess whether a program has had an effect on priority outcomes. Random assignment depends on the assumption of equality of groups.

- In *quasi-experimental studies*, the evaluator identifies a "comparison group"—that is, a community or population that is demographically similar to the target population, but is not receiving the program. Comparisons are made between the two groups. Like experimental designs, this type of design is used to assess whether a program has had an effect on priority outcomes, but depends for its validity on the ability to make the comparison between very similar groups.

- *Natural experiments* are studies that compare a naturally occurring event (not under the control of the evaluators or program planners) with a comparison condition. In order to identify the effect of the program/intervention, natural experimental designs require a comparison of a population of participants who receive the intervention and a similar population who do not (or groups varying in levels of treatment/intervention) (Craig et al.

2012). For example, comparing outcomes related to a new health regulation in different regions where there is no such regulation. This design represents an important option for program evaluation in an applied setting where randomizing participants to a treatment and control group is not possible for ethical or practical reasons.

- *Non-experimental designs* are also useful for process questions that can be addressed numerically. This type of design describes the situation without determining cause and effect. Participants are not *randomly* assigned to receive or not receive the intervention; thus, valid conclusions about cause and effect are very tenuous. Data are collected over time or looking back in time. For example, a descriptive design might address an evaluation question on program satisfaction using a survey over a single or multiple points in time. An example of a PRECEDE-PROCEED evaluation that used a non-experimental design is described in box 9.2.

BOX 9.2

Evaluation of a Hypertension Program Using a Single-Group Pretest/Post-Test Design

A published evaluation of a community-based hypertension program, designed for adults 40–59 years of age and living in the Philippines, was planned using the PRECEDE-PROCEED model (Calano et al. 2019). The program included four sessions delivered over a two-month period by nursing students and community health nurses. The sessions included taking blood pressure readings, health education sessions, motivational interviews, individualized lifestyle modification planning, and household visits.

The evaluation used a single-group pretest/post-test design to address two evaluation questions: (1) Was there was an increase in knowledge, adherence, and improved blood pressure scores of participants before and after the program, and (2) What was the magnitude of effect of the program on the knowledge, adherence and blood pressure scores? A total of 50 participants participated in the program. Data were analyzed using descriptive statistics and RM-MANOVA. Mean adherence, systolic blood pressure, and diastolic blood pressure significantly improved, attributing >25% of the change. Knowledge scores were also significantly higher following the program; however, this accounted for only 9% of the improvement. The authors conclude that the program is effective for adults in their community. They also suggest that the evaluation provides a framework for developing new programs or enhancing existing programs in Philippine communities.

Source: Excerpted from Calano, B.J.D., Cacal, M.J.B., Cal, C.B., Calletor, K.P., Guce, F.I.C.C., Bongar, M.V.V., & Macindo, J.R.B. (2019). Effectiveness of a community-based health programme on the blood pressure control, adherence and knowledge of adults with hypertension: A PRECEDE-PROCEED model approach. *Journal of Clinical Nursing, 28*(9–10), 1879–88. https://doi.org/10.1111/jocn.14787

Qualitative Designs

Qualitative designs address evaluation differently than quantitative approaches. For example, the objects of interest in a qualitative question might include staff experience in program implementation, the program process, cultural sensitivity of intervention materials, or unintended outcomes. The qualitative assessment might include descriptions of observations, participants or staff reactions to the program, and participants' experiences of how the program has affected them personally (Green and Kreuter 1999).

There are multiple traditions in qualitative inquiry, including biography, ethnography, realism, context analysis, phenomenology, heuristic inquiry, grounded theory, social constructivism, narrative inquiry, ethnomethodology, hermeneutics, case study, and many other approaches (Creswell and Poth 2018; Patton 2015; Savin-Baden and Major 2013; Thorne 2016). Describing all of these traditions goes far beyond the scope of this chapter and each has a literature of its own. Here we highlight three traditions used more frequently in program evaluation and suited to addressing evaluative questions—phenomenology, case study, and ethnography. All of these approaches are commonly used in mixed-method evaluations. We encourage readers to delve further into mixed-method designs by consulting additional introductory resources.[8]

- A **phenomenological study** describes the "lived experience" regarding a concept or phenomenon. The evaluation question(s) focuses on the perceived meaning of an experience, such as participation in an intervention or the effects of an intervention on a participant—for example, what it means to a patient to be part of a cancer survivor program (Creswell and Poth 2018).

- **Case studies** focus on a single case or multiple cases of a bounded system, such as a school classroom, community clinic, state public health department, or federal agency. For example, a case study evaluated the degree to which school districts promoted equitable access to emergency nutrition programming during the COVID-19 pandemic (McLoughlin et al. 2020). Case studies use detailed inquiry to examine the case(s) over time and with in-depth data collection and analysis. Case studies can be entirely qualitative, or they can combine qualitative and quantitative data (Yin 2018).

- **Ethnographic studies** focus on the description and interpretation of a cultural group, social group, or system. This approach has its roots in anthropology and involves prolonged observation, usually through participant observation in which evaluators immerse themselves into the day-to-day operations of a program. While ethnographic design *per se* is not commonly used in evaluation studies, many of the methods and techniques used, such as observation and interviews, have derived from this approach (Creswell and Poth 2018; Savin-Baden and Major 2013).

Quality of Evaluation Designs

The quality of the evaluation design used is a key consideration in ensuring the *credibility* and believability of findings. The way in which quality is determined differs for quantitative and qualitative designs. For quantitative evaluation, *reliability* refers to the repeatability of the findings (whether the results would be the same if the evaluation were done again, exactly as before). *Internal validity* refers to whether the program is the reason for the observed outcomes, rather than something else. It is applicable to the evaluation of programs in which you are trying to establish, with confidence, the causality of the intervention on the outcomes. *External validity* "refers to the degree to which findings from a study or set of studies can be generalized to and relevant for populations, settings, and times other than those in which the original studies were conducted" (Brownson et al. 2018; Green 2008; Green and Glasgow 2006; Green and Ottoson 2004).

A strong design protects against threats to internal validity such as selection bias, other events that occur in the setting (such as a policy change in the middle of the program evaluation), or the effects of participating in an evaluation. These threats are addressed by using an experimental design that randomly assigns participants to intervention and control groups and masks ("blinds") whether an individual knows whether he or she is in the intervention or control group. Because program evaluation takes place in practice settings, it is often not possible to assign participants (randomly or not) to treatment and control groups. Therefore, evaluation designs most often rely on quasi-experimental, non-experimental, and natural designs. A table illustrating quantitative designs most commonly used by evaluators is provided in Appendix E.

Most evaluators and researchers agree that the criteria for good quantitative design require translation or rethinking to be relevant for qualitative designs. In qualitative approaches, the criteria for a good design are ensuring that findings are *dependable*, *credible* (trustworthy), *transferable*, and *confirmable* (Miles et al. 2014). To accomplish this, the qualitative evaluator uses analytic strategies such as *triangulation*, confirming interpretations and conclusions from multiple sources, and "member checking" findings with participants. Using mixed methods helps to balance the strengths and weaknesses of a solely qualitative or quantitative approach. For example, a qualitative method can help to corroborate findings through triangulation and provide insight into understanding why an evaluand or intervention was (or was not) successful.

The tired and outdated argument that quantitative data are more credible than qualitative data misses the strengths and weaknesses of both approaches. There are times when policy-making bodies are moved to decisions about health problems by compelling stories, and other times when they act on the strength of numerical data. Stories can be more powerful than numbers and vice versa, depending on the question asked and the intended users.

Sampling

In an evaluation using a quantitative design, it will often be impossible to collect data from all those who receive the intervention (e.g., a neighborhood or community). In these cases, you must rely on a representative sample to collect the data from a portion of the population. This type of probability sample is achieved through a random selection of participants. Unfortunately, in program evaluation, a ***random sample*** is often not possible. Although ***convenience samples*** are often used (participants who are most easily reached, typically volunteers), they are considered to be biased because they are not representative of the target population. In these cases, the evaluator can perform statistical analyses to provide evidence whether the convenience sample represents the target population by comparing demographics and other key characteristics for which data are available on both the program population and the evaluation sample. Besides the comparability of the people's personal characteristics, the comparability of the experimental and non-experimental settings should be considered (Green 2008).

In qualitative studies, it also may not be feasible to collect data from all participants, and often it may not be desirable given the time and resources available. Qualitative inquiry uses ***purposive sampling*** versus random sampling. Here, the evaluator recruits participants with particular characteristics according to the evaluation question(s) being asked. There are two types of purposive sampling: (1) ***snowball sampling***, and (2) ***theoretical sampling***. In snowball sampling, the participants refer the evaluator to others in the target population who are then recruited into the evaluation, such as neighbors or friends. In theoretical sampling, the evaluator intentionally seeks out the specific types of participants, such as a particular age group or geographic location, whom the proposed program theory intends to benefit from the intervention (Morse 2011).

Multiple or Mixed Methods

The most common evaluation designs use multiple methods or mixed methods. That is because "There is rarely a single evaluation methodology that can fully capture all of the complexities of how programs operate in the real world" (Bamberger 2012, 3). *Multiple methods* evaluation is a broad category that refers to the use of any two different methods (either both qualitative or both quantitative *or* a mix of qualitative and quantitative). *Mixed methods* refers more specifically to using qualitative and quantitative methods together (e.g., rated items on a survey and interviews). In mixed methods the two forms of data are integrated, drawing on the combined strengths of each approach. This combination provides a deeper understanding than either quantitative or qualitative data alone

(Creswell and Poth 2018). A list of common methods for gathering quantitative and qualitative data, or both, is provided in table 9.5.

Sources of quantitative and qualitative data include existing materials or records, people, and observations. However, the methods used to access that information differ across these two inquiry paradigms. *Quantitative methods*, such as surveys, systematic observations, and program records, produce numerical data that quantifies events, knowledge, attitudes, behaviors, and health outcomes—for example, 50% of participants completed the program, yielding a 30% reduction in youth vaping or a 40% increase in self-esteem measures. *Qualitative methods*, such as in-depth interviews and ethnographic observation, systematically provide rich or "thick" descriptions of meaning, perception, or values, such as participant experiences accessing health care.

These methods work together in mixed methods. For example, quantitative methods can provide numerical ratings of an experience—30% of participants had limited access to fresh vegetables, as an example—while qualitative methods can provide an in-depth understanding of how participants perceive and dealt with their experience. Mixed methods can provide a broader appreciation for the range of responses to a program, and data on unintended outcomes (e.g., lack of access to fresh food worsened a chronic health condition), and expand the communication of evaluation findings to multiple stakeholders. For example, policy makers and community members may better understand and be able to use the descriptive stories from qualitative methods; funding agencies may require quantitative results to justify their investments.

TABLE 9.5. Selected techniques for gathering quantitative and qualitative data

Quantitative methods	Qualitative methods
• Survey (e.g., handout, phone, web-based, mail, with countable answers)	• Interviews (individual or group, in person, video, phone)
• Geographic mapping	• Participant observation / field notes
• Social network diagraming	• Case study
• Simulation, modeling	• Concept mapping
• Logs	• Debriefing sessions
• Registries or records	• Photovoice
• Web use statistics	• Drawing
• Program documents	• Journals or diaries

Source: Adapted from Centers for Disease Control and Prevention. (1999). Framework for program evaluation in public health. *Morbidity and Mortality Weekly Report, 48* (No. RR–11). https://stacks.cdc.gov/view/cdc/5204/cdc_5204_DS1.pdf

EVALUATION STEP 4: GATHER CREDIBLE EVIDENCE

According to the standards of program evaluation, the findings of an evaluation are intended to be used, not shelved. However, if stakeholders and intended users do not find the evaluation process or findings credible, it is highly unlikely that they will use the findings. In program evaluation, the concept of credible evidence includes the quality of evidence (e.g., internal and external validity, *trustworthiness, confirmability, transferability*). However, it is important to understand that credibility goes beyond the quality of evidence. Credibility, which goes beyond the quality of evidence, can be enhanced at every step in the evaluation process with genuine stakeholder involvement, observable sensitivity and cultural relatability of program staff and evaluators, relevant and answerable guiding questions, clear sources of evidence, an appropriate design and methods, and understandable findings. Use the checklist in Appendix C to ensure you are addressing the evaluation standards for this fourth evaluation step. Key concepts and actions that can help enhance the credibility of an evaluation are offered in table 9.6.

TABLE 9.6. Strategies to enhance evaluation credibility

Strategy	Practice considerations
Make valuing a transparent process.	• Program objectives and the questions derived from them are not necessarily neutral or "objective." • Work with stakeholders to develop objectives that contain a fair basis for judging whether the program is "good" or "successful." • The indicators of objectives need to reflect intent and be manageable, trackable over time, and useful for decision-making.
Consider the program evaluation standards at every step.	• Use checklists in Appendix C to consider and document application of standards. • When you cannot fully meet the standards, understand the trade-offs made among them. For example, if the feasibility standard predominates in sample selection, what are the implications for data accuracy?
Ensure the use of evaluation findings by presenting a balance of study strengths and weaknesses.	• All evaluations will likely have limitations. Be up-front about them. • Limitations may include an unrepresentative sample, low response rates, self-reported data, low participation rates, validity and reliability of quantitative measures, generalizability, or unanticipated events. • Explain how limitations may affect findings. For example, delays in data collection may make the findings less useful to decision-makers.
The learning organization integrates evaluation into its processes; evaluation is not an add-on or afterthought.	• The inquiry or learning process needs to be inherent in evaluation. • Evaluation needs to lead with education, not intimidation.

(continued)

TABLE 9.6. (*continued*)

Strategy	Practice considerations
Educate stakeholders about the importance of program process and outcomes.	• "...we want to be sure what the outcomes are outcomes *of*" (Weiss 1977, 10), that "of" being process. • Provide interim and process reports to keep stakeholders engaged throughout the evaluation.
Evaluation logistics need to be planned, managed, and accountable.	• Gain agreement on the evaluation intent, scope of work, team, tasks, budget, timeline, milestones, deadlines, and resources. • Establish an evaluation contract or agreement that spells out *what* is expected by *when* and *who* is responsible for it.

EVALUATION STEP 5: JUSTIFY CONCLUSIONS

The fifth step of the CDC's evaluation framework focuses on the conclusions of the evaluation. "The evaluation conclusions are justified when they are linked to the evidence gathered and judged against agreed-upon values or standards set by the stakeholders" (Centers for Disease Control and Prevention 1999, 18). According to the CDC framework, this step involves analysis, synthesis, and interpretation of findings, use of the standards of acceptability set by stakeholders earlier, and judgements about the value of the program. By having addressed these topics *before* the evaluation is implemented, you will be in a strong position to justify study conclusions. Be sure to consider the evaluations standards in this step, as seen in Appendix C.

At this point, it should come as no surprise that the work needed to justify conclusions isn't something that you do at the end of the evaluation. It is an integral part of the evaluation *planning* process that occurs in Phase 4 of PRECEDE-PROCEED prior to implementing the evaluation plan in Phases 5–8. In Step 5 of the evaluation, we focus on analytic strategies to justify conclusions effectively.

Methods of Analysis

To align evaluation questions with methods of analysis, your first task is to identify the kind of question being asked. Is it a quantitative or qualitative question? By their nature, qualitative questions are primarily exploratory, used to understand underlying reasons or motivations. In contrast, quantitative questions seek numbers to describe the array of participant responses and transform them into categories and statistics, such as quantifying knowledge, attitudes, behaviors, and health outcomes.

The most common types of questions in program evaluation focus on processes and outcomes. Common evaluation questions, their associated type of analyses, and examples of basic analytic strategies that are appropriate for process and outcome questions are listed in table 9.7.

TABLE 9.7. Examples of basic analytic strategies for process and outcome questions

Question	Strategy	Quantitative analytic examples	Qualitative analytic examples
Process evaluation			
What went on in the program?	Describe the program's features and context, and summarize results.	• Using descriptive statistics • Counting what is typical or unique	• Chronicling personal narrative(s) of events • Identifying relative amounts as "more" or "fewer"
Did the program follow what was planned? What were the facilitators and barriers to implementing the program?	Compare what was planned with what occurred. Identify the influences on implementation.	• Using descriptive statistics • Disaggregating data to identify multiple influences • Clustering data to identify like influences	• Chronicling personal narrative(s) of events • Coding data • Grouping data
Did the cost of the program stay within budget?	Describe the costs associated with implementing the program.	• Using descriptive statistics • Making comparisons with budget	• Describing participants' or staff's perceptions of program cost
Outcome/impact evaluation			
Were there changes in short-term, intermediate, or long-term/impact program outcomes?	Compare participants before and after the program. Compare participants and comparison/control group over time.	• Using analysis of variance • Using regression • Identifying commonalities and differences across demographic categories • Identifying deviant cases far from the mean	• Identifying participant patterns and similarities in meaning of perceptions about outcomes
Are there unexpected outcomes that occurred as a result of the program?	Describe any effects of the program that were unpredicted.	• Using descriptive statistics	• Chronicling personal narrative(s)
Economic evaluation			
What was the economic worth of the intervention?	Create a comparative analysis of two or more alternative interventions.	• Identifying cost-effectiveness ratio, cost per case averted, cost per life-year saved	• Describing participant/stakeholder perceptions of program value

Recommendations

Recommendations are the actions proposed for program stakeholders and decision-makers resulting from the evaluation. Recommendations go a step beyond stating whether the program objectives have been attained and whether the program has been effective. They provide specific action steps for consideration that focus on improving, continuing, expanding, reallocating, or terminating the program. Conclusions and recommendations need to be thought through carefully (not at the last minute) and informed by stakeholders. Recommendations that are based on insufficient evidence or not consistent with stakeholders' values can undermine the credibility of the evaluation (Centers for Disease Control and Prevention 1999, 22). Sharing preliminary findings with stakeholders early on to get their insights and ensure you have understood the context will help guide you in interpreting the data and making recommendations. The involvement and support of stakeholders throughout the process of developing recommendations is critical to determining the extent to which results are used and lessons shared. A number of resources can aid the evaluator in developing useful recommendations.[9]

EVALUATION STEP 6: ENSURE USE AND SHARE LESSONS LEARNED

Having worked through the previous steps of the evaluation framework, you should now have credible, justified evaluation findings in hand. But how will those findings get into the hands of intended users and inform program decision-making? It is a myth that the mere presence of findings ensures their use. The use of evaluation findings requires forethought and effort.

Again, the good news is that you've been working on and preparing for the use of evaluation findings in the previous phases of PRECEDE-PROCEED and steps in the CDC evaluation framework. Through your continual engagement with stakeholders, you know who the intended users are, along with their evaluation purposes and questions. They have identified what would be useful information to their decision-making, the kind of data collection methods that would be credible, and the kinds of analyses that would be understandable and actionable. Interim reports and feedback about the ongoing evaluation help keep intended users aware and involved in the program and the evaluation. With this level of preparation, intended users of the evaluation findings are more likely to be waiting for, even preparing to receive, the findings than surprised by an evaluation report plopped on their desk months after initial contact.

Plans for useful, ongoing feedback about the program and broader dissemination of findings need to be made in conjunction with stakeholders as early as possible in the evaluation planning. Timelines, milestones, and funding requirements need to consider when and how findings are reported. There may be issues of confidentiality, ownership of the data, negative findings, and data misuse to consider in the dissemination of findings. Most critically, the dissemination of findings needs to meet the standards of program evaluation: ***utility***, ***accuracy***, ***propriety***, ***feasibility***, and ***evaluation accountability***. It is unethical to "pick and choose" findings and turn them into a marketing report for program sponsors. All findings need to be considered and reported in line with the evaluation standards.

An evaluation report is a typical form of communication and there are accepted formats for how such reports should be constructed, including the background and purpose of the evaluation, a description of the program evaluated, the evaluation design and methodology, and findings, conclusions, and recommendations.[8] Beyond such formal reporting, multiple visual platforms are available to present findings creatively: informational or educational forums, media (television, radio, newspaper), personal contacts, electronic mailing lists, newsletters, videos, social media, and software applications. Evaluation findings need to be tailored in style, tone, message, source, and format for the intended users. Accurate evaluation findings that are incomprehensible and laced with unnecessary academic jargon, footnotes, and asides are not useful for informed decision-making.

Although the focus here has been on the use of evaluation findings, a word needs to be said about the potential for misuse of evaluation findings. Misuse could be intentional, such as not fully disclosing findings, or be unintentional, such as applying findings to contexts and programs dissimilar from those that were the subject of the evaluation. Those responsible for the evaluation and stakeholders need to be on guard for such potential misuse and face it with clarity. The use of evaluation findings is one of the standards by which evaluations are judged. The bottom line is: good evaluations facilitate the ethical use of findings; bad ones do not. While research findings may contribute to knowledge, evaluation findings are intended to contribute to accountability, informed decision-making and constructive action. They are intended to be useful in guiding action.

SUMMARY

Program evaluation is defined as "the systematic comparison of an object of interest with a standard of acceptability in order to provide evidence useful to informed decision-making." In too many instances, evaluation is something considered at the end—the end of planning or the end of the program. By working through Phases 1–4 of the PRECEDE-PROCEED model, evaluation will have been a forethought, not an afterthought, since key elements of evaluation are threaded throughout the PRECEDE-PROCEED planning process. The six steps in the CDC *Framework for Program Evaluation in Public Health* are conceptually aligned with the eight phases of the PRECEDE-PROCEED planning process and provide ready visualization of the evaluation process.

A last word about "Why evaluate?" Increasingly, the agency managing or funding the program may require evaluation to determine whether the program met its goals. This may be a necessary reason to evaluate, but it is not sufficient. PRECEDE-PROCEED is a planning tool designed to help people and communities globally to improve their health and well-being and address social issues. Evaluation is an essential part of public health because it is designed to let practitioners and stakeholders, including intended beneficiaries, know whether their efforts to improve health are working, and if not, to know what changes are needed to be successful. We hope that we have convinced you that thoughtful evaluation is a core source of evidence-based practice and, in turn, of practice-based evidence.

EXERCISES

1. Retrieve one program objective from both PRECEDE-PROCEED Phases 1 and 2 and three educational or ecological objectives from Phase 3. For each objective, identify an object of interest and two different standards of acceptability; explain the strengths and weaknesses of each standard.

2. Using a case example from a previous chapter or in one of the several chapters on applications in specific settings and populations that follow, explain what design you would use to answer questions posed by stakeholders and describe the methods you would use to collect data.

3. Using the checklist in Appendix C, provide a short answer for the ways in which each of the standards will be applied to the chosen case example for each of the six steps in the evaluation process.

Notes

1. For information about developing SMART objectives for evaluation, see https://www.cdc .gov/phcommunities/resourcekit/evaluate/smart_objectives.html, https://www.cdc.gov /dhdsp/evaluation_resources/guides/writing-smart-objectives.htm, or https://www.cdc .gov/tb/programs/Evaluation/Guide/PDF/b_write_objective.pdf. (Note to the user of these websites: these and other URL addresses such as the above can be easily accessed, without typing them, by using the website http://www.lgreen.net.)
2. The full set of 30 program evaluation standards are listed on the Joint Committee on Standards for Educational Evaluation website at http://www.jcsee.org/program

-evaluation-standards-statements. The book outlining the full set of standards, with case studies and supporting materials, is available for purchase (see Yarbrough et al. 2011).

3. For additional reading on how planning, implementation, and evaluation interact with each other and the context, see articles in Ottoson and Hawe (2009).

4. The terms "outcome evaluation" and "impact evaluation" are sometimes used interchangeably in the evaluation literature. In a previous edition of this book (Green and Kreuter 1999), impact evaluation was defined as "the assessment of program effects on intermediate objectives" and outcome evaluation was defined as the "effects of a program on ultimate objectives such as social benefits or quality of life." These distinctions were consistent with the medical use of the terms "process," "outcome," and "benefit." While there remain some inconsistencies in the way these terms are used in the literature, "impact evaluation" is now more commonly used to refer to long-term evaluation focusing on social impact or quality of life (the distal effects of an intervention), while "outcome evaluation" refers to a focus on short-term or intermediate outcomes that occur earlier in the causal chain (e.g., knowledge, behavior). In keeping with these developments, in this edition of PRECEDE-PROCEED we use "long-term outcome evaluation" or "impact evaluation" interchangeably to refer to changes in health status, social conditions or quality of life in the intended population. For a detailed discussion of outcome and impact evaluation, see Rossi et al. (2019) listed in the references.

5. For resources on logic models in public health, see https://www.cdc.gov/eval/tools/logic _models/index.html, https://www.wkkf.org/resource-directory/resources/2004/01 /logic-model-development-guide, and https://ctb.ku.edu/en/table-of-contents/overview /models-for-community-health-and-development/logic-model-development/main.

6. For a tale about the consequences of not connecting with all stakeholders to develop a logic model, see Lovato (2019). The book that contains this story has many other interesting stories about "failed evaluations."

7. Readers are encouraged to refer to Shadish et al. (2002), Rossi et al. (2019), and The Community Tool Box at https://ctb.ku.edu/en/table-of-contents/evaluate/evaluate -community-interventions/experimental-design/main, as well as other texts on research design and methods for further information about using a quantitative approach for program evaluation.

8. For an introductory resource on mixed methods, see Bamberger (2012) and https://www .interaction.org/wp-content/uploads/2019/03/Mixed-Methods-in-Impact-Evaluation -English.pdf.

9. For guidance on reporting, writing recommendations and supporting the use of evaluation results, see https://www.betterevaluation.org/en/rainbow_framework/report _support_use or https://www.cdc.gov/eval/materials/Developing-An-Effective -Evaluation-Report_TAG508.pdf.

References

Bamberger, M. (2012). Introduction to mixed methods in impact evaluation. *Impact Evaluation Notes, 3*(3), 1–38.

Bechar, S., & Mero-Jaffe, I. (2014). Who is afraid of evaluation? Ethics in evaluation research as a way to cope with excessive evaluation anxiety: Insights from a case study. *American Journal of Evaluation, 35*(3), 364–76. https://doi.org/10.1177/1098214013512555

Brownson, R.C., Fielding, J.E., & Green, L.W. (2018). Building capacity for evidence-based public health: Reconciling the pulls of practice and the push of research. *Annual Review of Public Health, 39*, 27–53. https://doi.org/10.1146/annurev-publhealth-040617-014746

Cashman, S.B., Adeky, S., Allen, A.J., Corburn, J., Israel, B.A., Montano, J., Rafelito, A., Rhodes, S.D., Swanston, S., Wallerstein, N., & Eng, E. (2008). The power and the promise: Working with communities to analyze data, interpret findings, and get to outcomes. *American Journal of Public Health, 98*(8), 1407–17.

Centers for Disease Control and Prevention. (1999). Framework for Program Evaluation in Public Health. *Morbidity and Mortality Weekly Report, 48*(No. RR–11). https://stacks.cdc.gov/view/cdc/5204/cdc_5204_DS1.pdf

Centers for Disease Control and Prevention. (2017, May 15). *A Framework for Program Evaluation*. Retrieved May 18, 2021, from https://www.cdc.gov/eval/framework/index.htm

Centers for Disease Control and Prevention. (2018, December 12). *Program Evaluation Framework Checklist for Step 1*. Retrieved May 18, 2021, from https://www.cdc.gov/eval/steps/step1/index.htm

Centers for Disease Control and Prevention. (n.d.) *Types of Evaluation*. National Center for HIV/AIDS, Viral Hepatitis, STD, and TB Prevention. https://www.cdc.gov/std/Program/pupestd/Types%20of%20Evaluation.pdf

Craig, P., Cooper, C., Gunnell, D., Haw, S., Lawson, K., Macintyre, S., Ogilvie, D., Petticrew, M., Reeves, B., Sutton, M., & Thompson, S. (2012). Using natural experiments to evaluate population health interventions: new Medical Research Council guidance. *Journal of Epidemiology and Community Health, 66*(12), 1182–6. https://doi.org/10.1136/jech-2011-200375

Creswell, J.W., & Poth, C.N. (2018). *Qualitative Inquiry and Research Design* (4th ed.). SAGE Publishing.

Donaldson, S.I., Gooler, L.E., & Scriven, M. (2002). Strategies for managing evaluation anxiety: Toward a psychology of program evaluation. *American Journal of Evaluation, 23*(3), 261–73. https://doi.org/10.1177/109821400202300303

Flicker, S. (2008). Who benefits from community-based participatory research? A case study of the Positive Youth Project. *Health Education and Behavior, 35*(1), 70–86. https://doi.org/10.1177/1090198105285927

Green, L.W. (2008). Making research relevant: if it is an evidence-based practice, where's the practice-based evidence? *Family Practice, 25*(Suppl. 1), i20–i24. https://doi.org/10.1093/fampra/cmn055

Green, L.W., & Glasgow, R.E. (2006). Evaluating the relevance, generalization, and applicability of research: issues in external validation and translation methodology. *Evaluation and the Health Professions, 29*(1), 126–53. https://doi.org/10.1177/0163278705284445

Green, L.W., & Kreuter, M.W. (1999). *Health Promotion Planning: An Educational and Ecological Approach* (3rd ed.). Mayfield Publishing Company.

Green, L.W., & Lewis, F.M. (1986). *Measurement and Evaluation in Health Education and Health Promotion*. Mayfield Publishing Company.

Green, L.W., & Ottoson, J.M. (2004). From efficacy to effectiveness to community and back: evidence-based practice vs. practice-based evidence. In Green, L.W., Hiss, R., Glasgow, R., et al (Eds.), *From Clinical Trials to Community: The Science of Translating Diabetes and Obesity Research*. National Institutes of Health.

Institute of Medicine. (2012). *An Integrated Framework for Assessing the Value of Community-Based Prevention*. National Academies Press.

Lovato, C.Y. (2019). A failed logic model: How I learned to connect with all stakeholders. In Hutchinson, K. (Ed.), *Evaluation Failures: 22 Tales of Mistakes Made and Lessons Learned* (pp. 65–9). SAGE Publishing.

McLoughlin, G.M., McCarthy, J.A., McGuirt, J.T., Singleton, C.R., Dunn, C.G., & Gadhoke, P. (2020). Addressing Food Insecurity through a Health Equity Lens: a Case Study of Large Urban School Districts during the COVID-19 Pandemic. *Journal of Urban Health, 97*, 759–75. https://doi.org/10.1007/s11524-020-00476-0

Miles, M.B., Huberman, A.M., & Saldaña, J. (2014). *Qualitative Data Analysis: A Methods Sourcebook* (3rd ed.). SAGE Publishing.

Morse, J.M. (2011). Purposive Sampling. In Lewis-Beck, M., Bryman, A.E., & Liao, T.F. (Eds.), *SAGE Encyclopedia of Social Science Research Methods*. SAGE Publishing.

Ottoson, J.M. & Hawe, P. (Eds.) (2009). *Knowledge Utilization, Diffusion, Implementation, Transfer, and Translation: New Directions for Evaluation* (No. 124). Jossey-Bass.

Patton, M.Q. (2008). *Utilization-Focused Evaluation*. SAGE Publishing.

Patton, M.Q. (2015). *Qualitative Research & Evaluation Methods: Integrating Theory and Practice* (4th ed.). SAGE Publishing.

Rossi, P.H., Lipsey, M.W., & Henry, G.T. (2019). *Evaluation: A Systematic Approach* (8th ed.). SAGE Publishing.

Savin-Baden, M., & Major, C.H. (2013). *Qualitative Research: The Essential Guide to Theory and Practice*. Routledge.

Shadish, W.R., Cook, T.D., & Campbell, D.T. (2002). *Experimental and Quasi-Experimental Designs for Generalized Causal Inference* (2nd ed.). Wadsworth Cengage Learning.

Shadish, W.R., Cook, T.D., & Leviton, L.C. (1991). *Foundations of Program Evaluation: Theories of Practice*. SAGE Publishing.

Task Force on Community Preventive Services. (2005). Understanding and using the economic evidence. In Zaza, S., Briss, S., Briss, P.A., & Harris, K.W. (Eds.), *The Guide to Community Preventive Services: What Works to Promote Health* (pp. 449–63). Oxford University Press.

Thorne, S. (2016). *Interpretive Description: Qualitative Research for Applied Practice*. Routledge.

Weiss, C.H. (1977). Between the cup and the lip. In Caro, F.G. (Ed.), *Readings in Evaluation Research* (pp. 115–24). Russell Sage Foundation.

Weiss, C.H. (1998). *Evaluation: Methods for Studying Programs and Policies* (2nd ed.). Prentice Hall.

Yarbrough, D.B., Shulha, L.M., Hopson, R.K., & Caruthers, F.A. (2011). *The Program Evaluation Standards: A Guide for Evaluators and Evaluation Users* (3rd ed.). SAGE Publishing.

Yin, R. (2018). *Case Study Research and Applications: Design and Methods* (6th ed.). SAGE Publishing.

Applications of PRECEDE-PROCEED in Specific Settings

Introduction to PRECEDE-PROCEED Applications

Having learned the foundations of PRECEDE-PROCEED in part I of the book (chapters 1 and 2) and the phases of the model in part II (chapters 3–9), we welcome you to part III: applications of PRECEDE-PROCEED in varied settings. Having provided application references and examples in small doses throughout the book, these coming chapters provide in-depth examples of how the model can work, phase by phase, in the varied circumstances of communities, worksites, schools, and health care settings and with varied applications in new communications technologies.

For chapters 10–14, we invited international authorities on public health and health promotion from major settings to reflect on their experience using the PRECEDE-PROCEED model in planning, implementing, and evaluating health policies and programs. They refer in these five chapters to the PRECEDE-PROCEED model's eight phases as they were named, visualized, and understood previously, as the present volume did not yet exist.

It is because of the applications presented in the following chapters and the bodies of research to which they refer that we have brought new understanding to the model in the preceding chapters of this book. While you will notice that Phases 1–3 and 6–8 are most comparable between this and previous publications of the model, it is Phases 4 and 5 that have evolved the most. Phase 4 continues to follow the assessments of Phases 1–3, but in this volume, Phase 4 brings to the forefront the *development* of not only intervention strategies, but development of implementation and evaluation strategies as well. Implementation of all these strategies are launched in Phase 4. Phase 5 now focuses on the process evaluation of interventions, and Phases 6–8 continue with the implementation of PROCEED tasks, including the evaluation of the short-term, intermediate, and long-term outcomes (previously named *impact* and *outcomes*).

Don't get lost in translation! The shifts in this volume's understanding, language, and visualization of PRECEDE-PROCEED grew out of the well-researched, detailed, and exemplary applications such as those to follow. Stick with the overarching ideas, assessments, and strategies in how PRECEDE-PROCEED and its evolution through five incarnations offer increasingly clearer pathways to planning, implementing, and evaluating programs and policies that contribute to the public's health. Join us at http://www.lgreen .net for a continuing discussion and over 1,200 examples of other PRECEDE-PROCEED applications. Perhaps, dear reader, you will develop applications that take PRECEDE-PROCEED to the next level of understanding. And perhaps you will be among those to pioneer innovative applications to the new challenges of global warming and pandemic diseases.

CHAPTER 10

Applications in Community Settings

•

Amelie G. Ramirez and Patricia Chalela

Learning Objectives

After completing the chapter, the reader will be able to:

- Understand that definitions of *community* in this context go beyond geography and recognize the term as identifying a group that shares not only distinctive characteristics, including special needs, but also laws, interests, norms, and values.
- Recognize how diverse racial, ethnic, physical, social, economic, and cultural characteristics affect community health and how the community's organization and the behaviors of the individual members shape it.
- Identify ways that the PRECEDE-PROCEED model has helped communities participate in health intervention planning and implementation and document and evaluate health outcomes.
- Become aware of and be prepared for the problems confronted by community health specialists in implementing the model and how they were resolved.

INTRODUCTION

In this chapter, we address how public health professionals use the PRECEDE-PROCEED model in **community** settings, particularly communities that are ethnically, racially, and socioeconomically diverse. Because of that complexity, it is essential that the interventions we develop fit the key aspects of the community in question. Communities come in all types and sizes, and the definition or designation of a community may have everything to do with geographic location (e.g., city, village, enclave, barrio, neighborhood) or little or nothing at all (e.g., the gay community, the Asian-American community). We may belong to a community designated by geography—a rural town in Nebraska or a metropolitan area like London, Singapore, or St. Louis—but we may also belong to an online school community with students identified by their enrollment but not the location of the school, the age of the enrollees, or grade level of the courses. Likewise, a person may belong to a religious community, a political party, or a community defined by age, race, ethnicity, gender or sexual orientation. Public health experts may be interested in communities made up of persons who share experiences (miners trapped underground for extended periods, people who live through disasters), who share the same culture (the Amish, Syrian refugees, or the Jewish diaspora), or who share the same diets, activities, or careers (vegetarians, runners, physicians). Community may be a place or location, or it may be a place defined by a shared history or sense of identity without boundaries (Institute of Medicine 2012). Sharing common beliefs, enjoying the same activities, propelled by the same sense of social responsibility, or experiencing a sense of belonging may, likewise, identify a very specific community—Holocaust survivors, for example, or school shooting survivors, or long-standing annual summer camp attendees.

The very diversity of communities themselves makes clear the need for the scaffolding that the stages of the PRECEDE model builds, such as the social assessment leading to and informing the subsequent epidemiological, behavioral, and environmental assessments that ultimately support constructing, implementing, and evaluating programs. If your public health practice is at the local level, you are most likely to be dealing with communities as geographic entities; if your office is at the state/provincial or national level, you are more likely to be dealing with aggregates of common interest across multiple communities, such as statewide advocacy coalitions concerned with air pollution or national governmental and voluntary associations devoted to the prevention of specific diseases such as COVID 19.

A definition of **community health** on which the public health field agrees eluded the discipline for many years. In its most simple form, it could be "the health status of a community" or "the well-being of a population that shares something in common." The search for a definition is briefly chronicled in an article by Goodman and colleagues (2014), who offer a definition broader than most, affirming public health practice as a distinct field and addressing its goals: "*Community health* is a multi-sector and multi-disciplinary collaborative enterprise that uses public health science, evidence-based strategies, and other approaches to engage and work with communities, in a culturally appropriate manner, to optimize the health and quality of life of all persons who live, work, or are otherwise active in a defined community or communities" (p. 60). This definition encapsulates several fundamental values in only 54 words: the collaborative nature of community work, the concept of cultural appreciation and competence, a definition of community beyond geographic distinctions, an acknowledgment of the integral role of science and of evidence-based methods, and the goal of optimizing health and quality of life of all persons in a community, not just some. As the PRECEDE-PROCEED planning model is examined in the context of community in the continuation of this chapter, consider how many of these values are encapsulated in the model.

THE PRECEDE-PROCEED MODEL IN COMMUNITY SETTINGS

The PRECEDE-PROCEED model for designing health programs gives planners (as presented in chapters 1–9) a framework to follow in identifying a community's needs, setting objectives for their resolution, creating or fashioning appropriate interventions based on theory and evidence-based practices, and pretesting the interventions with evaluation to produce practice-based evidence. In promoting analysis of the target community, the planning model imposes a systematic framework that aids priority setting and helps identify what resources, knowledge, or skills may be lacking in staff and the community. Therefore, it directs preparatory action and helps prevent compromising the program's impact. The model prioritizes examination of the characteristics of community and puts the focus on the population, ensuring relevance above and beyond the generic applicability of evidence-based practices or programs drawn from research in other places.

Based on PRECEDE's systematic planning approach for its foundation, the PROCEED phase recognizes not only the importance of the effective implementation of evidence-based practices but also emphasizes practice-based evidence, which is particularly relevant to this chapter's topic because it is locally developed and community-specific. Here we seek to explicate implementation's process, impact, and outcomes. Accordingly, we will discuss the PRECEDE-PROCEED model through studies and model applications, providing the boots-on-the-ground perspective of those who have worked across varied communities.

RECOGNIZING THE MODEL'S BIOETHICS

Underlying the PRECEDE-PROCEED model is respect for the four primary principles of bioethics: beneficence, nonmaleficence, autonomy, and justice, as laid out in table 10.1 (Centers for Disease Control and Prevention [CDC] 2018; Porter 2015). These principles imply that the proposed intervention will be undertaken with the intent of doing good; that is, the outcomes for the community will be beneficial, and the community's input through participation in the process will secure that objective with equitable distribution of resources commensurate with varied population segments' needs. If program planners can facilitate a process of participatory planning that enables planners and the community to see the social and health problems that affect the target populations through the same lens, they will more likely arrive at a program plan that is *relevant to local needs*, *appropriate to local culture and values*, and *consistent with resource possibilities*.

In chapter 2, it is recognized that the social context of communities from the community's perspective is a pragmatic and moral imperative, one that springs from not only respect but also the principles of **informed consent**. Likewise, following one of the foremost principles of biomedical ethics, planners, including community members, share proactively the intent *to do no harm*, either to participants or to the wider social community. Involving the community also ensures that the autonomy of the community to pursue remediation of health

TABLE 10.1. Methods PRECEDE-PROCEED uses to advance ethics principles and support public health essential services

| | Ethics Principles | | | |
	Autonomy	Beneficence	Nonmaleficence	Justice*
Description	Respecting persons	Working to ensure the well-being of others	Refraining from doing harm to others; protecting them from harm	Pursuing fairness
PRECEDE-PROCEED methods of securing ethical aims	• Engaging the participation of the community, indicating that participation is without coercion • Continual reevaluation and evolution	• Ensuring participatory processes, including participatory planning and evaluation • Continual reevaluation and evolution	• Ensuring participatory processes, including participatory planning and evaluation • Continual reevaluation and evolution	• Ensuring participation of the community through all phases, including planning, implementation, and evaluation • Continual reevaluation and evolution
Characteristics of outcomes using PRECEDE-PROCEED	• Empowering the community through inclusion, education, and mobilization	• Relevant to needs • Appropriate to local culture • Consistent with resource possibilities	• Orientation to prevention • Reduction of risk	• Impartial distribution of benefits from intervention • Incorporation of diversity • Most immediate and greatest needs met first • Sex, race, ethnicity, nativity, beliefs, and other differences are no reason for the denial of benefits

TABLE 10.1. (*continued*)

	Ethics Principles			
	Autonomy	**Beneficence**	**Nonmaleficence**	**Justice***
Public health essential services supported by PRECEDE-PROCEED†	• Informs, educates, and empowers people about health issues • Links people to needed personal health services and assures the provision of health care when otherwise unavailable • Evaluates the effectiveness, accessibility, and quality of personal and population-based health services	• Monitors health status to identify and solve community health problems • Diagnoses and investigates health problems and health hazards in the community • Develops policies and plans that support individual and community health efforts	• Enforces laws and regulations that protect health and ensure safety • Evaluates the effectiveness, accessibility, and quality of personal and population-based health services	• Monitors health status to identify and solve community health problems • Enforces laws and regulations that protect health and ensure safety • Evaluates the effectiveness, accessibility, and quality of personal and populations-based health services • Performs research for new insights and innovative solutions to health problems
Public health functions	• Policy development • Assurance	• Diagnosis • Policy development	• Assurance	• Assessment • Policy development • Assurance • System management

Sources: Selected data from Porter (2015) and the Centers for Disease Control and Prevention.

*Essential services supported by the pursuit of fairness are represented here by four of the Centers for Disease Control and Prevention's 10 essential services, but arguments could be made that justice encompasses all 10.

† These are drawn directly from the Centers for Disease Control and Prevention.

through this method makes it clear that community members engage in the project without coercion. Further, because the PRECEDE-PROCEED model seeks to delineate the critical role of social and environmental **determinants of health**, the principle of justice is at work. Under that principle, all benefits of health action, including beneficial interventions, are to be distributed impartially. All may eventually benefit, but direct and immediate beneficiaries are often the ones who need help the most or have been prioritized based on factual data collected. It affirms that despite differences in income, race or ethnicity, sex, place of birth, beliefs, or other characteristics, the benefits of an intervention will not be denied (Farquhar and Green 2015).

Beyond equality, the best PRECEDE-PROCEED applications seek to address a combination of social-behavioral and environmental factors—including lifestyle, lack of job opportunities, food deserts, unsafe neighborhoods, unhealthful exposures—and seek to help reduce factors that prevent disadvantaged groups from achieving the same level of health achieved by those whose lives are not marked by those deficits. During intervention planning and implementation, as workers engage communities in health education and improvement interventions and seek health equity, the planning data they collect must also include environmental and ecological factors, including identifying consequential health disparities and changing policies, practices, laws, and systems that present barriers to resources reaching across levels of the community for achieving health (Huff et al. 2015).

Calling PRECEDE-PROCEED a leading model for ethical health promotion, one health educator aligns with ethical practice the model's democratic and community-focused characteristics (Porter 2015): (1) its advancement of the ecological approach, (2) its persistent focus on populations rather than individuals, (3) its demand that health promotion be rooted in a democratic practice and rely on community involvement, (4) its focus on quality of life, and (5) its grounding in practice.

USING THE MODEL WITH COMMUNITIES

A planning model for a health intervention recognizes the relationships as points of action for planning, implementing, and evaluating the intervention. It identifies aims, actions, inputs and outputs, and ultimately outcomes. The PRECEDE-PROCEED model has been called a "particularly useful, widely applied, and easy-to-follow" planning model by Crosby and Noar (2017, S7). Its cohesive structure begins and ends in the same place: assessments of quality of life and health.

For the purpose of making the differences between populations of interest clear, the fourth edition of this book (Green and Kreuter 2005) drew a distinction between the terms *community interventions* and *interventions in the community*. The first was designated to refer to programs seeking to make a small, though potentially profound, change across an entire community; the second referred to programs or more targeted interventions that sought more intensive change in specific subpopulations within the community. These subpopulations could be, for example, any group having a specific illness (COVID-19, diabetes, AIDS, cardiovascular disease), young children, workers in a specific industry (e.g., coal mining, health care, farming), drug users, older adults, transgender teens, or churchgoers. Two examples follow.

One of the most well-known community interventions, as noted in previous chapters, was the historic North Karelia Project, a program launched in Finland in 1972 against newly recognized high rates of cardiovascular mortality (Puska 2002; Puska et al. 1988). Cooperating in the effort were the World Health Organization (WHO) and local and national experts and authorities. The tools in use were media campaigns, face-to-face community interaction (the organizers going out with "boots deep in the mud" to confer with local people in various segments of the population), and other activities coordinated with nongovernmental organizations, schools, and health and other services. Positive behavioral and other risk factor changes continued past the initial five-year study period to 1982, with men 30–59 years of age registering statistically significant reductions in smoking, the use of butter on bread, serum cholesterol levels, and systolic blood pressure. Though women were found to have increases in smoking that were not statistically significant, they did have statistically significant reductions in the use of butter on bread and systolic blood pressure. By the time of a reevaluation in 1995, men younger than 65 years of age had reduced coronary heart disease mortality by about 73% from statistics for 1967–1971 (preprogram years). In the decade preceding 2002, coronary heart disease mortality declined about 8% per year for both men and women (Puska 2002). Because the entire community was targeted, finding that 2% of the population lost weight during the early years of the project meant that 60,000 people benefited (Green and Kreuter 2005).

An example of interventions in the community (not necessarily community-wide) was work undertaken by nurse researchers at the University of North Carolina at Greensboro. These researchers wanted to understand the effects of several factors on health-related quality of life in a low-income (60% had a household income <$10,000/year) population of adult Hispanics with diabetes and low literacy (Hu et al. 2010). The researchers' review of the literature indicated that adults in this group experienced higher morbidity and mortality rates than those of non-Hispanic whites, and the prevalence of diabetes, cardiovascular disease risk factors, and complications from diabetes were higher in Hispanics than in non-Hispanic whites. To delineate quality of life in these patients, they used PRECEDE as a framework, studying 19 men and 40 women, 44.1% of whom rated their health as fair or poor. The investigators identified predisposing factors and behavior (age, body mass index, nutrition, physical activity) that explained 21% of variance and predicted quality of life ($p < .05$). In subsequent studies, some of these authors undertook more fact finding and interventions in Hispanic men and women with diabetes, offering programs meant to improve diabetes status and increase physical activity.

In a multicomponent approach, program planners incorporate more than a single factor in any intervention, usually constituting a program of interventions, with some directed at predisposing factors, some at enabling factors, and some at reinforcing factors. Falls among elders, for example, are complex. Not only do falls cause physical injuries, they can erode confidence, increase fear of falling, lead to long-term physical injuries, and actually raise the risk of early death (Robert Wood Johnson Foundation 2018). Programs that address the problem in multiple ways—offering physical exercise opportunities or instruction, providing education about hazards, modifying the person's environment or providing access to workers who can, optimizing medications, and supplementing the diet with vitamin D—are supported by strong evidence as being effective in reducing the risk of falling and the rate of falls in older adults (Gillespie et al. 2012; Goodwin et al. 2014). Another boon to these programs is that they can be effective in multiple settings, whether older adults live in care facilities or at home.

Another study conducted by the North Carolina investigators was a single-group diabetes intervention in a rural setting. Investigators enrolled 36 patients with diabetes and 37 family members to provide support in an educational program (Hu et al. 2014), achieving statistically significant changes in diabetes self-efficacy, systolic blood pressure, and health-related quality of life. Family members also netted benefits: they experienced a significant reduction in body mass index and improved knowledge of diabetes. The merits of seeking intensive change in a small, high-risk population are shared by community interventions—both promote health and provide prevention—but interventions in the community allow more interpersonal interaction, building relationships for ongoing collaboration, and can produce sustained effects if connected to the larger context of the community.

Within community intervention planning, the PRECEDE-PROCEED approach requires taking into consideration the larger context—that is, the multiple influences, or social determinants of health, that expand or limit opportunities and affect community and personal health behaviors. These are critical factors assessed in the early phases of planning. In a model with health and quality of life outcomes similar to those of PRECEDE-PROCEED planning, the Robert Wood Johnson Foundation undertook with the University of Wisconsin a project called "Building a Culture of Health, County by County." In it, social and economic factors (education, employment, income, family and social support, and community safety) make up 40% of what contributes to the ultimate health and quality of life outcomes. These are achieved particularly through health behaviors, such as diet and physical activity. Physical environment makes up another 10%, thereby, with social and economic variables, affecting half of the health factors critical to health outcomes, as seen in figure 10.1 (University of Wisconsin n.d.). Though the measurable extent of change for a given problem may vary from community to community, the influence can be very dramatic. Having community members participate in planning the intervention and interpreting the results helps ensure not only that interventions address issues important to members of the community but also that, once concluded, the intervention and evaluation of its results can be vetted and interpreted with the help of community members in the context of the cultural, social, and economic forces of their community.

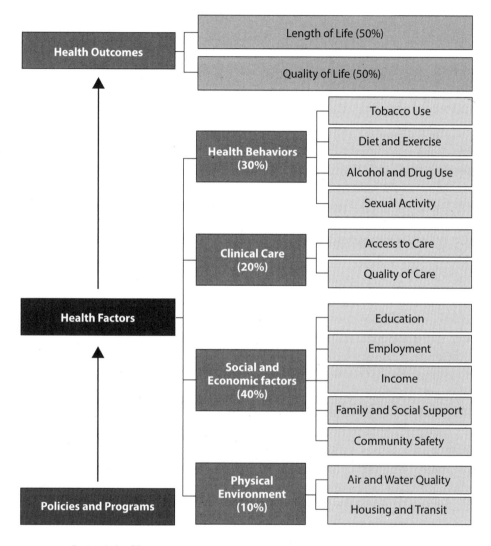

FIGURE 10.1. Factors in health outcomes. *Source:* County Health Rankings & Roadmaps. (2020). *County Health Rankings Model.* The University of Wisconsin Population Health Institute. http://www.countyhealthrankings.org

UNDERSTANDING THE UNIQUE NEEDS OF COMMUNITIES

Engaging the community in planning ensures that its residents, through their involvement, infuse their knowledge and culture into the intervention. Their collective aspirations, in fact, become its aims. Culture acts as an ordering force, which is based on a set of defining qualities, explicitly expressed or not, of community (Geertz 2000). It is not, as some might think of it, simply a compendium of characteristics to which an intervention should be tailored (Trickett et al. 2011).

Involving the community early in the planning process can itself be considered a form of intervention (Green and Kreuter 2005). Though some argue that participation by the community has to be present in every phase of an intervention, others disagree. Jerry C. Johnson, MD, who has been the leader of the Philadelphia Area Research Community Coalition, a 22-member alliance for health education, community work groups, community research projects, and other activities, told Weiner and McDonald (2013) that while participation in all phases of community-based participatory research (or assessment or evaluation) may be unrealistic, what is essential is participation in three areas: (1) determining the subject of research, (2) interpreting and giving advice about the results, and (3) disseminating the results within the community.

The PRECEDE-PROCEED approach has been used to create interventions for all types of communities: those defined by geography; those defined by race, ethnicity, or both; those who are underserved by health services; and those suffering with noninfectious chronic diseases, particularly cardiovascular disease, obesity, cancers, and other diseases. Many professionals and researchers work collaboratively and successfully with community members, but that does not mean that all members of the community will assess its needs in the same way.

Consider the work of Chicago investigators who used PRECEDE-PROCEED to perform formative research in a multiracial and multicultural population of elementary school-age children and their adult caregivers (Martin et al. 2016). They gained insights that helped them optimize the intervention.

Other practitioners and researchers seek community input sometimes exactly because they want to determine a ranking of priorities. Communities, as pointed out above, can consist of any of many collectivities of people, and this includes professions. The Institute for Health Promotion Research at the University of Texas Health Science Center at San Antonio created a national advisory committee of more than 300 experts to consult on the direction that Latino childhood obesity-related research should take (Ramirez et al. 2013). The 21-member committee included authorities on physical activity, behavioral science, nutrition, advocacy and public policy, school, and community . . . this group grew a network of more than 2,000 members! When the network was polled for direction, more than 300 network members responded, and the results indicated that their priorities should be initiatives directed at society, community, school, family, and individuals. Expanding the definition of *community* in this way includes a national network of researchers who are identifying their aspirations for the work in their field. This has the same benefits that come from assessing other types of communities (Weiner and McDonald 2013): those assessed become stakeholders in the process, and the potential for success is increased by their participation in the assessment because those contributing bring knowledge and identify service gaps. This planned approach enhances and empowers the community and can initiate and nurture collaborative relationships.

Such programs come in many shapes and sizes and engage with a community or multiple communities through different structures and with different purposes. Three such programs that were led in part by faculty at the University of Pennsylvania offer an opportunity to see a range of initiatives, as shown in table 10.2 (Weiner and McDonald 2013). The initiatives may arrive at their purpose, for example, through shared interests, relationships, or commitments; through surveys and interviews; or through convening one or more boards and prioritizing community needs or problems.

Each party is assessing the other, and sometimes small projects are a perfect path for test-driving the relationship. Because a history of distrust rooted

TABLE 10.2. Three examples of community-based participatory research by model

Model	Partners	Structure/ purpose	Building capacity/ sustainability	Elements of successful community-based participatory research relationships and lessons learned
Focused, single-issue collaboration	The community and academic environmental programs were partners.	A stakeholder advisory board of 15 people from the community was established to address environmental health problems.	"There should be money in it for the community. We need to incorporate them into grants."*	• Trust is essential and built on respect. • The program must address a community's problem. • Core resources (personnel) must be responsive to the community, including helping the community with health issues other than those targeted in the program. • Using a "community first" communication model means findings and other vital communications are shared first with the community. • It is much more difficult for policy makers to ignore communities' interests and concerns when they are shared by the university and the university is engaged with the community.

(continued)

TABLE 10.2. (*continued*)

Model	Partners	Structure/ purpose	Building capacity/ sustainability	Elements of successful community-based participatory research relationships and lessons learned
Targeted, area-based collaborative	This established community collaborative of multiple organizations included an academic health disparities program that wanted to reduce health disparities in the African-American community.	Part of the structure was the creation of education programs designed to meet community-defined priorities, including cancer and cardiovascular disease risk evaluation and cancer screening navigation.	Partners in the community work part-time paid positions and facilitate ongoing initiatives.	• Beginning with small projects allowed both sides to "test-drive" the relationship. • Having subcommittees as well as an executive committee ensured ongoing community input and collaboration.
Broad-based coalition	Twenty-two organizations, including, among others, three academic centers, a federal health center, a YMCA, a recreation center, grassroots organizations, a multipurpose center, and faith-based organizations, were participants.	The coalition was empowered to create core work groups, community health education projects, and research projects and training.	"You need to build in more capacity than you have in the grant" because "sustainability means leaving something behind when you leave."†	• Acknowledging and accepting distrust that exists and healing it by listening, following through, and persevering to work problems out ("staying at the table") are vital to establishing respect-generating relationships.

Source: Based on descriptions of programs in Weiner and McDonald (2013). All three programs are affiliated with the University of Pennsylvania.

* Edward Emmett, who was director of the Community Outreach and Engagement Core of the Center of Excellence in Environmental Toxicology and quoted in Weiner and McDonald (2013, p. 3).

† Joel Fein, MD, principal investigator on a Centers for Disease Control and Prevention-funded program to prevent violence, who was quoted in Weiner and McDonald (2013, p. 6). The program was affiliated with the coalition.

in racism and elitism existed between the University of Pennsylvania and the community, that distrust had to be overcome, according to Weiner and McDonald. Each successful interaction demonstrating reliability, ability, and truthfulness that resulted in a willingness to rely on one another could be considered an incremental increase in trust and a commensurate reduction in distrust, as evidenced by reductions in confrontation, blame, and overt frustration. These and other measures of trust can be identified in the amount of encouragement, productivity, and self-initiated activation that occurs across lines of distrust and begins to erase them. These programs were uniform in expressing the belief that trust is essential, and when distrust is present, it must be acknowledged, accepted, and healed.

INSIGHTS GAINED THROUGH COMMUNITY EPIDEMIOLOGICAL ASSESSMENT

Following the social needs assessment, investigators using the PRECEDE-PROCEED framework look at the epidemiological forces at work in characterizing the problem statistically and in causing the problem in a given community. Consider, for example, children who are members of minority groups of low income and at high risk of obesity. Among Latino children, determinants of obesity are complex, affected by the personal, social, and cultural strata to which they belong and by multiple environments, including those of the family, school, community, and larger society (Ramirez et al. 2013). Forces affecting Latino children disproportionately, however, include living in communities marked by food deserts, with diminishing access to low-cost fresh food. Latino parents report that physical activity is restricted because of unsafe neighborhoods and lack of recreational opportunities. These are some of the "pathogens" in the epidemic responsible for obesity in Latino children.

Furthermore, Latino adults suffer disproportionately from higher-than-average rates of chronic disease, some of which are linked to malnutrition. In a study of randomized controlled trials designed to promote better nutrition and appropriate exercise in a Latino population, researchers used a literature review to identify salient culturally sensitive determinants (Mier et al. 2010). Understanding Latino cultural values and incorporating the following components were found to be critical: (1) bilingual and bicultural materials and facilitators, (2) family-based activities, (3) program literature written at an appropriate reading level, and (4) social support.

CONSIDERING EDUCATION AND RECOGNIZING RELATIONSHIPS IN THE COMMUNITY ECOLOGY

As indicated in the Guinea worm eradication example highlighted in chapter 1, health planners or researchers working in a community have to consider how the education of the community can strongly influence its acceptance and willingness to participate in a health initiative. In minority communities, the cost of disenfranchisement may have been losses in educational achievement or a separation from the mainstream that leaves the community at a disadvantage. Perhaps an immigrant community clings to rural customs and beliefs that isolate it further and that even engender greater discrimination against it. Conversely, perhaps government or nonprofit organizations within a community offer services that foster growth in community capacity and engagement. These relationships affect how interventions will work and how accurately they reflect the issues upon which the program will intervene.

Aboriginal communities and Torres Strait Islanders were the focus of Australian investigators who initiated a pilot study after learning that though these populations composed 2.8% of the national population, they represented 6% of vehicular fatalities (Hunter et al. 2017). In particular, children under the age of four years from these First Nation communities were also four times more likely than children from the majority population to die of a road-related injury. Researchers were also concerned about evidence that indicated that as few as 49% of Australians restrained children in a car seat appropriate for their size or age. Using PRECEDE-PROCEED, researchers worked to identify predisposing, enabling, and reinforcing factors for Australians' use of car restraints.

In the results, 83% of children in the study were found to be restrained properly. The study, with strong local representation, had several lessons: safety and safety programs should address issues of affordability, including the cost of fitting car seats safely in cars. In the end, especially through the focus group process, families in childcare centers became seen as communities, grandparents and peers were forces in the car safety universe, care centers could add impetus to messaging, and parents took their car safety responsibility seriously: "We have rules in my car," one said, and another reported, "I wouldn't let him in the car [without a car seat] 'cos he's the number one thing in my world" (p. 7). In the simplest terms, the PRECEDE-PROCEED Model helped translate that Aboriginal problem into four simple questions: What's the problem? Who has it? Why them? What can we do about that problem?

Churches have been communities of interest in many published studies employing the PRECEDE-PROCEED model. Two studies found that similar values in faith communities supported nutrition and energy balance interventions, though the intervention populations differed (Buta et al. 2011; Parker and Fineberg 2013). "Fostering African American Improvement in Total Health! (FAITH!)," a PRECEDE-PROCEED and theory-based health intervention in Baltimore, was a church-based initiative designed to educate the community about good nutrition practices and reducing health risks by changing dietary practices (Buta et al. 2011; Parker and Fineberg 2013). Investigators in San Antonio made partners of Latino church leaders, and together they addressed childhood obesity. Reinforcing factors in these Baltimore and San Antonio projects included church family social support and Biblical reminders that the body was God's temple. Some of the themes in these programs will be echoed later when we examine a church-based health ministry in the African-American community to appreciate process evaluation.

What is important to understanding the value of the PRECEDE-PROCEED model in planning for some other interventions in Latino and African-American communities is that programs designed to "lift all boats" will be insufficient in reversing the trajectory from obesity to chronic illness and diminished quality of life (Parker and Fineberg 2013). That is because entrenched disparities from long-term social and economic disadvantage, including discrimination and poverty, still control the environment. They are evident in the presence of dangerous streets and unsafe public parks and the absence of markets that offer affordable fresh food and schools that provide a generous supply of age-appropriate books.

IDENTIFYING ADMINISTRATIVE ISSUES AND INFLUENCING POLICIES IN COMMUNITIES

Key stakeholders who have conscientiously engaged the community in the PRECEDE-PROCEED procedures (after assessing the social needs and taking into consideration epidemiology, environment, education, and ecology) must then take stock of their organization's alignment with the aims or objectives of the implementation (described in full in chapter 8). That is critical because harnessing predisposing, reinforcing, and enabling characteristics *of the administration* will be critical to help create, maintain, and sustain that initiative. Accordingly, a realistic understanding of the organizational strengths and weaknesses is a practical and critical part of the planning process.

Following best practices usually is characterized by involving external individuals or organizations and transparency. These may include:

- instituting a governing board from a panel composed of academics, experts outside of academics, and community members, thereby creating a team of external evaluators to help keep the intervention on track;
- ensuring that all training required of managers, coordinators, and others is executed properly;
- having members of participating communities assume positions on an intervention's governing board, assume volunteer or paid positions with the staff, or create or assemble a network that supports the achievement of major aims;
- providing a modicum of training, supervision, coordination, and other preparation and support to help build a sense of ownership in the community and well serves the longevity of the program.

In an analysis of survey results from the Community Tracking Study Household Survey, Yamada et al. (2015), with PRECEDE-PROCEED, found specific enabling, predisposing, and reinforcing factors (given, respectively, in the list below) that adversely affected health care access for the elderly. The health inequality resulted from:

- disparities in health care access;
- perceived needs for health care that went unmet;
- a generally perceived delay in securing health care.

Among the enabling factors were increases in drug prices and out-of-pocket payments that imposed a financial burden, especially on persons 65 years of age and older. Those factors also imposed an increase in poverty or an increase in out-of-pocket payments, both of which could result in deterioration of health status. The authors concluded that policy makers must address such issues to make health care more affordable for the elderly and reduce the inequality of access to and use of health care services.

IMPLEMENTING AND EVALUATING PROCESSES IN COMMUNITIES

Process evaluation, as noted in chapter 9, is the first step of the PROCEED Phases 5–8. It accompanies initial and trial implementation and precedes full program implementation and impact evaluation, as seen in figure 10.2. Evaluating the procedure of implementing the program works to guarantee that the procedure selected for the intervention is (1) followed and therefore feasible, and (2) adaptable, ensuring any necessary adjustments are made. This evaluation prevents harm, reduces risks, identifies any barriers to protocol adherence, and provides insight to needed modifications. Furthermore, process evaluation will allow researchers to interpret more fully the eventual impact evaluation (Gielen et al. 2008). Careful monitoring will answer key questions for program managers.

Though researchers and community members no doubt would consider assessing the implementation of their interventions challenging enough, it is harder still to imagine conducting a process evaluation in the midst of a disaster. Nonetheless, that is what was recommended by two physicians who served as members of complementary federal health response teams (a disaster medical assistance team and a team from the US Public Health Service Commissioned Corps) who responded 48 hours after Hurricane Rita made landfall in September 2005 (Rios and Cullen 2006). Conditions treated included oxygen-dependent pulmonary disease; cardiovascular disease (acute myocardial infarction, complex congestive heart failure); mood, mental, or developmental disorders (bipolar disorder, schizophrenia, and autism); and other illnesses (e.g., asthma, Alzheimer's disease, and ectopic and high-risk pregnancy). They believed the

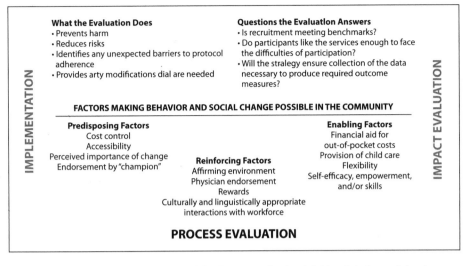

What the Evaluation Does
- Prevents harm
- Reduces risks
- Identifies any unexpected barriers to protocol adherence
- Provides arty modifications dial are needed

Questions the Evaluation Answers
- Is recruitment meeting benchmarks?
- Do participants like the services enough to face the difficulties of participation?
- Will the strategy ensure collection of the data necessary to produce required outcome measures?

IMPLEMENTATION

IMPACT EVALUATION

FACTORS MAKING BEHAVIOR AND SOCIAL CHANGE POSSIBLE IN THE COMMUNITY

Predisposing Factors
Cost control
Accessibility
Perceived importance of change
Endorsement by "champion"

Reinforcing Factors
Affirming environment
Physician endorsement
Rewards
Culturally and linguistically appropriate
interactions with workforce

Enabling Factors
Financial aid for
out-of-pocket costs
Provision of child care
Flexibility
Self-efficacy, empowerment,
and/or skills

PROCESS EVALUATION

FIGURE 10.2. Process evaluation in communities. Process evaluation is initiated during early implementation and before impact evaluation. Evaluation helps those conducting interventions in communities prevent harm and reduce risks, along with other safety measures, and answers questions about meeting trial benchmarks. Careful monitoring and evaluation (observation, surveys, and key interviews) will answer important questions and identify predisposing, reinforcing, and enabling factors that affect behavior and social change in the community. Potential factors are listed here. Illustration by Beth Allen.

tool could help teams like theirs reach their health-related goals in the future for evacuees seeking shelter.

One researcher has pointed out that Green and Kreuter have not exempted themselves from process evaluation in developing the PRECEDE-PROCEED model (Porter 2015). They augmented the model by adding PROCEED to its antecedent PRECEDE in 1991, building on the framework that was introduced and refined in the 1970s and 1980s. Bartholomew et al. (1988; 2011) and their successors at the University of Texas School of Public Health in Houston (Fernández et al. 2005) and Maastricht University in the Netherlands (Kok and Mesters 2011) have built on PRECEDE-PROCEED in elaborating on the range of evidence and theoretical options for "mapping" interventions quantitatively (with surveys, audits, counts of services provided) or qualitatively (review of contracts, interviews with personnel, consumer reports). Workplaces, schools, and health care settings constitute communities of other kinds, and applications of and lessons from the model in these settings are described and analyzed in the next three chapters (chapters 11–13) and in the applied settings and channels of the final section of this book.

Aspects of other community planning models have been integrated into PRECEDE-PROCEED over the course of its evolution through five editions of this book and nearly five decades of application, including *A Behavioral Model of Families' Use of Health Services* (Anderson 1968) and a planning model sponsored by the Centers for Disease Control and Prevention called the Planned Approach to Community Health (PATCH) based on the principles of PRECEDE-PROCEED (Green and Kreuter 1992) and applied across numerous states. Other models combined with PRECEDE-PROCEED by Green and collaborators have included Intervention Mapping (Bartholomew et al. 1998), Pooling Information about Prior Interventions (D'Onofrio 2001), Multilevel Approaches Toward Community Health (MATCH) (Institute of Medicine 2012), and the Six-Step Program Development Chain Model (Sussman 2001). Researchers have embraced the step-wise process of Intervention Mapping (Kok and Mesters 2011; Tramm et al. 2012), and Fernández and the coauthors in this volume (chapter 6) and elsewhere (Fernández et al. 2005; Fernández et al. 2009) find it a workable framework for identifying health determinants and selecting approaches for addressing them.

EVALUATING IMPACT IN COMMUNITIES

Determining whether an intervention is having the intended impact is only part of the evaluation. Evaluators must also determine whether unexpected negative consequences are occurring simultaneously. In minority communities, planners must address these key questions (Trickett et al. 2011): do these community interventions (1) come to grips with the nature of health inequalities, (2) acknowledge and challenge their complexity with complex solutions, and (3) deal with the multicausal nature of health inequalities? Insights to those basic questions are key to effective program planning.

If investigators or health planners were to identify what fundamentally makes their research or health promotion interventions meaningful or impactful, it is likely to be distilled to identifying which programs actually prompt action and contribute to health. In an examination of 30 studies undertaken as part of a Ghanaian-Dutch program, Kok and colleagues (2016) used Contribution Mapping to evaluate systematically which of the studies would be used to meet national health goals within 12 months of ending the program.

The evaluation revealed, for example, that implementation of a tuberculosis program that overcame financial and transport barriers to obtaining treatment helped reveal the high prevalence of HIV and hepatitis C not only among prisoners but also among guards. Counseling, education, and treatment were provided; health services improved; national health insurance was extended to the prisoners; and the prison itself (a 17th-century colonial fortress) was eventually closed.

Six features of the research that were successfully used were noted for contributing to the success of the programs:

- identifying a fit with national research goals,
- empowering researchers to initiate their own use of the transportation or financial support arrangements,
- engaging potential key users during proposal preparation,
- introducing new practices as part of the implementation,
- engaging potential key users in interpreting results and proposing improvement recommendations, and
- distributing printed reports of findings in a targeted way.

In addition, three characteristics were deemed integral to successfully moving the findings to action: (1) having a vision of what should be done and who should do it; (2) holding a formal position that allowed setting the project on a course for action; and (3) recognizing that powerful systems, structures, and dynamics nurtured some actions and constrained others. Analyses of this type in communities where members participate in some or all aspects of the research—in Latino communities, for example (Mier et al. 2010), or in African-American, Asian, and other communities—are warranted so that factors contributing broadly to their success and the key characteristics related to taking action and implementing them can be identified and tested.

EVALUATING OUTCOMES IN COMMUNITIES

In addition to the indicators for both "quality of life" and "health" as ultimate outcome goals in the application of the PRECEDE-PROCEED model, initiatives are increasingly expected to track policy contributions related to important *intermediate outcomes* (Ottoson et al. 2013). Accordingly, the PRECEDE-PROCEED model acknowledges the reality that, globally, communities are social-ecological units in which health-related behaviors are influenced by interpersonal and community networks as well as governing policies.

The *Salud America!* program integrated evaluation on multiple layers to ensure meaningful evaluation and to introduce early career investigators to the potential inherent in policy change, as seen in box 10.1 (Ottoson et al. 2013; Ramirez et al. 2013). In another instance, a South Texas researcher and her colleagues pursued policy venues and informal surveying in order to educate policy makers, eventually becoming known as subject matter experts and making policy recommendations to officials (Mier et al. 2013). They were working in Hidalgo County, near the Texas-Mexico border, where the population in 2016 was 91.8% Latino, 57.6% had completed high school or less, and the median annual income was $32,489 for men and $26,545 for women. Their message indicated that (1) a disproportionate number of Mexican-American children were affected by obesity and, (2) those children were unable to meet levels of recommended physical activity. Though Mier and colleagues (2013) did not report following the PRECEDE-PROCEED model specifically, they endorsed ecologic models in this project and in their other work emphasizing the importance of incorporating salient cultural values and characteristics in program planning (2010).

COMMUNITY IMPLEMENTATION

Procedures in the early phases of PRECEDE engage community members in the intervention, which helps in building their trust. The iterative nature of these

---

BOX 10.1

PRECEDE-PROCEED Tackles Outcomes: "Policy contribution is not a straight line in time or tasks"

Salud America!, created by the Institute of Health Promotion Research at The University of Texas Health Science Center at San Antonio, offered researchers an opportunity to apply to participate in a group of 20 for individual grants of a maximum of $75,000 for up to two years, all with the aim of reducing Latino childhood obesity. After completion of their projects, investigators learned about the Policy Contribution Spectra framework (with public, policy, and science/evaluation parts) and its usefulness in acquainting investigators with the potential policy contributions of their work. Full descriptions of the year-long work with investigators is reported elsewhere.

In the last phase of the PRECEDE-PROCEED process, investigators make a final determination of how project outcomes aligned with what the community wanted or needed. Interim determinations are an ongoing part of the process throughout. The researchers of *Salud America!* produced those final reports, but also learned to embrace the next step: seeking policy change. In these endeavors, outcomes are often measured not in months, but in years.

The investigators talked to lawmakers, promoted awareness of Latino childhood obesity, and moved forward collaboratively to mobilization. Ottoson et al. (2013) make it clear that the "policy contribution is not a straight line in time or tasks," but it is "multidirectional, multifaceted, and multileveled" (pp. S288, S287). It is important to encourage those new to policy endeavors to see them as extensions of other community involvement, including visiting lawmakers at state capitols, pressing a table or graph into the hand of a voter, or simply informing a friend or relative of changes in statistics affecting the homeless. These corollaries are not so very different from endeavors to sway votes on health care, health access, or nutrition.

assessments gives planners multiple opportunities to address any concerns raised by community members. During early phases of *Salud America!*, those who were overwhelmed could override any moderator in order to refocus the conversation on understanding immigration policy uncertainty, the threat of racial profiling, and migratory issues (Ottoson et al. 2013).

During implementation and the evaluations of the PROCEED phases, modifications can be made as the program examines the processes of implementation and their impact. It is important to remember that without subgroup input and analyses, the evaluation may miss unique findings relevant to, and known only to, subgroups who may be at greater risk.

CHALLENGES OF MODEL IMPLEMENTATION IN COMMUNITIES

Some of the challenges that face the health program planner include the following:

- Interventions are a team sport. They are by nature collaborative and culturally supportive. Problems can occur when plans focus too much on individuals or decision-making lies in too few hands. Planners should strive for relevance and usefulness to the population and should aim for making the plan practical and actionable to policy makers and other researchers (Green et al. 2009). Without consideration of "community or organizational conditions in which people live, grow, work, and play" (Trickett et al. 2011, p. 1411), sustainability will likely be lost.

- Fluidity, flexibility, and functionality are hallmarks of the PRECEDE-PROCEED model, and these characteristics are especially relevant to communities because of the growing diversity that characterizes them (Yang et al. 2015).

- Using the PRECEDE-PROCEED planning model with other theoretical models can add complexity, but also can bolster the potential for impact.

- Some argue that planners too often fail to develop or thoroughly describe health promotion interventions systematically (Kok and Mesters 2011). The consequences can then be that other practitioners face barriers to replication or implementation because descriptions of elements, particularly of methods, are absent or inadequate. This can be daunting to under-resourced programs in low-income communities of color or rural communities seeking to implement evidence-based programming.

SUMMARY

The PRECEDE-PROCEED model has been globally employed with success in the design, implementation, and evaluation of health promotion programs and practices in a wide range of community health issues, settings and populations. Its acceptance and ongoing application since its introduction decades ago are indications of its practicality, its easy-to-understand approach, and its welcome integration of diagnostic planning and process evaluation and other perspectives that emphasize the value of *practice-based evidence*. This, in turn, has complemented the demand for more *evidence-based practice*. That integration helps planners avoid the pitfalls of assuming that research-sourced evidence can adequately represent the realities of communities, cultures, and settings other than those in which their evidence was produced. It also gives communities not just access to locally relevant data, but also public respect and credibility through the collection and use of that relevant data.

Systematic planning is essential to creating cohesive programs, from social diagnosis through to evaluation of outcome, but rigidity is not the aim, nor should it be a price that must be paid for a systematic approach (Corcoran 2011). When initiatives are planned comprehensively not only *for* and with the community, but also *by* the community—that is, representatives of the community own with other planners the plan, the context in which it is created, the identification of the goals, and the implementation and evaluation—the community is more likely to benefit and realize the changes it wants most to see.

EXERCISES

Think about a specific health problem you would like to address in a community setting (i.e., school, neighborhood, or ethnic group)—for example, childhood obesity in a mostly Latino low-income neighborhood. Residents in this neighborhood work mostly in construction, landscaping activities, and housekeeping. They have limited access to healthful foods with only one grocery store within five miles; there are multiple fast food restaurants, and several are located within one mile of the school area. Families have limited access to active spaces (trails, parks, and recreation facilities), and the neighborhood has safety issues with broken street lights, street dogs, and reports of gang-related activities. Based on this description, construct the PRECEDE-PROCEED model diagram and detail your observations or assumptions about the first four phases.

Phases 1 and 2 will help you identify the goal and objectives of your intervention program:

1. Describe the demographic characteristics of the community and identify the key stakeholders to be involved in your plan to address this community health problem—for example, teachers, parents, or church leaders (Phase 1—Social Assessment).

2. Select five key stakeholders to be part of your Community Advisory Committee (CAC) to guide the intervention you would like to implement, and briefly describe why you selected them (Phase 1).

3. Describe the strategies to conduct a community needs assessment and identify community priorities (i.e., focus groups, key informant interviews, and key topics to include) (Phase 1).

4. Review the literature and draft a one-page summary of the epidemiology of childhood obesity in Latinos to present to the CAC (i.e., childhood obesity-related morbidity and mortality and the behavioral and socio-environmental risk factors that influence the health issue you want to address, which is, in this example, childhood obesity in a mostly Latino neighborhood) (Phase 2—Epidemiological Assessment).

To access data on this topic, please visit *Salud America!* It is a national network organized to promote Latino health equity and to perform research in healthy families and schools, healthy neighborhoods and communities, and healthy and cohesive cultures:

- Healthy Families and Schools: https://salud-america.org/issues/healthy-families-schools/
- Healthy Neighborhoods and Communities: https://salud-america.org/issues/healthy-neighborhoods-communities/
- Healthy and Cohesive Cultures: https://salud-america.org/issues/healthy-cohesive-cultures/

Phases 3 and 4 will help you plan and design your intervention.

5. List the predisposing (i.e., knowledge, attitudes, beliefs), reinforcing (i.e., influence of the social environment), and enabling (i.e., availability of resources, accessibility of services, state and local policies) factors affecting childhood obesity in this neighborhood (Phase 3—Behavioral and Environmental Assessment).

6. Think about what factors determine the feasibility of implementing the program to address childhood obesity in this neighborhood, including the resources available, associated organizations, and other invested stakeholders. Also, consider what national, state, and local policies or programs serve to lessen this health problem (i.e., community parks, farmers markets,

community gardens, local schools' food policies, fit programs sponsored by the Special Supplemental Nutrition Program for Women, Infants, and Children [WIC], and other initiatives) (Phase 4—Administrative and Policy Assessment).

References

Anderson, R. (1968). *A Behavioral Model of Families' Use of Health Services* (Research Series 25). University of Chicago Center for Health Administration Studies.

Bartholomew, L.K., Parcel, G.S., & Kok, G. (1998). Intervention mapping: A process for developing theory and evidence-based health education programs. *Health Education and Behavior, 25*(5), 545–63. https://doi.org/10.1177/109019819802500502

Bartholomew, L.K., Parcel, G.S., Kok, G., Gottlieb, N.H., & Fernández, M.E. (2011). *Planning Health Promotion Programs: An Intervention Mapping Approach* (3rd ed.). Jossey-Bass.

Buta, B., Brewer, L., Hamlin, D.L., Palmer, M.W., Bowie, J., & Gielen, A. (2011). An innovative faith-based healthy eating program: From class assignment to real-world application of PRECEDE-PROCEED. *Health Promotion Practice, 12*(6), 867–75. https://doi.org/10.1177/1524839910370424

Centers for Disease Control and Prevention. (2018). The Public Health System and the 10 Essential Public Health Services. Atlanta: Centers for Disease Control and Prevention. Retrieved October 10, 2019, from https://www.cdc.gov/publichealthgateway/publichealthservices/essentialhealthservices.html

Corcoran, N. (2011). *Working on Health Communication.* SAGE Publishing.

Crosby, R., & Noar, S. (2017). What is a planning model?: An introduction to PRECEDE-PROCEED. *Journal of Public Health Dentistry, 71*(Suppl. 1), S7–S15. https://doi.org/10.1111/j.1752-7325.2011.00235.x

D'Onofrio, C. (2001). Pooling information about prior interventions: A new program planning tool. In Sussman, S. (Ed.), *Handbook of Program Development for Health Behavior Research and Practice* (pp. 158–200). SAGE Publishing.

Farquhar, J. & Green, L.W. (2015). Community intervention trials in high-income countries. In Detels, R., Gulliford, M., Abdool Karim, Q., and Tan, C.C. (Eds.), *Oxford Textbook of Public Health* (6th ed., Vol. 2, pp. 516–27). Oxford University Press. https://doi.org/10.1093/med/9780199661756.003.0112

Fernández, M., Gonzales, A., Tortolero-Luna, G., Partida, S., & Bartholomew, L. (2005). Using intervention mapping to develop a breast and cervical cancer screening program for Hispanic farmworkers: Cultivando la salud. *Health Promotion Practice, 6*(4), 394–404. https://doi.org/10.1177/1524839905278810

Fernández, M., Gonzales, A., Tortolero-Luna, G., Williams, J., Saavedra-Embesi, M., Chan, W., & Vernon, S.W. (2009). Effectiveness of Cultivando La Salud: A breast and cervical cancer screening promotion program for low-income Hispanic women. *American Journal of Public Health, 99*(5), 936–43. https://doi.org/10.2105/AJPH.2008.136713

Geertz, C. (2000). *Available Light: Anthropological reflections on philosophical topics.* Princeton University Press.

Gielen, A., McDonald, E., Gary, T., & Bone, L. (2008). Using the PRECEDE-PROCEED model to apply health behavior theories. In Glanz, K., Rimer, B., & Viswanath, K. (Eds.), *Health Behavior and Health Education* (4th ed., pp. 407–33). Jossey-Bass.

Gillespie, L.D., Robertson, M.C., Gillespie, W.J., Sherrington, C., Gates, S., Clemson, L., & Lamb, S.E. (2012). Interventions for preventing falls in older people living in the community. *Cochrane Library, 12*(9), CD007146. https://doi.org/10.1002/14651858.CD007146.pub3

Goodman, R.A., Bunnell, R., & Posner, S.F. (2014). What is "community health"?: examining the meaning of an evolving field in public health. *Preventive Medicine, 67*(Suppl. 1), S58–S61. https://doi.org/10.1016/j.ypmed.2014.07.028

Goodwin, V.A., Abbott, R.A., Whear, R., Bethel, A., Ukoumunne, O.C., Thompson-Coon, J., & Stein, K. (2014). Multiple component interventions for preventing falls and fall-related injuries among older people: systematic review and meta-analysis. *BMC Geriatrics 14*, 15. https://doi.org/10.1186/1471-2318-14-15

Green, L., Glasgow, R., Atkins, D., & Stange, K. (2009). Making evidence from research more relevant, useful, and actionable in policy, program planning, and practice: Slips "twixt cup and lip". *American Journal of Preventive Medicine, 37*(6 Suppl. 1), S187–S191. https://doi.org/10.1016/j.amepre.2009.08.017

Green, L., & Kreuter, M. (1992). CDC's planned approach to community health as an application of PRECEDE and in inspiration for PROCEED. *Health Education Journal, 23*(3), 140–7. https://doi.org/10.1080/10556699.1992.10616277

Green, L., & Kreuter, M. (2005). *Health Program Planning: An Educational and Ecological Approach* (4th ed.). McGraw-Hill.

Hu, J., Wallace, D.C., McCoy, T.P., & Amirehsani, K.A. (2014). A family-based diabetes intervention for Hispanic adults and their family members. *The Diabetes Educator, 40*(1), 48–59. https://doi.org/10.1177/0145721713512682

Hu, J., Wallace, D.C., & Tesh, A.S. (2010). Physical activity, obesity, nutritional health and quality of life in low-income Hispanic adults with diabetes. *Journal of Community Health Nursing, 27*(2), 70–83. https://doi.org/10.1080/07370011003704933

Huff, R.M., Kline, M.V., & Peterson, D.V. (Eds.) (2015). *Health Promotion in Multicultural Populations: A Handbook for Practitioners and Students*. SAGE Publishing.

Hunter, K., Keay, L., Clapham, K., Brown, J., Bilston, L.E., Lyford, M., Gilbert, C., & Ivers, R.Q. (2017). "He's the number one thing in my world": Application of the PRECEDE-PROCEED model to explore child car seat use in a regional community in New South Wales. *International Journal of Environmental Research and Public Health, 14*(10), E1206. https://doi.org/10.3390/ijerph14101206

Institute of Medicine. (2012). *An Integrated Framework for Assessing the Value of Community-Based Prevention*. National Academies Press.

Kok, G., & Mesters, I. (2011). Getting inside the black box of health promotion programmes using intervention mapping. *Chronic Illness, 7*(3), 176–80. https://doi.org/10.1177/1742395311403013

Kok, M.O., Gyapong, J.O., Wolffers, I., Ofori-Adjei, D., & Ruitenberg, J. (2016). Which health research gets used and why?: an empirical analysis of 30 cases. *Health Research Policy and Systems, 14*(1), 36. https://doi.org/10.1186/s12961-016-0107-2

Martin, M.A., Floyd, E.C., Nixon, S.K., Villalpando, S., Shalowitz, M., & Lynch, E. (2016). Asthma in children with comorbid obesity: Intervention development in a high-risk urban community. *Health Promotion Practice, 17*(6), 880–90. https://doi.org/10.1177/1524839916652845

Mier, N., Ory, M.G., & Medina, A.A. (2010). Anatomy of culturally sensitive interventions promoting nutrition and exercise in Hispanics: A critical examination of existing literature. *Health Promotion Practice, 11*(4), 541–54. https://doi.org/10.1177/1524839908328991

Mier, N., Smith, M.L., Irizarry, D., Carillo-Zuniga, G., Lee, C., Trevino, L., & Ory, M.G. (2013). Bridging research and policy to address childhood obesity among border Hispanics: A pilot study. *American Journal of Preventive Medicine, 44*(3 Suppl. 3), S208–S214. https://doi.org/10.1016/j.amepre.2012.11.013

Ottoson, J.M., Ramirez, A.G., Green, L.W., & Gallion, K.J. (2013). Exploring potential research contributions to policy: The Salud America! experience. *American Journal of Preventive Medicine, 44*(3 Suppl. 3), S282–S289. https://doi.org/10.1016/j.amepre.2012.11.025

Parker, L., & Fineberg, H. (2013). Building strategies and leadership for change: The obesity epidemic in Latino children. *American Journal of Preventive Medicine, 44*(3 Suppl. 3), S292–S293. https://doi.org/10.1016/j.amepre.2012.12.001

Porter, C. (2015). Revisiting Precede–Proceed: A leading model for ecological and ethical health promotion. *Health Education Journal, 75*(6), 753–64. https://doi.org/10.1177/0017 896915619645

Puska, P. (2002). Successful prevention of non-communicable diseases: 25 year experiences with North Karelia Project in Finland. *Public Health Medicine, 4*(1), 5–7.

Puska, P., Leparski, E., Lamm, G., Heine, H., Pereira, J., Pisa, Z., & Thelle, D. (1988). *Comprehensive cardiovascular community control programmes in Europe.* World Health Organization Regional Office for Europe.

Ramirez, A., Gallion, K., Despres, C., & Adeigbe, R. (2013). Salud America!: A national research network to build the field and evidence to prevent Latino childhood obesity. *American Journal of Preventive Medicine, 44*(3 Suppl. 3), S178–S185. https://doi.org/10.1016 /j.amepre.2012.12.005

Rios, L., & Cullen, T. (2006). A disaster medical assistance team operates a hurricane evacuation shelter with U.S. public health service support. *Preventing Chronic Disease, 3*(2). http://www.cdc.gov/pcd/issues/2006/apr/05_0239.htm

Robert Wood Johnson Foundation. (2018, March 26). *Multi-component fall prevention interventions for older adults.* County Health Rankings and Roadmaps. Retrieved April 1, 2018, from https://www.countyhealthrankings.org/take-action-to-improve-health/what-works -for-health/strategies/multi-component-fall-prevention-interventions-for-older-adults

Sussman, S. (2001). The six-step program development chain model. In Sussman, S. (Ed.), *Handbook of Program Development for Health Behavior Research and Practice.* SAGE Publishing.

Tramm, R., McCarthy, A., & Yates, P. (2012). Using the PRECEDE-PROCEED model of health program planning in breast cancer nursing research. *Journal of Advanced Nursing, 68*(8), 1870–80. https://doi.org/10.1111/j.1365-2648.2011.05888.x

Trickett, E., Beehler, S., Deutsch, C., Green, L., Hawe, P., McLeroy, K., Miller, R.L., Rapkin, B.D., Schensul, J.J., Schulz, A.J., & Trimble, J.E. (2011). Advancing the science of community-level interventions. *American Journal of Public Health, 101*(8), 1410–9. https://doi.org/10.2105 /AJPH.2010.300113

University of Wisconsin Population Health Institute. (n.d.) *What is health?* County Health Rankings and Roadmaps. Retrieved April 1, 2018, from http://www.countyhealthrankings .org/what-is-health

Weiner, J., & McDonald, J. (2013). Three models of community-based participatory research. *LDI Issue Brief, 18*(5), 1–7.

Yamada, T., Chen, C.C., Murata, C., Hirai, H., Ojima, T., Kondo, K. & Harris, J.R. (2015). Access disparity and health inequality of the elderly: Unmet needs and delayed healthcare. *International Journal of Environmental Research and Public Health, 12*(2), 1745–72. https:// doi.org/10.3390/ijerph120201745

Yang, H.J., Ho, M.K., & Kuo, L.H. (2015). A model for programming planning in emerging technology promotion. *Recent Researchers in Engineering Education,* 142–9. Retrieved February 27, 2018, from http://www.wseas.us/e-library/conferences/2015/Salerno/EDU /EDU-21.pdf

CHAPTER 11

Applications in Occupational Settings

•

Paul Terry, Nico Pronk, and Shelley Golden

Learning Objectives

After completing the chapter, the reader will be able to:

- Integrate the PRECEDE-PROCEED model and data from health risk assessments, health care claims data, and organizational development surveys (i.e., employee satisfaction, engagement, and perceived organizational support) in workplace health program planning.
- Describe the most effective strategies to engage workplace-based stakeholders (e.g., CEO, CFO, managers, employees, wellness champions) in the planning, implementation, and evaluation processes.
- Identify evidence-based "best practices" in workplace health promotion and how best practices scorecards can be applied to advancing the planning and evaluation elements of the PRECEDE-PROCEED model.
- Use tenets of the social-ecological framework to show how both the voice of the employee and the business case for workplace health improvement can be equally represented in program planning.
- Explain how complex systems science complements the PRECEDE-PROCEED model when evaluating and implementing programs or policies in occupational settings.

INTRODUCTION

Considering the genesis and growth of worksite health promotion, those who were trained in the use of the PRECEDE-PROCEED model and who are now working in occupational settings are likely experiencing hindsight bias—the "I knew it all along" phenomenon. Even though it may have taken decades longer than the model's originators, Green and Kreuter, anticipated, planners of worksite wellness are finally embracing the social-ecological principles associated with the model. As with most public health interventions over the past decades, worksite wellness programs between the 1980s and 2000 were primarily designed to reduce individual health risk factors by supporting improvements in personal lifestyles (Golden and Earp 2012). Perhaps the most prescient aspect of the PRECEDE-PROCEED model was its "knowing all along" that social and environmental factors profoundly mitigate (or enhance) the success of individual behavior change.

Today, "building a culture of health" is a broadly accepted catchphrase (HERO 2016). Health educators formerly focused on designing individual risk reduction programs and perhaps community programs, using at least participatory methods, are now actively engaged in assessing and intervening in organizational and environmental policies that influence a population's health (Goetzel et al. 2014a; Green and Allegrante 2011; Kent et al. 2016; O'Donnell 2005; Pronk 2014; Terry et al. 2013).

In the nascent stages of the worksite wellness movement, very few companies employed a comprehensive approach that paid deliberate attention to both policy and programs and the balance between social and individual responsibility for health that the model demands (Green and Cargo 1994). Indeed, most programs were a piecemeal amalgam of health assessments, biometric screenings, and health education classes. In 2004, fewer than 9% of employers reported using a comprehensive approach that integrated assessments, planning, interventions, and evaluations (Linnan et al. 2008). Subsequently, worksite wellness became a $4 billion industry (Mattke et al. 2012), with most employers indicating support for employee wellness (AON Hewitt et al. 2016; Mattke et al. 2013; Willis Towers Watson 2017). Still, a 2016 survey found that while 83% of companies with over 200 employees offered wellness programs, only 13% had comprehensive programs (Kaiser Family Foundation 2016).

With these modest investments, it is not surprising that studies of the effectiveness of worksite wellness have produced inconsistent results. For many years, a primary goal of employer-sponsored wellness programs was to contain rising health care costs and increase employee productivity. Several well-designed studies affirmed the oft-touted 3:1 return on investment (ROI) from wellness (Baxter et al. 2014; Goetzel et al. 2001), while others indicated only marginal financial and health benefits (Jones et al. 2018; Mattke et al. 2013).

As the field of worksite wellness has matured, the value proposition to employer-sponsored programs has broadened in ways that can be better informed by PRECEDE-PROCEED. Planning for health promotion is increasingly more in tune with the broader business, social, and environmental problems a company is trying to solve. Where safer, healthier, less stressed, and more productive employees were the promise of wellness in past decades (Alderman et al. 1980; McLeroy et al. 1984; Gottlieb et al. 1992; Stainbrook and Green 1987; Task

Force on Community Preventive Services 2010; Terry et al. 2010), a movement from "wellness" to "well-being" is afoot, with ambitions for worksite wellness that highlight the value of a more engaged workforce. Though "engagement" may be a catchphrase that is surpassing a "culture of health" as a worksite wellness imperative, its meaning is a work in progress. Employee engagement is purportedly about happier, more psychologically resilient, and financially secure workers who are finding their life's purpose, who have work that induces "flow," and who enjoy a work pace that enables work-life balance. Engagement is more recently thought to be more likely in a workplace that enables an authentic connection with communities and contributes to the sustainability of the planet (Quelch 2016; Terry 2017).

As with ROI research, studies aiming to ratify this contemporary value proposition showed early mixed results (Lovato et al. 1993). A survey of 2,320 consumers 23 years later suggests employees view worksite wellness as a valuable employee benefit, with 47% considering it a "good business investment" and 43% indicating wellness programs make them "feel better about the company" (AON Hewitt et al. 2016). On the other hand, another survey indicates more than 60% are dissatisfied with their employer's wellness offerings (Willis Towers Watson 2017). As this chapter will argue, these differences are likely attributable to planning. Is the program driven by a plan? Is the plan relevant to the company's priorities? Was it developed using the participatory planning principles of PRECEDE-PROCEED? A consultant involved with the survey that uncovered employee dissatisfaction with wellness addresses these questions succinctly: "Employers that listen to their employees and formulate strategies that take their needs into account will have the most success redesigning existing programs and introducing new ones" (Shelly Wolff, phone interview, February 10, 2018).

Health promotion program planners love a captive audience, and most people spend 58% of their adult lives in the workplace. It is not merely the amount of time spent there; rather, it is the prospect of the workplace harboring safety hazards, toxic exposures, or dispiriting managers versus its potential for protecting and promoting well-being that makes the workplace such a compelling setting for health promotion practice (World Health Organization 2018). As was described in chapter 1, it is not only the concentration of people, but the context and controllability of the environment that bestows the application of PRECEDE-PROCEED with such enormous promise in occupational settings. Relative to other venues for public health and health promotion practice, such as schools, communities, or health care settings, health promotion in the workplace has been a lower priority for the public health education profession. This may partly explain why the literature is relatively sparse for the use of PRECEDE-PROCEED in occupational settings. There is, however, a more compelling explanation and a more urgent opportunity for workplace-based program planners. Of the many "best practices" that researchers have been codifying in worksite health promotion, one of the most commonly accepted but most underutilized best practices is strategic planning (Grossmeier et al. 2016; Hartwell et al. 1988; Weaver et al. 2018).

This chapter aims to summarize how PRECEDE-PROCEED has been successfully applied in workplace settings. We will highlight the need to increase strategic planning generally and, more specifically, show how each step in PRECEDE-PROCEED can inform improvements in the worksite health promotion process. Even with the best-laid plans, worksites are complex ecosystems, so this chapter will also summarize the tenets of complexity theory and review the social-ecological model to deepen the reader's appreciation for a robust planning framework. This chapter presents studies from years past and current company programs that together offer practice-based evidence about what best predicts success.

A goal of this chapter is to elicit more widespread use of PRECEDE-PROCEED in occupational settings in order to reconcile commonly accepted "best practices" from other settings against the varied, emerging, and often untested goals for worksite health promotion described above. Accordingly, this chapter will show how PRECEDE-PROCEED provides a cogent planning framework that connects to core principles in workplace program design, draws on best practices, and uses planning tools like health assessments and best practices scorecards to build and support the use of practice-based evidence for a workplace health promotion strategy (Goetzel et al. 2014a; Green 2008).

A REVIEW OF PRECEDE-PROCEED APPLICATIONS IN THE WORKPLACE

Workplace health promotion studies based on the PRECEDE-PROCEED model have been designed and conducted for a wide range of behavioral and environmental challenges, such as reducing heart disease (Bailey et al. 1994; Sun and Shun 1995); tobacco use (Bibeau et al. 1988; Bertera et al. 1990; Sun and Shun 1995); managing weight (DeJoy et al. 2012); controlling blood pressure and hyperlipidemia (Bertera 1990a); increasing breast self-exams (Chie et al. 1993); and reducing exposures to pesticides (Quandt et al. 2001) and blood-borne infections (DeJoy et al. 1995). Formal training in the use of the PRECEDE-PROCEED model in workplace settings increases a learner's readiness to apply each of the components in the model to improve employee wellness program offerings (Ottoson 1995). For example, maintaining employee participation and sustaining behavior change is a recurrent challenge in worksite wellness. Drawing on the diagnostic elements in the PRECEDE-PROCEED model, a "preprogram diagnostic interview" model was developed to ensure that both individual and environmental factors were being used to prevent dropouts from the program and reduce behavioral relapse (Lovato and Green 1990).

In some landmark studies, the PRECEDE-PROCEED model has been featured as it influenced the intervention planning (Bertera 1990b; Chie et al. 1993; DeJoy et al. 1995; Sun and Shun 1995). For example, the model was used to examine the differences between white-collar and blue-collar workers and their smoking rates (which averaged 54.6%) in China; the study showed that enabling and predisposing factors were strong predictors of smoking behavior (Sun and Shun 1995). Similarly, an intervention strategy designed to reduce nurse exposure to blood-borne pathogens such as HIV/AIDS was based on the PRECEDE-PROCEED model and, accordingly, included both environmental (protective devices) and behavioral (performance feedback) components (DeJoy et al. 1995). Another study that focused on reducing cardiovascular disease risk did a factor analysis of predisposing, enabling, and reinforcing factors to better predict healthful lifestyle choices among urban employees in China (Chiou et al. 1998).

Worksite-based studies also commonly use the PRECEDE-PROCEED model to guide an intervention's evaluation (Bailey et al. 1994; Bertera 1993; Bibeau et al. 1988; Schecter et al. 1997). A case study example of work-site studies is found in box 11.1. With a focus on the participatory research tenets of the model, one study with Latino farmworkers showed how regulatory barriers were as relevant to the intervention plan as modifiable behaviors in reducing the risks of pesticide exposure (Quandt et al. 2001). Herbert and White (1996) focused on the principles of community mobilization in reducing higher-than-average heart disease rates in worksites in Canada. The PRECEDE-PROCEED model served as the organizing framework for the evaluation of the worksite data derived from health risk assessments (HRAs), wellness committees, and program interventions (Herbert and White 1996). Similarly, in a weight management research project, DeJoy and colleagues (2012) discussed how the PRECEDE-PROCEED model informed their systematic evaluation of the effects of environmental changes in a Georgia workplace on body weight and perceived organizational support.

WHAT IS THE PROBLEM IN *YOUR* WORKPLACE?: PRECEDE-PROCEED PHASES 1–3

As was emphasized in earlier chapters, beginning with the end in mind is a central tenet of effective planning; in the case of workplace health promotion, it will verify that one size does not fit all when it comes to designing your program. Not only is there significant variation in the problems an employer is trying to solve, key human resources priorities for a company will likely change over time. In a

BOX 11.1
The DuPont Company: The PRECEDE-PROCEED Model's Seminal Worksite Case Study

The DuPont Company, a mining and manufacturing company with 80,000 employees in 85 locations, was an early adopter of the PRECEDE-PROCEED model. In 1987, DuPont introduced a comprehensive, extensively researched worksite wellness program based on the model. Dr. Robert Bertera was the program developer and researcher leading DuPont's program, which was recognized with the Society for Public Health Education's Excellence Award. Bertera received his doctorate at Johns Hopkins University during the time that Dr. Larry Green was at Hopkins teaching such future leaders about the PRECEDE-PROCEED model.

In a series of studies, Bertera was among the first worksite health promotion researchers to show the significant relationships between employee health risks and higher health care costs and absenteeism (Bertera 1990a; 1990b; 1991; 1993). Consistent with the PRECEDE-PROCEED model, DuPont's planning process was data-driven, with detailed analysis of morbidity and mortality data and surveys of employees and organizational leaders. Based on these inputs and a combination of learning experiences, environmental supports, and recognition, programs were developed with specific objectives aimed at reductions in tobacco use and better prevention and control of high blood pressure and hyperlipidemia.

Based on initial pilot studies, a 7% reduction in blue-collar workers' absenteeism (compared to non-pilot sites) was one of the early indicators of success for DuPont's programs. After a two-year study period comparing 7,178 program participants with 7,101 non-participating employees, Bertera reported risk level improvements in six of the seven risk factors targeted. The percent of high-risk employees, those with three or more risk factors, decreased by 14%, and the number of self-reported sick days decreased by 12% in the participation group (Bertera 1993).

weak economy with high unemployment rates, employers usually focus on cost containment, and worksite health programs may be supported primarily if a near-term return on investment seems assured. In a strong economy, with keen competition for talent, health and well-being initiatives that solve for employee engagement, happiness, and loyalty may take precedence.

Does your worksite wellness program have a vision statement and a mission? And, just as importantly, does your wellness program's mission align seamlessly with the mission statement of the company? Phases 1, 2, and 3 of PRECEDE ensure that your program is responsive to the unique problems *your* organization is trying to solve. Recall that the term "program" in this book is intended to include the full range of components required to bring about the intended changes in health and social outcomes. In short, a program awaits a clear vision. Your program planning should account for the dynamic forces occurring in the company, your community, and the nation. As stated in chapter 1, "Complexity is the price one pays for embracing an ecological approach to health planning." Later in this chapter, we review complexity theory and systems thinking that, like this social diagnosis stage, heighten our cultural awareness through participatory approaches to planning and increase our sensitivity to other contextual characteristics of the workplace.

Phase 1: What Is Relevant to Your Company's Stakeholders?: Social Assessment and Situational Analysis

Who are the stakeholders you need to engage within workplace health planning? Who best understands the organizational context that can enable a program to thrive, and what resources should you draw on to accomplish the first phases of PRECEDE that demand ardent cultural awareness? And what principles can guide you in working through the PRECEDE stages? Building on a scoping review article by Nico Pronk, table 11.1 summarizes PRECEDE planning steps and positions them alongside established worksite health promotion best practices principles and program elements. Pronk (2014) examined the most commonly cited articles featuring elements of best practices in worksite wellness. By organizing the 44 elements he found according to their definitions, he identified nine planning principles embedded within them (Pronk 2014; Fonarow et al. 2015) For example, Phase 1 of PRECEDE involves conducting a social assessment and situational analysis; table 11.1 shows Pronk's related findings that keeping a program "relevant" is a principle behind several best practices elements. These include programs that are mission-driven, accessible, and tailored to the needs of employees and their families and communities.

Determining a program's relevance requires the full participation of all stakeholders. As described in chapters 1 and 2, research shows that the successful engagement of those who are the subject of a change is directly tied to their involvement in deciding what needs changing. In a workplace setting, you might think of employees as the customers of your program and the employer, most often via their human resources department, as the retailer of the employee wellness products and services. When the needs of all workplace wellness stakeholders are equitably balanced, the situational analysis proffers equal attention to the work environment as it does to employee behaviors, as indicated in PRECEDE's Phase 2. To date, the payer for worksite wellness has been the employer and, accordingly, the business case for worksite wellness has been that of delivering an ROI to the employer by focusing on changing employee behavior (Goetzel et al. 2001; Mattke et al. 2012). As suggested above, in a flush economy, the employee may be the more influential stakeholder and the case for wellness may increasingly relate to creating an environment highly conducive to worker satisfaction (Flynn et al. 2018).

TABLE 11.1. Aligning the PRECEDE-PROCEED model with principles of worksite wellness program design and best practices elements used in worksite health promotion planning

PRECEDE-PROCEED model elements	Worksite wellness program design principles	Worksite wellness best practices elements
Phase 1: Social Assessment and Situational Analysis. Use of a participatory approach to planning and collecting insights into the cultural and social circumstances unique to that population. Not only do the kinds of social and business performance problems a workplace experiences offer a barometer of the workplace culture, they also illuminate critical social and economic determinants.	*Relevance:* Programs apply to the needs and interests of workers and their families, a critical factor in long-term engagement of employees. *Compliance:* Elements that ensure a health management program meets regulatory and ethical requirements and safeguards individual-level data.	Program connected to company mission, vision, and business objectives. Easily accessible program options. Effective program options (evidence-informed). Tailored programmatic solutions for individuals. Multiple program delivery options and modalities. Ensuring ergonomic and safety standards are met (e.g., OSHA). Ensuring regulatory requirements are met (e.g., HIPAA, ADA, GINA, EEOC). Ensuring appropriate ethical standards are met such as equity across the workforce, equal access to services and resources.
Phase 2: Epidemiological Assessment. Identify the specific health goals or problems that may contribute to, or interact with, the social goals or problems noted in Phase 1 and identify determinants of health in the genetics, behavioral patterns, and environment of the population.	*Leadership:* Set the vision for the program, assign accountability, ensure structural support for the program, engage leaders throughout the organization.	Assessment of health risks with feedback: health assessments, biometric screenings. Organizational commitment to a healthy culture (mission and vision) of leadership. Adequate resourcing. Strategic plan with goals and objectives. Leadership engagement. Multi-level leadership. Assigned program accountability.

TABLE 11.1. (*continued*)

PRECEDE-PROCEED model elements	Worksite wellness program design principles	Worksite wellness best practices elements
Phase 3: Educational and Ecological Assessment. "The ecological approach inherently recognizes context and the educational approach recognizes that each place has its own history, has learned its own traditions, enables people to perform their responsibilities, and reinforces its own way of doing things." (chapter 1)	*Comprehensiveness:* Elements that include health education, supportive physical and social environments, integration of the worksite program in to the organization's structure, linkage to related programs, and worksite health screening.	Supportive physical and psychosocial work environments and organizational policies. Multilevel programming: individual, group, management/organizational, environmental, policy. Organizational environmental and policy assessment. Integration of programs and vendors: linkages to EAPs, work-life balance, disease management, case management, return-to-work, FMLA, occupational safety and health, occupational medicine, ergonomics.
Predisposing factors: A person's or population's knowledge, attitudes, beliefs, values, and perceptions that facilitate or hinder motivation for change.	*Partnership:* Efforts designed to integrate with multiple stakeholders, including individual workers, organized labor, community organizations, vendor companies, and other internal partners.	Participatory practices. Worker involvement and representation.
Reinforcing factors: Rewards received and the feedback the learner receives from others following the adoption of a behavior—may encourage or discourage continuation of the behavior.	*Engagement:* Promote respect throughout the organization, build trust, facilitate program co-ownership through participatory principles, ensure worker representation in decision-making processes. Provide meaningful incentives that leverage intrinsic motivation and fit the company culture, and create a workplace environment in which health programs thrive.	Wellness champions network. Meaningful and relevant participation incentives. Human-centered culture. Health and wellness committee engagement.
Enabling factors: The skills, resources, or barriers that can help or hinder the desired behavioral changes as well as environmental changes.	*Comprehensiveness:* Elements that include health education, supportive physical and social environments, integration of the worksite program into the organization's structure, linkage to related programs, and worksite health screening.	Awareness and education programs. Behavior change programs. Supportive physical and psychosocial work environments and organizational policies.

(*continued*)

TABLE 11.1. (*continued*)

PRECEDE-PROCEED model elements	Worksite wellness program design principles	Worksite wellness best practices elements
Phase 4: Administrative and Policy Assessment and Intervention Alignment. Ensuring the program has the policy, organizational, and administrative capabilities and resources to make this program a reality.	*Leadership and Communication:* Set appropriate organizational policies to support health, and support the program via needed resources. Provide a formal communication strategy that includes a branding approach for program visibility, ongoing communications using multiple delivery channels, and targeted and tailored messaging designed to reach specific subgroups.	Adequate resourcing. Program branding. Year-round comprehensive program communications.
Phase 5: Implementation. The program components and interventions needed to affect the changes specified in previous phases.	*Implementation:* Provide a planned, coordinated, and fully executed implementation of health management programs, including ongoing monitoring and designated staff with clearly delineated accountabilities.	Operations work plan. Implementation management system. Population triage, segmentation.
Phases 6–8: Process, Impact, and Outcome Evaluation. All four phases of PRECEDE may be viewed as formative evaluation in which diagnostic and assessment data serve to set program priorities, goals, objectives and targets, and also as baseline measures for later summative evaluation. In the PROCEED component and Phases 5–8, this prior information serves as the source of baseline data for monitoring implementation and progress.	*Data-Driven and Compliance:* Ongoing measurement, evaluation, reporting, and analytics. Data represent the program experience and can drive continuous program improvement. Elements that ensure a health management program meets regulatory and ethical requirements and safeguards individual-level data.	Continuous improvement model. Measurement and evaluation. Data-driven. Analysis and reporting. Regulatory compliance: HIPAA, GINA, ADA, PPACA, state law.

Phase 2: Epidemiological Assessment and the Need for Multi-Level Leadership

Phase 1 of PRECEDE focused on a vision responsive to the problems a workplace is trying to solve. In Phase 2, the challenge of translating this vision into achievable objectives and desired outcomes continues. In Phases 2 and 3, program planners collect data and continue with formative evaluations aimed at understanding what factors, particularly health-related issues, are contributing to company and employee problems. As previewed above, these are likely a combination of behavioral factors like current employee health risks or social interactions, along with environmental factors outside an individual employee's control, like the built environment or workplace policies that influence health or happiness.

New to this step of the PRECEDE-PROCEED model is genetic testing, which, due to genetic nondisclosure laws and Equal Employment Opportunity Commission (EEOC) protections, will be used judiciously in workplaces (Terry 2017a). These combinations of factors should be examined as to whether, how, and why they contribute to the problems identified in Phase 1. As shown in table 11.1, leadership at multiple levels is germane to assessing these factors effectively as well as the organizational commitment and resources available to address these problems.

The worksite wellness tools most commonly used for collecting data needed for Phase 2 are computer-based HRAs, biometric screenings, and best practices scorecards (Anderson et al. 2014; Goetzel and Terry 2013; Roemer et al. 2013; Terry 2013). Where biometric screenings offer objective health data, HRAs offer self-reported data from individual employees about their lifestyle practices and physical and emotional health. Scorecards are company self-assessments usually completed by stakeholders from the human resources and wellness program staff (HERO 2018b; CDC 2019). Phase 2 of PRECEDE-PROCEED examines behavioral, genetic, and environmental contributors to the problems identified in Phase 1, and most scorecards contain most of the elements summarized under the "best practices" column in table 11.1. The results of a self-rating after completing a scorecard enable companies to compare their environment and health programs to national reference data. The CDC and Health Enhancement Research Organization (HERO) scorecards are the two most commonly used that are freely available (CDC 2019; HERO 2018a). Ideally, it is a combination of these individual and cultural data that informs PRECEDE Phase 2, but the wherewithal to collect and analyze such integrated data has largely been confined to very large organizations. One survey showed that nearly 80% of those companies responding obtained data via HRAs, but only about 40% of companies conducted a culture audit or had data available related to employee engagement or productivity (Weaver et al. 2018). It is rarer still to find organizations that have analyzed their individual health data alongside data about their environment and culture (Flynn et al. 2018; Grossmeier et al. 2016).

Having a strategic plan and written objectives is considered a best practice and is, therefore, a standard question asked in scorecards. Of particular significance, per the aims of this chapter, is the dearth of good planning in worksite wellness. Over 1,800 companies have completed the HERO scorecard developed in cooperation with Mercer (HERO 2018b). One study of HERO scorecard users found that 44% of companies reported that they had no written strategic plan and only 25% of companies had a multi-year strategic plan. And, just as inopportunely, of those who had a written plan, fewer than half (47%) felt that their strategic planning had been effective (HERO 2018b). In another HERO study of 205 organizations who responded to scorecard questions about strategic planning, of those who had no written objectives, only 6% reported significant employee health risk improvement and 22% reported slight improvement. In contrast, 21% of organizations with written objectives reported significant improvement and 49% reported slight improvement (Hunt 2017).

One of the most common contextual factors influencing Phase 2 planning is simply the size of the organization and the time and resources available for investing in planning and executing a wellness strategy. An analysis of the kinds of planning activities reported by companies, organized by company size, is provided in table 11.2 (HERO 2018b). Larger organizations are more likely to have both an annual plan and a long-term plan, albeit this is still fewer than a third of all companies. The measurable objectives monitored by companies also vary according to company size. But metrics about program participation, changes in health risks, and improvements in clinical outcomes remain the most common factors organizations are trying to improve. Notably, smaller companies are more likely than larger companies to measure success according to employee satisfaction, engagement and productivity, and performance impacts. It may be these variables are deemed more controllable by small organizations or, conversely, that large organizations see these factors as a Pandora's box they are reluctant to open.

Phase 3: Educational and Ecological Assessment and the Need for Comprehensiveness

Visit the website of any workplace large enough to have one and you can almost always find the "About Us" tab. It may be the best place to start when you are ready to embark on Phase 3 of PRECEDE-PROCEED, for it is here that you will get a sense of the organization's vision and core values. The problems and root causes of the problems you have identified in the first phases now need to be put in the context of how the organization views itself. If the "About Us" section of the website includes an "Our History" tab, all the better. Understanding the organization's stories, markers of success, and leadership philosophy are absolutely germane to the task of mobilizing resources to solve organizational problems. Too often, worksite health and well-being initiatives are lost on organizational leaders and employees alike because they aren't strategically aligned with the day-to-day core purpose of the company. Based on two independent surveys of employers and a general population of working adults, McCleary and colleagues (2017) found that nearly 60% of employees believed employers should be involved with improving the health of their employees. However, half as many employees as employers reported that wellness programs were available in their companies, and fewer than half of employees felt that their workplace was conducive to good health. Phase 3 examines the factors that can make a program a company priority by affecting change in the health outcome objectives, versus the program becoming invisible.

TABLE 11.2. Use of strategic planning elements according to company size (HERO Scorecard)

The HERO Health and Well-being Best Practices Scorecard in collaboration with Mercer®			
	Fewer than 500 employees	500–4,999 employees	5,000 or more employees
Formal, written, strategic plan for health and well-being			
Have a long-term plan (2+ years) only	9%	13%	19%
Have an annual plan only	26%	23%	24%
Have both a long-term and annual plan	9%	19%	31%
Don't have a formal plan	57%	45%	26%
Number of respondents	265	361	196
Measurable objectives included in health and well-being strategic plan (among employers with a plan)			
Participation in health and well-being programs	85%	90%	90%
Changes in health risks	50%	59%	73%
Improvements in clinical measures/outcomes	34%	47%	52%
Absenteeism reduction	19%	19%	23%
Productivity/performance impact	27%	15%	25%
Financial outcomes measurement (medical plan cost or other health)	44%	52%	57%
Winning health and well-being program awards	43%	40%	38%
Recruitment/retention	35%	24%	15%
Employee satisfaction/morale and engagement	65%	62%	53%
Customer satisfaction	20%	19%	24%
None of the above	3%	4%	3%
Number of respondents	115	197	146

Predisposing, Enabling and Reinforcing Factors in the Workplace

Predisposing Factors. Perhaps as troubling as sponsoring a worksite wellness program that few employees know about is investing in one where those who would benefit the most use it the least. There are countless factors that predispose employees to participate in offerings like yoga, fitness, cooking classes, or mindfulness meditation versus, say, a financial well-being class. An analysis of the first year of a comprehensive wellness program at the University of Illinois showed that less healthy, lower-income wage earners were less likely to participate in wellness than higher-wage earners (Jones et al. 2018). This is consistent with other research showing that lower-wage workers were, ironically, less likely to take advantage of financial incentives to participate in worksite wellness (Sherman and Addy 2018). As Maslow's hierarchy of needs would have it, if basic needs are unmet, other wellness goals may seem superfluous. One recent survey found that one-quarter of workers reported difficulty paying for food, heat, and housing, the same percentage said they had decreased their retirement plan contributions and 43% had decreased other savings (Fronstin and Greenwald 2018). Another study showed that financial worries about the costs of health care were the top financial concern of consumers, with 30% of employees saying their "level of debt is ruining the quality of their life" (AON Hewitt et al. 2016). Clearly, understanding what predisposes a population to engage in wellness requires a keen understanding of what is relevant to employees' daily lives.

Enabling Factors. As the planning phases above have emphasized, programs are most likely to be deemed relevant when they are co-created with stakeholders. Enabling full participation in planning, like enabling behavior change, is a function of removing barriers and improving skills. One worksite-based randomized controlled trial was designed to compare the effectiveness of a traditional approach to worksite wellness to a consumer-directed approach. Traditional wellness meant health coaching, group programs, and educational campaigns were offered to employees according to the population's most prevalent health risks. The consumer-directed approach involved coaching and educating employees about how to assess their needs, values, and priorities independently to find resources. Called the Activate Study, the findings were consistent with the proverb "Give a man a fish, and you feed him for a day. Teach a man to fish, and you feed him for a lifetime"—that is, employees who were coached in self-management skills were as likely to improve in health risk scores as those coached on risk reduction behaviors. Equally as importantly, those who were coached in activation skills were significantly more likely to report being confident in their self-management ability going forward (Harvey et al. 2012; Terry et al. 2011).

Reinforcing Factors. The wellness provisions of the Affordable Care Act (ACA) ratified the use of financial incentives to encourage and reinforce employees to achieve and maintain low health risks such as maintaining healthy weight and blood pressure and not smoking (Affordable Care Act 2010). Ever since the provisions were enacted, there has been debate about the fairness and effectiveness of financial incentives related to participation in programs or tied to health outcomes. It has been necessary to remind those less familiar with worksite wellness that the incentive program is not the wellness program (Terry 2019). Research on the use of financial incentives consistently shows that money can motivate short-term participation, but it is less clear that such extrinsic rewards will evoke sustainable behavior change (Terry 2017b; Terry 2019a; Volpp 2008; Volpp et al. 2011). The more promising reinforcing factors are intrinsic motivators that support healthy choices over the long term, such as the following.

Context Matters: The Role of the Social-Ecological Model and Complex Systems Science

The first three phases of PRECEDE help planners understand the complex interplay of factors that produce the health landscape of a worksite. As such, they overlap with the principles and approaches of social-ecological models and complex system science. The social-ecological model is a tool used in public health to identify the determinants of a specific health issue in a population. It views health as determined by an interplay of characteristics and actions of individuals; the people with whom they interact; the places where they live, work, and play; and the institutions and policies that provide the political, legal, and economic scaffolding of their lives. This interplay is depicted as a series of concentric circles, as shown in figure 11.1, representing different levels of health influence.

One way to think about applying social-ecological models to worksite wellness, consistent with PRECEDE-PROCEED, is to view the workplace as a microcosm in which all ecological levels operate. This approach conceptualizes key worker factors, like educational background, workstyle, and extraversion, as interacting with supervisory characteristics, like supervisory and co-worker support; job characteristics, like required overtime or employee autonomy; and workplace environment factors, like safe working conditions and company policies to influence health. The PRECEDE-PROCEED model becomes a tool to guide planners in identifying aspects of the workplace across a host of ecological levels that deserve consideration when planning worksite wellness initiatives.

Social-ecological models highlight not only different levels of analysis, but also the interplay of factors across those levels, and are thus understood to also be a systems approach to health. The workplace itself, the staff, the relationships, and the associated dynamic interactions with people, products, environments, and (micro)cultures represent a complex social system (Pronk and Narayan

2016). Based on this, complex systems science may, using either quantitative (e.g., systems modeling) or qualitative (e.g., systems mapping) methods, elucidate important factors and relationships influencing the desired outcomes of workplace wellness programs. System modeling uses mathematical or computational efforts to create a virtual laboratory in which different scenarios may be tested or evaluated. Systems mapping, on the other hand, may be used to better "see" the system as a whole. This may be accomplished by creating a visual in which many factors are shown along with the direction of their interactions. An example of a systems stock-and-flow map applied to understanding and preventing chronic disease is offered in figure 11.2. The flow shows the progression to disease and the stocks illustrate opportunities for interventions. Such visualizations can facilitate dialogue among stakeholders during the program planning process.

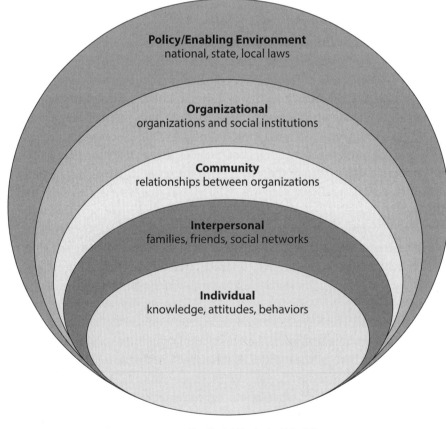

Policy/Enabling Environment
national, state, local laws

Organizational
organizations and social institutions

Community
relationships between organizations

Interpersonal
families, friends, social networks

Individual
knowledge, attitudes, behaviors

FIGURE 11.1. The Social-Ecological Model.

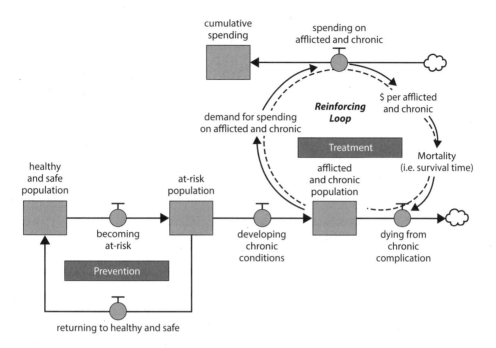

FIGURE 11.2. Stock and Flow Map created by the Georgia Health Policy Center to understand and prevent chronic disease. *Source:* Georgia Health Policy Center, Andrew Young School of Policy Studies. (n.d.) *Systems Thinking.* Georgia State University. https://ghpc.gsu.edu/tools-frameworks/systems-thinking/

Best Practices that Build a Culture of Health and Reinforce Healthful Behaviors

In a study by Flynn using the HERO scorecard, company responses to best practices variables were organized into low, medium, and high responses (Flynn 2014). Best practices such as leadership support, employee involvement, a supportive environment, health policies, programs, resources, and rewards were aggregated to identify those companies considered to have higher organizational support (incorporating both enabling and reinforcing factors) for employee wellness. The following list of best practices components are commonly examined to predict program success:

- A company mission/vision statement that supports a healthful workplace culture;
- Senior leaders who consistently articulate the value and importance of health;
- The presence of policies that support employee health and well-being;
- A built environment that supports well-being;
- Senior leaders who support well-being;
- Employee involvement in decisions about well-being program content;

- Use of wellness champion networks to support well-being programs;
- Support for mid-managers and supervisors in attempts to improve well-being.

The results showed that "companies that report a higher level of organizational support not only have an overall higher score on the HERO Scorecard but also have higher scores within each section of the scorecard [see box 11.2]. In other words, the companies that provide a greater degree of organizational support are stronger in all best practices areas" (Flynn 2014).

BOX 11.2
The L.L. Bean Company: A Planning Phases Case

The L.L. Bean case study is one of nine "Promoting Healthy Workplaces" studies from Johns Hopkins University that profiles American companies with exemplary stories to tell about their employee health and well-being initiatives. These are available at the website of the Institute for Health and Productivity Studies (Institute for Health and Productivity Studies 2018). Where all of the companies profiled by the Institute use the first phases of the PRECEDE-PROCEED model, L.L. Bean stands out relative to the data collection and analysis needed in steps one, two, and three of the model. As much as the L.L. Bean company conjures iconic images of fit employees conquering the great outdoors, the reality is that most jobs there, like at most workplaces, are sedentary (Freundlich 2015).

As part of the planning process for the L.L. Bean program, called "Healthy Bean," planners examined health risk and biometric assessment data from 4,000 employees and found their call centers were experiencing the highest risk levels, with 71% with high blood pressure, 67% obese, and 11% living with diabetes. Importantly, their situational analysis did not stop with health risk data analysis. After a pilot of an exercise and weight management initiative with 24 obese employees, program planners found that emotional issues were a significant negative predisposing factor (or, said another way, the lack of a positive emotional reaction to healthy eating), which served as an impediment to participation.

Based on initial data collection, the wellness program staff partnered with the L.L. Bean Employee Assistance Program (EAP) staff and developed an additional social assessment focused on mental, emotional, and financial well-being issues. This additional round of data collection showed that providing help for emotional, family stress, and financial issues was as vital to enabling relief from a sedentary job as were the diet and exercise activities originally offered. Their pilot program and educational assessments also showed program planners that group and individual counseling sessions to discuss body image issues and support realistic goal-setting were important reinforcing factors for improving program results. These learnings from the educational and ecological assessments were vital to the eventual positive improvements in cardiovascular and emotional health at L.L. Bean (Institute for Health and Productivity Studies 2018).

WHAT IS *YOUR* PLAN?: PRECEDE-PROCEED PHASES 4 AND 5: ADMINISTRATIVE AND POLICY ASSESSMENT, INTERVENTION ALIGNMENT, AND IMPLEMENTATION

As should be evident from the list of 44 best-practice components listed in table 11.1, there is now a veritable laundry list of tools, tactics, and methods that, based on evidence to date, are contributors to success in worksite wellness. Phases 4 and 5 of PRECEDE-PROCEED ask that you sort through the laundry and, based on the assessments conducted thus far, urge you to surface those items that fit your organization best, given the size and shape of the problems you are trying to solve. Borrowing from the insights in chapter 1, a "best practice" is one that is presumed to be effective across cultures and socioeconomic conditions, regardless of historical precedent in social customs, laws, and policies. It gets its "best" reputation on the basis of the strength of evidence in highly controlled randomized research trials. Note that many best practice components in table 11.1 relate to tailoring strategies according to employee preferences, but also to the unique values and goals of the organization.

The evidence informing Phases 4 and 5, then, is derived both from health education literature and from within the company. Or, more succinctly, "the pathway to better evidence-based practice is through more practice-based evidence." As an aside, in a journal article that profiled Lawrence Green, a co-editor of this book and the source for that quote, Green mused that he has espoused his belief in the essential role of "practice-based evidence" so often that someone may well engrave it on his tombstone (Green and Terry 2015).

Most human resources departments are not staffed with health educators, and most companies lack the resources to develop a long-range strategy, much less customize and develop a comprehensive program. As indicated earlier, only 13% of companies surveyed in 2016 had comprehensive wellness programs. Based on this same survey by the Kaiser Family Foundation, most companies take a centralized approach to implementation. The following list shows the percent of companies surveyed that offer each of these best practices components (Kaiser Family Foundation 2016).

- Employee screenings with follow-up – 70%
- Health education – 64%
- Supportive physical and social environment – 64%
- Links to related employee services – 50%
- Integration of health promotion into organization's culture – 47%

A noteworthy study that took a centralized approach to planning and coordination but also respected the cultural differences at decentralized locations occurred at Johns Hopkins University and School of Medicine (JHM). On behalf of their more than 50,000 employees, JHM developed a five-year strategic plan designed to "support a healthy workplace throughout JHM" (Safeer et al. 2018). The JHM program developers based their plan on the social-ecological model by organizing their intervention strategies within the environmental, organizational, interpersonal, and individual-level influences from the model. The CDC scorecard was used to determine a first-year baseline for JHM overall, as well as at 12 JHM locations, and scorecards were completed a year later to assess progress toward best practices overall and at the 12 sites respectively.

Consistent with the PRECEDE-PROCEED model, each location decided what part of their scorecard they would try to improve during the year based on their unique circumstances, values, and priorities. Eleven of the 12 locations showed improvements in their scorecards from year one to year two. There were striking similarities between the findings at JHM using the CDC scorecard and those based on using the HERO scorecard, especially related to the importance of organizational support. To wit, "the entity with the highest improvement in total score from baseline to year two was also the most improved entity in the organizational supports score. In contrast, the only entity that did not improve their score in the organizational support section was consequently the only entity that did not improve their total score from year one to year two" (Safeer et al. 2018, e103). Universities are thought to have egalitarian cultures, so it is not surprising that principles of participatory research and the social-ecological framework feature prominently in their program planning. The success at JHM affirms the importance of aligning worksite health promotion interventions and administrative supports, as does the exemplary case from the University of Michigan below.

The University of Michigan: An Exemplary Case of Phase 1, Participatory Assessment, and Phases 4 and 5, Administrative and Policy Assessment, Intervention Alignment, and Implementation

Two organizational websites that offer open access to a plethora of cases and planning resources that relate to PRECEDE-PROCEED Phases 4 and 5 are the HERO and the CDC Workplace Health Resource Center (CDC 2019; HERO 2019). From HERO's website, the University of Michigan's MHealthy program stands out with respect to its intentional alignment of their policy assessment with their interventions and administrative supports. The MHealthy program has institutionalized a wellness champion network with over 585 staff and faculty members who strive to create a sense of community via worksite activities. Though there is a strong centralized wellness team responsible for guidance and resources, the champions ensure that programs are tailored at the site level based on local-level needs. Champions are trained to use ACES, an acronym that means "announce, complete, execute, and share—to engage, connect, and build support with their colleagues" (MHealthy 2017, 2).

The MHealthy planning process involves the frequent use of stakeholder groups who attend advisory committees. That input is augmented with a Voices of the Staff initiative. Eight teams of "voices," representing a total of about 200 employees, meet monthly to "share concerns and interests of staff in areas of health and well-being, work/life integration, diversity, equity and inclusion, climate, parking and transportation" (MHealthy 2017, 4). Strong executive leadership keeps wellness relevant on campus, as MHealthy is a presidential initiative and the business case for wellness is part of their Leaders Creating a Culture at Its Best workshop. The "U-M Philosophy of Well-Being" is a "view of health and well-being, which includes mental and emotional, environmental, occupational, social, intellectual, spiritual, and physical dimensions" (MHealthy 2017, 5). A 2016 Culture of Health Survey at U-M found that two-thirds of employees agreed or strongly agreed that their supervisors supported their health and well-being, and nearly two-thirds agreed that MHealthy contributed to the university being a great place to work (Grossmeier 2017).

IS *YOUR* PLAN WORKING?: PRECEDE-PROCEED PHASES 6–8: PROCESS, IMPACT, AND OUTCOME EVALUATION

There is little question that well-designed worksite health promotion programs work (Goetzel et al. 2014b; Pronk and Allen 2009; Soler et al. 2009; Task Force on Community Preventive Services 2010; Terry et al. 2011). The more pressing question in the context of PRECEDE-PROCEED is whether *your* health and well-being initiative is meeting your goals—or, said another way, is able to answer: "What has your program done for me lately?" The evaluation step in Phase 6 is as much about continuously improving the program to address unresolved or emergent problems as it is about documenting results against initial aims. Worksite wellness best practices, as delineated throughout this chapter, can guide you in designing a program that is evidence-based. For example, Terry, Seaverson, Grossmeier and Anderson (2008) examined nine quality components and the use of best practices in 22 companies (representing 767,640 employees). Their findings indicated that those companies with the highest indices based on nine best practices measures had significantly better program outcomes than companies with lower indices. Specifically, companies better at best practices such as leadership support, strategic planning, and comprehensive communications achieved higher health assessment completion rates, intervention enrollment rates, and health behavior change than companies with a lesser commitment to these best practices.

This chapter has emphasized the primacy of a comprehensive approach in predicting program success, but, as table 11.1 is intended to convey, it is not simply executing a long laundry list of practices that delivers results. Instead, it is the alignment of interventions, policies, and administrative data that enables improvements in outcomes. HERO scorecard data is used in table 11.3 to show the overlaps between companies that report that they have policies in place to support wellness and those that report they changed their physical environments to undergird the policy. You can see, for example, that only 23% of companies that say they have policies in place to support physical activity are also able to report that they have incorporated changes into their workplace that make getting more active easier for employees. Companies are doing better in the area of healthful eating, with 51% of companies who report that they have nutrition improvement policies also having environmental supports in place such as healthful food in vending machines or healthful snacks at meetings (HERO 2018a).

TABLE 11.3. Aligning workplace programs and policies (HERO Scorecard data, 2016)

Program: Supports Healthy Eating		Policy Support	
		Yes	No
Physical Environment	Yes	51%	16%
	No	8%	26%

Program: Supports Physical Activity		Policy Support	
		Yes	No
Physical Environment	Yes	23%	45%
	No	6%	27%

Program: Supports Stress Management		Policy Support	
		Yes	No
Physical Environment	Yes	20%	16%
	No	10%	54%

If we put the results of the nine quality components study alongside the progress related to better alignment of policies and programs reflected in table 11.3, there is cause for optimism that program planning can be increasingly informed by good evidence. Nevertheless, such an evidence-based program may fail to achieve your aims if it does not also consider evidence garnered from your established and maturing program. Another study by Terry and colleagues used both individual-level data (n = 205,672 employees) and company-level data (n = 55 companies) to demonstrate how one size does not fit all when it comes to best practices (Terry et al. 2013). By examining best practice components separately, this study showed how each component influenced program participation and outcomes. What's more, this study analyzing best practices showed how each component differentially influenced cohorts based on age and gender. For example, it is commonly believed that women and older employees are more likely to participate in wellness programs. This study, however, showed striking differences in both gender and age at the company level. Some companies had women and elders less likely to enroll in programs, while at other companies women and elders were more than twice as likely to enroll in programs. The researchers behind the study surmised that health promotion should consider the limitations of the "herd effect" in program design.

Social Learning Theory holds that we imitate others like us. The study analyzing best practices showed that such observational learning or role modeling (Bandura 2004) is amplified in organizations where there is a critical mass of certain age or gender cohorts. When many in the "in-group" are participating, it can have a snowballing effect. Just as critically, the study indicated the inverse is also likely.

In chapter 1, we noted that the educational approach to planning has both empirical and philosophical underpinnings. The empirical data from the Terry et al. (2013) study affirms that empirically measured changes in knowledge and action can shape the social and environmental capacity and systems in any community or workplace. Accordingly, a one-size-fits-all worksite wellness program can reinforce disparities, where programs tailored to the unique contexts of a culture can foster inclusivity and higher engagement.

With respect to the philosophical tenets of PRECEDE-PROCEED and how the practice-based evidence such as that discussed above should guide program improvements, we underscore the admonitions in chapter 1 that we must remain committed to the principles of informed consent, active participation, and engagement of those we serve, and ensuring our own cultural sensitivity and competence as we create health enhancing programs. Showing such a commitment can start as simply as asking employees what they value and how things are going with your wellness program. Where answers will likely vary dramatically across companies, as well as between locations within a company, at the national level there is cause for optimism that worksite wellness is becoming ever more volitional and culturally competent. A national survey found that attitudes about employer-sponsored health and wellness programs are increasingly positive in recent years, with nearly 70% of employees saying wellness programs help them get and stay healthy. Broader wellness objectives are also being met, given that nearly 70% say the programs are a reason to stay with their company and 74% believe the programs improve their company's reputations (AON Hewitt et al. 2016).

There are indications that millennials will be more interested in health and well-being initiatives than were the generations who offered the proving grounds for worksite wellness. For example, where 35% of baby boomers say they would like their managers to be very or somewhat active in promoting wellness, 57% of millennials favor such management support (AON Hewitt et al. 2016). Just as the Terry et al. (2013) study showed how sensitivity to gender and age differences is needed in program planning, generational differences offer another frontier for more sophisticated planning in workplace health promotion (AON Hewitt et al. 2016). In the spirit of the PRECEDE-PROCEED model, if our planning also accounts for differences by industry type, organizational size, educational levels, income, and race, and if we adjust our evidence-based practices according to what we learn from such practice-based evidence, then we can be assured that Dr. Green's tombstone will be well attended indeed.

Dell, Inc. "Well at Dell": An Exemplary Evaluation Case, Phases 6–8

The Health Project is the organization that sponsors the C. Everett Koop National Health Awards, prizes that recognize excellence in worksite health promotion programs. This is arguably the most results-oriented recognition program in worksite wellness, and the open access website at The Health Project has cataloged award winners going back to the 1994 inception of the Koop Award (The Health Project 2018).

Dell, Inc. launched their "Well at Dell" program in 2004 and won the Koop Award in 2013. In keeping with the evaluation step in PRECEDE-PROCEED, Dell put systems in place to produce evaluation data that could be applied toward continuous program improvement (Well at Dell 2013). First, Dell selected best-in-class providers of wellness services who shared their belief in a data-driven culture. They then required their providers to attend an annual training session to understand Dell's culture and program priorities. Second, Dell empowered their 40,000 employees (called "team members") with data management tools that enabled ongoing support for health care and wellness decision-making. Finally, true to the data-oriented culture of a computer company, Dell focused on a "know your numbers" campaign that featured annual employee goal-setting in weight, exercise, blood pressure, and smoking abstinence. Financial incentives, by way of health insurance premium differentials, encouraged participation. Individual coaching was freely available for team members who fell short of their goals.

Given that these evaluation and monitoring practices are accompanied by comprehensive wellness program offerings, it is not surprising that more than 80% of team members and 45% of spouses or domestic partners had participated in "Well at Dell." A four-year span of repeated health survey measures showed a 7% increase in the number of participants at low risk and a 5% decrease in the number of participants at high risk. These improvements in health risks were associated with an annual increase in return on investment from wellness programming of 1.86:1 to 2.21:1 during that reporting period (Well at Dell 2013).

SUMMARY

Best practices in planning, implementing, and evaluating a worksite wellness program align well with the phases of PRECEDE-PROCEED. Strategic planning embeds worksite wellness in organizational objectives and leadership practices, tools such as HRAs and scorecards provide data for monitoring and evaluating progress, and PRECEDE-PROCEED's emphasis on stakeholder participation builds support from all levels of an organization, ensuring that worksite wellness programs are appropriate and responsive to organizational culture and employees' needs. The literature on worksite wellness programs provides many examples of successful programs that share these features, instilling optimism that more organizations will adopt thoughtfully planned and implemented programs of their own.

EXERCISES

1. Much of the evolution of workplace-based health promotion derived from the *business* case for improving employee health was exemplified at DuPont. If you started over and wanted to build the *employee* case, how could the PRECEDE-PROCEED model support the case?

2. Lifestyle change and culture change are, of course, keenly interrelated. Name examples from workplace settings, such as at L.L. Bean, where individual health choices are profoundly mitigated, for good or for bad, by the environment.

3. Considering the health promotion planning and evaluation practices that led to the "Well at Dell" program at Dell, Inc., what elements of their case best advance the business case at the corporate executive level?

4. Considering the health promotion planning and evaluation practices that led to the MHealthy program at the University of Michigan, what components of their case best advance the employee's case at the shop floor level?

References

Affordable Care Act. (2010). *Read the Affordable Care Act*. HealthCare.gov. Retrieved February 2, 2019, from https://www.healthcare.gov/where-can-i-read-the-affordable-care-act/

AON Hewitt, National Business Group on Health, and The Futures Company. (2016). *Consumer Health Mindset Study 2016*. http://www.aon.com/attachments/human-capital -consulting/2016-Consumer-Health-Mindset.pdf

Alderman, M., Green, L.W., & Flynn, B.S. (1980). Hypertension control programs in occupational settings. *Public Health Reports 95*(2), 158–63. Reprinted in Parkinson, R. et al. (Eds.), *Managing Health Promotion in the Workplace*. Mayfield Publishing Co.

Anderson, D.R., Seaverson, E.L.D., & Terry, P.E. (2014). Health assessment. In O'Donnell, M.P. (Ed.), *Health Promotion in the Workplace* (4th ed., pp. 409–38). American Journal of Health Promotion.

Bailey, P.H., Rukholm, E.E., Vanderlee, R., & Hyland, J. (1994). A heart health survey at the worksite: The first step to effective programming. *AAOHN Journal 42*(1), 9–14. https:// journals.sagepub.com/doi/pdf/10.1177/216507999404200103

Bandura, A. (2004). Health promotion by social cognitive means. *Health Education and Behavior, 31*(2), 143–64. https://doi.org/10.1177/1090198104263660

Baxter, S., Sanderson, K., Venn, A., Blizzard, C.L., & Palmer, A.J. (2014). The relationship between return on investment and quality of study methods in workplace health promotion programs. *American Journal of Health Promotion, 28*(6), 347–63. https://doi.org/10.4278 /ajhp.130731-LIT-395

Bertera, R.L. (1990a.) The effects of workplace health promotion on absenteeism and employment costs in a large industrial population. *American Journal of Public Health, 80*(9), 1101–5. https://doi.org/10.2105/ajph.80.9.1101

Bertera, R.L. (1990b.) Planning and implementing health promotion in the workplace: A case study of the Du Pont Company experience. *Health Education Quarterly, 17*(3), 307–27. https://doi.org/10.1177/109019819001700307

Bertera, R.L. (1991). The effects of behavioral risks on absenteeism and health-care costs in the workplace. *Journal of Occupational and Environmental Medicine, 33*(11), 1119–24. https://doi.org/10.1097/00043764-199111000-00006

Bertera, R.L. (1993). Behavioral risk factor and illness day changes with workplace health promotion: two-year results. *American Journal of Health Promotion, 7*(5), 365–73. https:// doi.org/10.4278/0890-1171-7.5.365

Bertera, R.L., Oehl, L.K., & Telepchak, J.M. (1990). Self-help versus group approaches to smoking cessation in the workplace: eighteen-month follow-up and cost analysis. *American Journal of Health Promotion, 4*(3), 187–92. https://doi.org/10.4278/0890-1171-4.3.187

Bibeau, D.L., Mullen, K.D., McLeroy, K.R., Green, L.W., & Foshee, V. (1988). Evaluations of Workplace Smoking Cessation Programs: A Critique. *American Journal of Preventive Medicine, 4*(2), 87–95. https://doi.org/10.1016/S0749-3797(18)31202-9

Centers for Disease Control and Prevention (CDC). (2019, January 30). *Worksite Health ScoreCard*. Retrieved on February 26, 2019, from https://www.cdc.gov/workplacehealth promotion/initiatives/healthscorecard/index.html

Chie, W.C., Cheng, K.W., Fu, C.H., & Yen, L.L. (1993). A study on women's practice of breast self-examination in Taiwan. *Preventive Medicine, 22*(3), 316–24. https://doi.org/10.1006 /pmed.1993.1026

Chiou, C.J., Huang, Y.H., Ka, J.K., Chun, F.J., & Huang, H.Y. (1998). Related factors contributing to the healthy lifestyle of urban employees through the PRECEDE model. (Chinese). *Kaohsiung Journal of Medical Sciences, 14*(6), 339–47.

DeJoy, D.M., Wilson, M.G., Padilla, H.M., Goetzel, R.Z., Parker, K.B., Della, L.J., & Roemer, E.C. (2012). Process evaluation results from an environmentally focused worksite weight management study. *Health Education and Behavior, 39*(4), 405–18. https://doi.org/10.1177 /1090198111418109

DeJoy, D.M., Murphy, L.R., & Gershon, R.M. (1995). The influence of employee, job/task, and organizational factors on adherence to universal precautions among nurses. *International Journal of Industrial Ergonomics, 16*(1), 43–55. https://doi.org/10.1016/0169-8141 (94)00075-E

Flynn, J.P., Gascon, G., Doyle, S., Matson Koffman, D.M., Saringer, C., Grossmeier, J., Tivnan, V., & Terry, P. (2018). Supporting a culture of health in the workplace: A review of evidence-based elements. *American Journal of Health Promotion, 32*(8), 1755–88. https://doi.org /10.1177/0890117118761887

Flynn, J.P. (2014). *Understanding Organizational Support.* HERO Employee Health Management Best Practices Scorecard In Collaboration With Mercer©: Annual Report 2014 (pp. 12–13). Retrieved February 26, 2019, from https://hero-health.org/publication/hero-scorecard -2014-progress-report/

Fonarow, G.C., Calitz, C., Arena, R., Baase, C., Isaac, F.W., Lloyd-Jones, D., Peterson, E.D., Pronk, N., Sanchez, E., Terry, P.E., Volpp, K.G., Antman, E.M., & American Heart Association. (2015). Workplace wellness recognition for optimizing workplace health: a presidential advisory from the American Heart Association. *Circulation, 131*(20), e480–97. https:// doi.org/10.1161/CIR.0000000000000206

Fronstin, P., & Greenwald, L. (2018). *Workers Rank Health Care as the Most Critical Issue in the United States.* Retrieved May 18, 2021, from https://www.ebri.org/docs/default-source /ebri-issue-brief/ebri_ib_459_wbs-24sept18.pdf?sfvrsn=531b3e2f_4

Freundlich, N. (2015, June 30). *Overcoming obstacles to wellness: Reaching call center workers at LL Bean.* Institute for Health and Productivity Studies, Johns Hopkins University. Retrieved February 18, 2018, from https://www.jhsph.edu/research/centers-and-institutes /institute-for-health-and-productivity-studies/ihps-blog/overcoming-obstacles-to -wellness-reaching-call-center-workers-at-ll-bean

Goetzel, R.., & Terry, P.E. (2013). Current State and Future Directions for Organizational Health Scorecards. *American Journal of Health Promotion, 5/6,* 11–12. https://doi.org/10.4278 /ajhp.27.5.tahp

Goetzel, R.Z., Guindon, A.M., Turshen, J., & Ozminkowski, R.J. (2001). Health and productivity management: Establishing key performance measures, benchmarks, and best practices. *Journal of Occupational and Environmental Medicine, 43*(1), 10–17. https://doi.org/10.1097 /00043764-200101000-00003

Goetzel, R.Z., Henke, R.M., Mosher, R., Benevent, R., Tabrizi, M.J., Kent, K., Smith, K., Roemer, E.C., Grossmeier, J., Mason, S.T., Gold, D.B., Noeldner, S.P., & Anderson, D.R. (2014a). The predictive validity of the HERO Scorecard in determining future health care cost and risk trends. *Journal of Occupational and Environmental Medicine, 56*(2), 136–44. https://doi.org /10.1097/JOM.0000000000000081

Goetzel, R.Z., Henke, R.M., Tabrizi, M., Pelletier, K.R., Loeppke, R., Ballard, D.W., Grossmeier, J., Anderson, D.R., Yach, D., Kelly, R.K, McCalister, T., Serxner, S., Selecky, C., Shallenberger, L.G., Fries, J.F., Baase, C., Isaac, F., Crighton, K.A., Wald, P., . . . Metz, R.D. (2014b). Do workplace health promotion (wellness) programs work? *Journal of Occupational and Environmental Medicine, 56*(9), 927–34. https://doi.org/10.1097/JOM.0000000000000276

Golden, S.D., & Earp, J.A. (2012). Social ecological approaches to individuals and their contexts: twenty years of health education & behavior health promotion interventions. *Health Education and Behavior, 39*(3), 364–72. https://doi.org/10.1177/1090198111418634

Gottlieb, N.H., Lovato, C.Y., Weinstein, R.P., Green, L.W., & Eriksen, M.P. (1992). The implementation of a restrictive worksite smoking policy in a large decentralized organization. *Health Education Quarterly, 19*(1), 77–100. https://doi.org/10.1177/109019819201900106

Green, L.W., & Allegrante, J.P. (2011). Healthy people 1980-2020: raising the ante decennially or just the name from public health education to health promotion to social determinants. *Health Education and Behavior, 38*(6), 558–62. https://doi.org/10.1177/10901981114 29153

Green, L.W. (2008). Making research relevant: if it is an evidence-based practice, where's the practice-based evidence? *Family Practice, 25*(Suppl. 1), i20–i24. https://doi.org/10.1093/fampra/cmn055

Green, L.W., & Cargo, M. (1994). The changing context of health promotion in the workplace. In O'Donnell, M. (Ed.), *Health Promotion in the Workplace* (2nd ed., pp. 497–524). Delmar Publishers, Inc.

Green, L., & Terry, P.E. (2015). "What's past is prologue": views from Dr. Lawrence Green. *American Journal of Health Promotion, 29*(3), TAHP2–8.

Grossmeier, J., Fabius, R., Flynn, J., Noeldner, S., Fabius, D., Goetzel, R., & Anderson, D. (2016). Linking Workplace Health Promotion Best Practices and Organizational Financial Performance: Tracking Market Performance of Companies With Highest Scores on the HERO Scorecard. *Journal of Occupational and Environmental Medicine, 58*(1), 16–23. https://doi.org/10.1097/JOM.0000000000000631

Grossmeier, J. (2017). The Art of Health Promotion: Linking research to practice. *American Journal of Health Promotion, 31*(6), 515. https://doi.org/10.1177/0890117117735957

Hartwell, T.D., Wilensky, G., McFadden, D.W., Dunlop, B.D., Piserchia, P.V., Richardson, J.E., Kroner, B., Lovato, C., & Green, L.W. (1988). *Evaluation of Worksite Health Enhancement Programs: A Monograph*. Research Triangle Institute.

Harvey, L., Fowles, J.B., Xi, M., & Terry, P.E. (2012). When activation changes, what else changes? The relationship between change in Patient Activation Measure (PAM) and employees' health status and health behaviors. *Patient Education and Counseling, 88*(2), 338–43. https://doi.org/10.1016/j.pec.2012.02.005

Health Enhancement Research Organization (HERO). (2016). *Defining a Culture of Health: Key Elements That Influence Employee Health and Well-Being*. Retrieved February 20, 2018, from https://hero-health.org/wp-content/uploads/2016/09/CoH-Definition-and-Elements_final-v2.pdf

Health Enhancement Research Organization (HERO). (2018a). *All Resources*. Retrieved February 19, 2018, from https://hero-health.org/resources/all-resources/

Health Enhancement Research Organization (HERO). (2018b). *The HERO Health and Well-Being Best Practices Scorecard, In Collaboration with Mercer©: 2018 Progress Report*. Retrieved February 26, 2019, from https://hero-health.org/wp-content/uploads/2018/12/6009559-HB-2018-HERO-Scorecard-Progress-Report_final.pdf

Health Enhancement Research Organization (HERO). (2019). *HERO Scorecard*. Retrieved February 26, 2019, from https://hero-health.org/hero-scorecard/

Herbert. R., & White, R. (1996). Healthy hearts at work: Prince Edward Island Heart Health Program CSC Worksite Pilot Project. *Canadian Journal of Cardiovascular Nursing, 7*(2), 12–18.

Hunt, N. (2017, March 6). *Strategic Planning as a Fundamental Step for Achieving Outcomes*. Health Enhancement Research Organization. Retrieved February 22, 2018, from https://hero-health.org/blog/strategic-planning-as-a-fundamental-step-for-achieving-outcomes

Institute for Health and Productivity Studies, Johns Hopkins University. (2018). *Promoting Healthy Workplaces*. Johns Hopkins Bloomberg School of Public Health. Retrieved February 18, 2018, from https://www.jhsph.edu/research/centers-and-institutes/institute-for-health-and-productivity-studies/projects/current-projects/promoting-healthy-workplaces/

Jones, D., Molitor, D., & Reif, J. (2018). *What Do Workplace Wellness Programs Do? Evidence from the Illinois Workplace Wellness Study*. University of Illinois and NBER. Retrieved February 13, 2018, from https://www.nber.org/programs-projects/projects-and-centers/workplace-wellness?page=1&perPage=50

Kaiser Family Foundation. (2016, September 14). *2016 Employer Health Benefits Survey*. Retrieved February 19, 2018, from https://www.kff.org/report-section/ehbs-2016-summary-of-findings/

Kent, K., Goetzel, R.Z., Roemer, E.C., Prasad, A., & Freundlich, N. (2016). Promoting Healthy Workplaces by Building Cultures of Health and Applying Strategic Communications. *Journal of Occupational and Environmental Medicine, 58*(2), 114–22. https://doi.org/10.1097/JOM.0000000000000629

Linnan, L., Bowling, M., Childress, J., Lindsay, G., Blakely, C., Pronk, S., Wieker, S., & Royall, P. (2008). Results of the 2004 national worksite health promotion survey. *American Journal of Public Health, 98*(8), 1503–9. https://doi.org/10.2105/AJPH.2006.100313

Lovato, C., & Green, L.W. (1990). Maintaining employee participation in workplace health promotion programs. *Health Education Quarterly, 17*(1), 73–88. https://doi.org/10.1177/109019819001700108

Lovato, C., Green, L.W., & Stainbrook, G. (1993). The benefits perceived by industry in supporting health promotion programs in the worksite. Harvard Symposium on Worksite Health Promotion. In Opatz, J.P. (Ed.), *Economic Impact of Worksite Health Promotion* (pp. 3–31). Human Kinetics Publishers.

McCleary, K., Goetzel, R., Roemer, E.C., Berko, J., Kent, K., & De La Torre, H. (2017). Employer and Employee Opinions about Workplace Health Promotion (Wellness) Programs: Results of the 2015 Harris Poll Nielsen Survey. *Journal of Occupational and Environmental Medicine, 59*(3), 256–63. https://doi.org/10.1097/JOM.0000000000000946

McLeroy, K.R., Green, L.W., Mullen, K.D., & Foshee, V. (1984). Assessing the effects of health promotion in worksites: A review of the stress program evaluations. *Health Education Quarterly, 11*(4), 379–401. https://doi.org/10.1177/109019818401100401

Mattke, S., Schnyer, C., & Van Busum, K.R. (2012). *A Review of the U.S. Workplace Wellness Market*. RAND Corporation. https://www.rand.org/pubs/occasional_papers/OP373.html.

Mattke, S., Liu, H., Caloyeras, J.P., Huang, C.Y., Van Busum, K.R., & Khodyakov, Shier V. (2013). *Workplace Wellness Programs Study: Final Report*. RAND Corporation. Retrieved February 23, 2019, from https://www.rand.org/content/dam/rand/pubs/research_reports/RR200/RR254/RAND_RR254.pdf

MHealthy. (2017). *University of Michigan Case Study: MHealthy Creating a Culture of Health*. Retrieved February 26, 2019, from https://hero-health.org/publication/culture-of-health-case-study-university-of-michigan/

O'Donnell, M.P. (2005). A simple framework to describe what works best: improving awareness, enhancing motivation, building skills, and providing opportunity. *American Journal of Health Promotion, 20*(1), Suppl. 1–7 following 84, iii.

Ottoson, J.M. (1995). Use of a conceptual framework to explore multiple influences on the application of learning following a continuing education program. *Canadian Journal for the Study of Adult Education, 9*(2), 1–18.

Pronk, N.P. (2014). Best practice design principles of worksite health and wellness programs. *ACSM's Health & Fitness Journal, 18*(1), 42–6. https://doi.org/10.1249/FIT.0000000000000012

Pronk, N.P., & Allen, C.U. (2009). A culture of health: creating and sustaining supportive organizational environments for health. In Pronk, N.P. (Ed.), *ACSM's Worksite Health Handbook* (2nd ed.). Human Kinetics Publishers.

Pronk, N.P., & Narayan, K.M. (2016). The application of systems science to addressing obesity at the workplace: Tapping into unexplored potential. *Journal of Occupational and Environmental Medicine, 58*(2), 123–6. https://doi.org/10.1097/JOM.0000000000000648

Quandt, S.A., Arcury, T.A., Austin, C.K., & Cabrera, L.F. (2001). Preventing occupational exposure to pesticides: using participatory research with Latino farmworkers to develop an intervention. *Journal of Immigrant and Minority Health, 3*(2), 85–96. https://doi.org/10.1023/A:1009513916713

Quelch, J., & Boudreau, E. (2016). *Building a culture of health: A new imperative for business*. Springer International Publishing. https://doi.org/10.1007/978-3-319-43723-1

Roemer, E.C., Kent, K.B., Samoly, D.K., Gaydos, L.M., Smith, K.J., Agarwal, A., Matson-Koffman,

D.M., & Goetzel, R.Z. (2013). Reliability and validity testing of the CDC Worksite Health ScoreCard: an assessment tool to help employers prevent heart disease, stroke, and related health conditions. *Journal of Occupational and Environmental Medicine, 55*(5), 520–6. https://doi.org/10.1097/JOM.0b013e31828349a7

Safeer, R., Bowen, W., Maung, Z., & Lucik, M. (2018). Using the CDC Worksite Health ScoreCard to assess employer health promotion efforts: A case study at Johns Hopkins Medicine. *Journal of Occupational and Environmental Medicine, 60*(2), e98–e105. https://doi.org/10.1097/JOM.0000000000001206

Schecter, J.H., Green, L.W., Olsen, L., Kruse, K., & Cargo, M. (1997). Application of Karasek's Demand/Control Model in a Canadian occupational setting including shift workers during a period of reorganization and downsizing. *American Journal of Health Promotion, 11*(6), 394–9. https://doi.org/10.4278/0890-1171-11.6.394

Sherman, B, & Addy, C. (2018). Low-wage workers and health benefits use: Are we missing an opportunity? *Population Health Management, 21*(6), 435–7. https://doi.org/10.1089/pop.2017.0191

Soler, R.E., Leeks, K.D., Razi, S., Hopkins, D.P., Griffith, M., Aten, A., Chattopadhyay, S.K., Smith, S.C., Habarta, N., Goetzel, R.Z., Pronk, N., Richling, D.E., Bauer, D.R., Buchanan, L.R., Florence, C.S., Koonin, L., MacLean, D., Rosenthal, A., Koffman, D.M., . . . Task Force on Community Preventive Services. (2009). A systematic review of selected interventions for worksite health promotion: the assessment of health. *American Journal of Preventive Medicine, 38*(Suppl. 2), S237–62. https://doi.org/10.1016/j.amepre.2009.10.030

Stainbrook. G., & Green, L.W. (1987). Measurement and evaluation methods for worksite stress-management programs. In Murphy, L.R., & Shoenbaum, T.F. (Eds.), *Worksite Stress Management: Conceptual and Practical Issues* (pp. 109–147). National Institute for Occupational Safety & Health.

Sun, W., & Shun, J. (1995). Smoking behavior amongst different socioeconomic groups in the workplace in the People's Republic of China. *Health Promotion International, 10*(4), 261–6. https://doi.org/10.1093/heapro/10.4.261

Task Force on Community Preventive Services. (2010). Recommendations for worksite-based interventions to improve workers' health. *American Journal of Preventive Medicine, 38*(Suppl. 2), S232–6. https://doi.org/10.1016/j.amepre.2009.10.033

The Health Project. (2018). *C. Everett Koop National Health Awards*. Retrieved February 18, 2018, from http://thehealthproject.com/

Terry, P.E. (2013). Organizational Health Scorecards. *American Journal of Health Promotion, May/June issue*, 1.

Terry, P.E. (2017). Best practices in health promotion: The joy of chasing the uncatchable. *American Journal of Health Promotion, 31*(5), 375–7. https://doi.org/10.1177/0890117117725444

Terry, P.E. (2017a). Preserving employee privacy in wellness. *American Journal of Health Promotion, 31*(4), 271–3. https://doi.org/10.1177/0890117117715043

Terry, P.E. (2017b). Incentives and Big E engagement. *American Journal of Health Promotion, 31*(6), 462–4. https://doi.org/10.1177/0890117117737221

Terry, P.E. (2019). On voluntariness in wellness: Considering organizational health contingent incentives. *American Journal of Health Promotion, 33*(1), 9–12. https://doi.org/10.1177/0890117118817012

Terry, P.E. (2019a). Incentives, mandates and taxes: When doing more equates to learning more. *American Journal of Health Promotion, 33*(2), 166–9. https://doi.org/10.1177/0890117119825684

Terry, P.E., Fowles, J.B., Xi, M. & Harvey, L. (2011). The ACTIVATE study: results from a group randomized controlled trial comparing a traditional worksite health promotion program with an activated consumer program. *American Journal of Health Promotion, 26*(2), e64–e73. https://doi.org/10.4278/ajhp.091029-QUAN-348

Terry, P.E., Grossmeier, J., Mangen, D., & Gingerich, S. (2013). Analyzing best practices in employee health management: how age, sex, and program components relate to employee engagement and health outcomes. *Journal of Occupational and Environmental Medicine, 55*(4), 378–92. https://doi.org/10.1097/JOM.0b013e31828dca09

Terry, P.E., Seaverson, E.L., Grossmeier, J., & Anderson, D.R. (2008). Association between nine quality components and superior worksite health management program results. *Journal of Occupational and Environmental Medicine, 50*(6), 633–41. https://doi.org/10.1097/JOM.0b013e31817e7c1c

Terry, P.E., Seaverson, E.L., Staufacker, M.J., & Gingerich, S.B. (2010). A comparison of the effectiveness of a telephone coaching program and a mail-based program. *Health Education and Behavior, 37*(6), 895–912. https://doi.org/10.1177/1090198110367876

Volpp, K., Asch, D., Robert, G.R., & Loewenstein, G. (2011). Redesigning employee health incentives—lessons from behavioral economics. *New England Journal of Medicine, 365*(5), 388–90. https://doi.org/10.1056/NEJMp1105966

Volpp, K.G., John, L., Troxel, A., Norton, L., Fassbender, J., & Loewenstein, G. (2008). Financial incentive-based approaches for weight loss: a randomized trial. *Journal of the American Medical Association, 300*(22), 2631–7. https://doi.org/10.1001/jama.2008.804

Weaver, G., Mendenhall, B.N., Hunnicutt, D., Picarella, R., Leffelman, B., Perko, M., & Bibeau, D.L. (2018). Performance against WELCOA's Worksite Health Promotion Benchmarks Across Years Among Selected US Organizations. *American Journal of Health Promotion, 32*(4), 1010–20. https://doi.org/10.1177/0890117116679305

Well at Dell. (2013). *Dell, Inc.* The Health Project. Retrieved February 18, 2018, from http://thehealthproject.com/winner/dell-inc/

Willis Towers Watson. (2017, November 17). *2017/2018 Global Benefits Attitudes Survey: The employee voice: more security, more flexibility, more choices.* Retrieved April 25, 2021, from https://www.willistowerswatson.com/en-US/Insights/2017/11/2017-global-benefits-attitudes-survey

World Health Organization. (2018). *Global strategy on occupational health for all: The way to health at work. Recommendation of the second meeting of the WHO Collaborating Centres in Occupational Health, 11–14 October 1994, Beijing, China.* Retrieved February 22, 2018, from http://www.who.int/occupational_health/publications/globstrategy/en/index2.html

CHAPTER 12

Applications in School Settings

Planning Efforts to Help Schools Prevent Noncommunicable Diseases:
Integrating Local, State, National, and International Resources

•

Lloyd J. Kolbe, Holly Hunt, and Faten Ben Abdelaziz

Learning Objectives

After completing the chapter, the reader will be able to:

- Describe the modern school health program, its various components, and how health and education agencies together can plan, implement, and evaluate efforts to help schools improve both public health and education.
- Identify and employ relevant public health surveillance systems to monitor efforts that can help schools measurably improve both public health and education.
- Identify and employ available online resources that local, state, national, and international organizations can integrate to help schools improve both public health and education.

INTRODUCTION AND PURPOSES

Primary and secondary schools worldwide enroll about 1.5 billion young people each year (UNESCO n.d.b.).[1] For example, within the United States, about 130,000 public and private schools in more than 13,000 school districts employ 6 million teachers and staff to educate and nurture 55 million prekindergarten through twelfth grade (PK-12) students every school day, usually for 13 of the most formative years of their lives (USED n.d.a.). In each nation, modern school health programs that include multiple components could substantially improve both the health and education of successive generations of young people and the consequent productivity of the adults they eventually will become (Kolbe 2019).[2]

The findings and conclusions in this chapter are those of the authors and do not necessarily represent the views, decisions, or policies of the institutions with which they are affiliated.

Such programs are especially important for low- and middle-income communities and nations (Bundy et al. 2006; Bundy 2011; Macnab et al. 2014).

Recent research suggests that healthier children learn better and that more educated adults live healthier, more productive, wealthier, and longer lives. Growing evidence suggests that well-planned school health programs improve various indicators of student health. In addition, recent evidence suggests school health programs improve various indicators of academic performance, including student attendance, mood, concentration, memory, classroom behavior, academic effort, school engagement, standardized tests/education skills, grade-point average, grade advancement, literacy, and school completion (CDC 2017c; Kolbe 2019; Michael et al. 2015; Rasberry et al. 2017).

Relevant health and education agencies can plan, implement, and evaluate school health programs to improve measurably both health and education objectives. These plans can be developed ideally across local schools, school districts, states/provinces, nations, and international jurisdictions (Cameron et al. 2007). A wide variety of organizations across these jurisdictions have developed continuously evolving resources. These resources are commonly available through the Internet.[3] Many of these resources continue to evolve over time and, thus, are often denoted in the references as "n.d."—that is, no date. They can be used to help health and education practitioners collaboratively plan, implement, and evaluate school health programs within their own jurisdictions.

The purpose of this chapter is to offer practitioners and researchers—as well as faculty and students in various colleges and universities that train these professionals—a scientifically credible and practical model to help them:

- Plan, implement, and evaluate school health programs that can achieve specific measurable health and education objectives within local schools, school districts, states/provinces, and nations.

- Integrate the evolving efforts and resources that have been developed to help achieve such objectives across the above jurisdictions.

- Describe for interested health and education organizations—as well as for parents, students, and policymakers—how such objectives can realistically be achieved within their own jurisdictions.

This chapter focuses on three elements. First, it focuses on planning school health programs to prevent and control one category of health problems: the noncommunicable diseases (NCDs) also known as chronic diseases. The four main types of NCDs are cardiovascular diseases (like heart attacks and stroke), cancers, chronic respiratory diseases (such as chronic obstructed pulmonary disease and asthma), and diabetes. These diseases cause nearly three-quarters of all deaths in the world and comprise some of the most serious and costly health problems that increasingly afflict every community (WHO 2018b). The planning process described in this chapter to prevent NCDs, however, can also be used to plan school health programs that can prevent other serious health problems (e.g., Chaney et al. 2000; Howatt et al. 1997; Taylor et al. 1999).

Second, the chapter focuses on the United States as an example of one nation's efforts, within the context of broader international efforts to improve school health programs across many nations. The chapter thus does not summarize the good work conducted in many other individual nations to improve school health programs, though citations note exemplary reviews of some of them.

Third, several planning models can be employed, alone or in combination with each other, to help plan school health programs. Such models include the US Centers for Disease Control and Prevention (CDC)'s School Health Index (CDC 2018k) and the Intervention Mapping model (e.g., Belansky et al. 2011; 2013). This chapter focuses primarily on the PRECEDE-PROCEED model, which has been used widely in the United States and internationally during the past four decades (Green et al. 2022).[4] Principles of PRECEDE-PROCEED are very consistent with the principles of the New Framework for Impact and Accountability that the World Health Organization (WHO) is using to complete its *Thirteenth General Program of Work 2019-2023* (WHO 2018d).[5]

BUILDING HEALTH AND EDUCATION PARTNERSHIPS

Before developing a plan to improve school health programs, planners are urged to invite potential key partners to participate in the planning, implementation, and evaluation process. School health programs can be most effective, efficient, and sustainable when interested government and nongovernment health, education, and other organizations work together within their respective jurisdictions (Kolbe et al. 2015). Health agencies have described how they can improve health by improving education (CDC 2016a; Frieden 2010; WHO 2011; 2014b; 2015; 2016a). Conversely, education agencies have described how they can improve education by improving health (ASCD n.d.c.).[6] The PRECEDE-PROCEED planning process can help foster:

- Meaningful participation of key partners in the planning process;
- Flexibility to enable partners to address the specific nature of the student population that they serve, and the specific interests of participating partners; and
- Scalability to enable school health programs to be effective across local schools, school districts, states, nations, and international jurisdictions.

The CDC offers an example of what a national organization can do to help schools prevent NCD risk behaviors across jurisdictions in the United States (Kolbe et al. 2004). The CDC maintains two school health websites that describe a wide variety of available resources that can be used across jurisdictions to improve school health programs (CDC 2018a; 2018f). The CDC also provides support for states and large city school districts to monitor the prevalence of student risk behaviors that cause NCDs and other serious health problems (CDC 2018r). In addition, the CDC monitors the implementation of school health policies and practices that can reduce those behaviors (CDC 2017m; 2017n). Further, the CDC provides support for many states and several national nongovernmental organizations to help schools prevent NCDs (CDC 2017a; 2018f).

More than one hundred other national organizations in the United States independently implement efforts to improve school health programs throughout the country, often through their state-level, if not local-level, affiliates (Kolbe 2015). These national organizations include education organizations (e.g., NASBE n.d.a.), health organizations (e.g., ASTHO n.d.a.), school health organizations (e.g., ASHA n.d.), and organizations that focus on specific school health components, such as school health services (e.g., AAP n.d.), as well as other relevant organizations (e.g., RWJF n.d.). For example, the National Association of Chronic Disease Directors (NACDD) has developed many school health resources (NACDD n.d.b.), including guides to help:

- health professionals understand how to work with the education sector (NACDD 2013).
- education professionals understand how to work with the health sector (NACDD 2009).
- state health departments that do not have dedicated funding for school health programs (NACDD 2012).
- local health departments work with local school districts and schools (NACDD 2017a).

In addition, the Alliance for a Healthier Generation (AHG n.d.b.) and Action for Healthy Kids (AHK n.d.), respectively, help schools across the United States prevent student obesity and consequent NCDs, and the County Health Rankings and Roadmaps (CHRR) offers a range of resources that can help partner agencies work together (CHRR n.d.a.; n.d.b.; n.d.c.; 2018).

Various international organizations help improve school health programs within and across many nations, including WHO Headquarters (e.g., WHO n.d.i.; n.d.n.), WHO Regional Offices (e.g., WHO/EMRO 2010), UNESCO (2016; 2017a; n.d.a.), UNICEF (n.d.), World Bank (n.d.), World Food Program (WFP n.d.), Save the Children (n.d.), International School Health Network (ISHN 2018), and

Partnership for Child Development (PCD n.d.), among others. These and other international organizations work together as part of the Focusing Resources on Effective School Health (FRESH) Partnership to improve school health programs within and across nations (FRESH Partnership n.d.).

LESSONS FROM THE PAST: SOME EXAMPLES OF RESEARCH ABOUT THE EFFECTIVENESS OF SCHOOL HEALTH PROGRAMS TO PREVENT NONCOMMUNICABLE DISEASE (NCD) RISKS

During the last half of the 20th century, researchers found that a relatively small number of risk behaviors—including tobacco use, physical inactivity, unhealthful diets, and harmful alcohol use—contributed to unhealthy metabolic/ physiological conditions, including overweight/obesity, raised blood pressure, raised blood glucose, and raised cholesterol. These, in turn, contributed to NCDs (Bauer et al. 2014; WHO n.d.d.; 2013). These risk behaviors usually are established during childhood and adolescence, frequently are interrelated, and are difficult to change after they have been established (Kann et al. 2018). Accordingly, schools could do much to help young people establish lifelong healthful behaviors. As summarized in box 12.1 (p. 327), from the 1970s through the 1990s, the US National Institutes of Health (NIH) funding progressively developed and evaluated the effectiveness of school health programs to prevent NCD risks.

In summary, PRECEDE-PROCEED has been used in the past to provide evidence about the effectiveness of school health programs to reduce NCD risks among relatively small numbers of students in research studies. As described in the following sections, PRECEDE-PROCEED can be used in the future to help plan, implement, and evaluate broader efforts to help schools implement evidence-informed, if not evidence-based, interventions (Kumah et al. 2019), and increasingly more practice-based evidence, that can prevent NCDs among large numbers of students within and across jurisdictions.[7]

PLANNING FOR THE FUTURE: AN OVERVIEW OF THE PRECEDE-PROCEED MODEL

Various types of logic models can be used by partner organizations to collaboratively plan, implement, and evaluate efforts designed to improve the well-being of their populations (CDC 2018b; WKKF 2004). As depicted in table 12.1 (p. 328), PRECEDE-PROCEED is a logic model that can be employed with and for schools at two specific stages.

BOX 12.1

Guided by the PRECEDE-PROCEED Model, NIH Progressively Developed and Evaluated School Health Programs to Prevent Noncommunicable Disease (NCD) Risks

During the 1970s through the 1990s, the US National Institutes of Health (NIH) began funding a series of randomized-controlled trials (RCTs) to determine whether school health programs could prevent the establishment of NCD risk behaviors (Stone et al. 1989). During the same time period, Green had published early iterations of the PRECEDE-PROCEED model that were being used to plan and evaluate interventions in various settings—including community, health care, occupational, and school settings—to reduce a wide range of health risk behaviors (e.g., Green 1974). NIH provided support for the American Health Foundation to test the effectiveness of a school health intervention called "Know Your Body" (KYB) to prevent the establishment of NCD risk behaviors among elementary school students. KYB employed PRECEDE-PROCEED to plan school interventions that included a health education curriculum, parental activities, and a health risk screening assessment that could help each student modify her or his personal risk profile of health behaviors and physiological conditions that contribute to NCDs. Field trials in three large cities found that KYB improved health knowledge, reduced cigarette smoking, reduced blood pressure, and improved blood cholesterol (Bush et al. 1989; Resnicow et al. 1992; Walter 1989), but KYB did not improve other NCD risk behaviors and associated conditions (Resnicow et al. 1993).

As another example, NIH provided support for Bogalusa Heart Study researchers to test the effectiveness of a school health program to reduce NCD risk behaviors and associated conditions among elementary school students (Berenson et al. 1991). The program applied the PRECEDE-PROCEED model to develop a health education curriculum, parent and family activities, school lunches, and physical education classes that supported healthy behaviors. RCTs of the program found that students in intervention schools improved their knowledge about NCD risk behaviors and improved their blood cholesterol. Students who selected healthier lunches showed the greatest improvements in blood cholesterol, and boys improved their physical fitness (Arbeit et al. 1992).

As a third example, NIH then provided support for researchers at five universities to collaboratively develop and assess the effectiveness of a Child and Adolescent Trial for Cardiovascular Health (CATCH) intervention to reduce NCD risk behaviors among students in nearly 100 elementary schools across four states (Perry et al. 1990). Although CATCH researchers did not apply the PRECEDE-PROCEED model, they similarly helped teachers to implement a school health education curriculum; school food service personnel to provide less fat and sodium in school meals; school physical education teachers to provide more vigorous physical activity; and parents to provide more physical activity and healthier foods. The RCT of CATCH found that intervention schools were able to reduce student energy intake from fat in school lunches; reduce daily student energy intake from fat; increase the intensity of physical activity in school physical education classes; and increase the amount of daily vigorous physical activity (Luepker et al. 1996).

TABLE 12.1. PRECEDE-PROCEED Model for planning, implementing, and evaluating efforts to help schools improve health, education, and other outcomes

(A) First Stage: PRECEDE (*Working from right to left, identify appropriate and available indicators to be achieved in each phase*)

Phase 4	Phase 3	Phase 2B	Phase 2A	Phase 1
Implementation inputs	← Educational and ecological processes	← Genetic, behavioral, and environmental impacts	← Health and education impacts	← Quality of life outcomes

(B) Second Stage: PROCEED (*Working from left to right, monitor and improve the extent to which indicators in each phase improve over time*)

Phase 5	Phase 6	Phase 7B	Phase 7A	Phase 8
Implementation inputs	→ Educational and ecological processes	→ Genetic, behavioral, and environmental impacts	→ Health and education impacts	→ Quality of life outcomes
Examples of inputs	Examples of processes	Examples of indicators	Examples of indicators	Examples of indicators
Every Student Succeeds Act	*Predisposing processes:*	*Health:*	*Health:*	Self-reported physical health, self-reported mental health, tertiary education, employment, income/wealth
Individuals with Disabilities Education Act	(1) Health education	Tobacco use, alcohol use, dietary habits, physical activity, overweight/obese	Illness and premature deaths from cardiovascular disease, cancer, diabetes, and chronic respiratory diseases	
Patient Protection and Affordable Care Act	(2) Social and emotional climate			
	Reinforcing processes:			
Pro-Children Act	(3) Family engagement			
Healthy, Hunger-Free Kids Act	(4) Community involvement			
	Enabling processes:	*Education:*	*Education:*	
	(5) Physical environment	Mood, classroom behavior, academic effort, concentration, memory	School attendance, standardized/tests, education skills, secondary school completion	
	(6) Nutrition environment and services			
	(7) Physical education and physical activity			
	(8) Health services			
	(9) Counseling, psychological, and social services			
	(10) Employee wellness			

TABLE 12.1. (*continued*)

Phase 5	Phase 6	Phase 7B	Phase 7A	Phase 8
	Indicator systems/ data	Indicator systems/ data	Indicator systems/ data	Indicator systems/ data
	CDI	CDI	CDI	BLI
	FRESH	GSHS	CHRR	CDI
	SABER	GYTS	SDG	CHRR
	NASBESHPPS	HBSC	WHS	QLI
	SHPPS	STEPS		SDG
	SHP	YRBSS		

Examples of Indicator Systems
- BLI: Better Life Index (Organisation for Economic Co-operation and Development [OECD], http://www.oecdbetterlifeindex. org/#/11111111111)
- CDI: Chronic Disease Indicators (Centers for Disease Control and Prevention [CDC], https://www.cdc.gov/cdi/index.html)
- CHRR: County Health Ranking and Roadmaps—Social and Economic Factors (CHRR, https://www.countyhealthrankings.org/explore -health-rankings/measures-data-sources/county-health-rankings-model/health-factors/social-and-economic-factors)
- FRESH: Core and Thematic Indicators to Support FRESH (United Nations Educational, Scientific and Cultural Organization [UNESCO], http://hivhealthclearinghouse.unesco.org/sites/default/files/resources/FRESH_M%26E_CORE_INDICATORS.pdf and http://hivhealth clearinghouse.unesco.org/sites/default/files/resources/FRESH_M%26E_THEMATIC_INDICATORS.pdf)
- GSHS: Global School-Based Student Health Survey (World Health Organization [WHO], http://www.who.int/ncds/surveillance/gshs/en/; CDC, https://www.cdc.gov/gshs/)
- GYTS: Global Youth Tobacco Survey (WHO, http://www.who.int/tobacco/surveillance/gyts/en/)
- HBSC: Health Behavior in School-Aged Children (WHO/EURO, http://www.euro.who.int/en/health-topics/Life-stages/child-and -adolescent-health/health-behaviour-in-school-aged-children-hbsc)
- SABER: School Health and School Feeding (World Bank, http://saber.worldbank.org/index.cfm?indx=8&pd=9&sub=0)
- SDG: UN Sustainable Development Goals Monitoring Framework (Sustainable Solutions Development Network, http://indicators .report/indicators/)
- SHP: School Health Profiles (CDC, https://www.cdc.gov/healthyyouth/data/profiles/index.htm)
- STEPS: STEPwise approach to noncommunicable disease risk factor surveillance (STEPS) (WHO, http://www.who.int/ncds/surveillance /steps/riskfactor/en/)
- SHPPS: School Health Policies and Practices Study (CDC, https://www.cdc.gov/healthyyouth/data/shpps/index.htm)
- QLI: Quality of Life Indicators (European Union, http://ec.europa.eu/eurostat/statistics-explained/index.php/Quality_of_life_indicators _-_measuring_quality_of_life#Framework)
- WHS: World Health Statistics data visualization dashboard (WHO, http://apps.who.int/gho/data/node.sdg.3-4)
- YRBSS: Youth Risk Behavior Surveillance System (CDC, https://www.cdc.gov/healthyyouth/data/yrbs/index.htm)

As depicted by table 12.1(A), the first stage is the planning stage, during which program planners and their collaborators and evaluators work sequentially from *right to left* columns:

- In Phase 1, to specify indicators of "quality of life outcomes" their schools might help achieve;

- In Phase 2, to plan to improve specific indicators of (2A) longer-term, then (2B) shorter-term "health and education impacts" that contribute to these outcomes;

- In Phase 3, to plan to improve specific indicators of "educational and ecological processes" that contribute to these impacts; and,

- In Phase 4, to plan to improve specific indicators of "implementation inputs" that contribute to these processes.

The first stage is designed to "precede" program implementation. PRECEDE is the acronym for Predisposing, Reinforcing, and Enabling Constructs in Educational Diagnosis and Evaluation.

As depicted by table 12.1(B), the second stage is the evaluation stage, during which program planners and evaluators then work sequentially from *left to right* columns in Phases 5, 6, 7, and 8 to monitor and improve the achievement of indicators specified in the planning stage. The second stage is designed to "proceed" with program implementation and evaluation. PROCEED is the acronym for Policy, Regulatory, and Organizational Constructs in Educational and Environmental Development.

Next depicted by table 12.1, beneath each phase (column) are examples of inputs, processes, or indicators that can be used to plan and monitor the respective phases.

Finally, as depicted by table 12.1, the examples in each phase (except input examples) are various US and international indicator surveillance systems. Data from these systems often can be used across jurisdictions to identify, monitor, and improve achievements in each phase.

Partner organizations can apply the PRECEDE-PROCEED model to help schools improve both the health and education of their students by implementing each of the six steps outlined below.

Step One: Social Assessment to Improve Quality of Life Outcomes (Table 12.1, Phases 1 and 8)

In Phase 1, organization partners can conduct a **social assessment** to identify quality of life outcomes within their own jurisdiction that school health programs can help improve. Illustratively, by helping to reduce the impact of NCDs in the jurisdiction, school programs can help (1) increase the average length and quality of life of the population in that jurisdiction; (2) increase the economic productivity of those who otherwise would become ill, disabled, and die from NCDs; (3) decrease the costs of health care that otherwise will be needed for those afflicted by these diseases; and (4) by both increasing economic productivity and decreasing health care costs, make additional economic resources available to improve education, employment, housing, economic development, and other needs in that jurisdiction.

In the United States, one of the four goals of Healthy People 2020 (HP 2020)—the nation's health objectives for the year 2020—was to promote "quality of life, healthy development, and health behaviors across all life stages" (USDHHS n.d.h.). The development of indicators to monitor quality of life in the United States is evolving (CDC 2016b; USDHHS n.d.g.). HP 2020 tracked two health-related quality of life and wellness objectives, including the proportion of adults who self-report good or better (1) physical health, and (2) mental health (USDHHS n.d.i.). At the time of this writing, the United States is developing HP 2030 national health objectives and projected metrics for their accomplishment and measurement (USDHHS n.d.c.).

The CDC and other organizations within the United States have jointly developed a comprehensive set of 124 Chronic Disease Indicators (CDI) and a website (Holt et al. 2015; CDC 2018c; 2020b)[8] that provides online national-, state-, and metropolitan-level data about overarching conditions that can be used to monitor quality of life outcomes, such as life expectancy at age 65 (in Step One). Some Chronic Disease Indicators also can be used to monitor specific chronic diseases, such as diabetes (in Step Two below); chronic disease risk factors, such as tobacco use (in Step Three below); and school component processes, such as school physical activity (in Step Four below).

Internationally, several organizations have developed indicator systems to monitor quality of life outcomes within and across nations, including the United Nations Development Program (UNDP n.d.), European Union (EU 2018), Organization for Economic Cooperation and Development (OECD n.d., 2020), Social Progress Imperative (SPI n.d.), and Sustainable Development Solutions Network (Helliwell et al. 2018).

Well-planned school health programs could help improve the above quality of life indicators within jurisdictions by helping to reduce the impact of NCDs, as outlined in the next step.

Step Two: Epidemiological Assessment A to Improve Longer-Term Health and Education Impacts (Table 12.1, Phases 2A and 7A)

In Phase 2A, partners can conduct an **epidemiological assessment A** to identify longer-term health and education outcomes that their school health programs could improve, including a reduction in illnesses and deaths from specific NCDs. In 2016, NCDs caused 71% of all deaths worldwide—78% of these deaths occurred in low- and middle-income nations—and generated an enormous burden of illness, disability, and health care costs in each nation (WHO 2018b). For example, in the United States, about two-thirds of all deaths are caused by NCDs (Holt et al. 2015). Because 60% of all US adults have at least one NCD, while 42% have two or more, the treatment of these diseases consume the majority of all healthcare costs (Bauer et al. 2014; Buttorff et al. 2017). The US HP 2020 includes numerous long-term national chronic disease health impact objectives and indicators, including objectives to reduce deaths respectively from cardiovascular diseases, cancer, diabetes, and asthma (USDHHS n.d.b.; n.d.d.; n.d.j.; n.d.m.).

To strengthen international efforts to reduce the burden of NCDs, WHO developed a Global Action Plan for the Prevention and Control of Noncommunicable

Diseases 2013–2020 (WHO 2013). The WHO plan provides a logic model road-map and a menu of policy options that can help interested nations attain nine NCD global targets, including a 25% reduction in premature deaths from NCDs by 2025. Each nation can monitor progress toward these global targets by using 25 global indicators. School health programs could substantively help achieve five of the nine global targets by monitoring and achieving four of the 25 global indicators, including reductions in tobacco use, harmful alcohol use, physical inactivity, and overweight/obesity (as further described in Step Three below). To help each nation achieve the global NCD targets, the WHO has developed WHO Tools to Prevent and Control Noncommunicable Diseases (WHO 2014d), an NCD Global Monitoring Framework (WHO n.d.l.), a compilation of NCD Pro-files for each nation (WHO 2014c), a global status report on NCDs (WHO 2014a), and reviews of progress in each nation (WHO 2018b).

In 2014, the WHO established the Global Coordination Mechanism on the Prevention and Control of Noncommunicable Diseases to facilitate and enhance coordination of activities, multistakeholder engagement, and action across sec-tors at local, national, regional, and global levels (WHO n.d.c.). The Global Coor-dination Mechanism maintains an interactive, online Knowledge Action Portal that enables interested individuals and communities to work with each other across sectors and borders to prevent NCDs (WHO n.d.j.).

In 2015, the United Nations (UN) launched the broader UN 2030 Agenda for Sustainable Development (UN 2015), which includes a UN Global Plan of Action to improve the well-being of all people in each nation by 2030.[9] The Global Plan includes 17 Sustainable Development Goals (SDGs) (UN 2020) to be measured in each nation by common indicators (UN n.d.a.; n.d.b.; SDSN n.d.a.), including indicators for SDG Goal #3 (Good Health and Well-Being) and for SDG Goal #4 (Quality Education). National data for these indicators are being generated for each nation (Bertelsmann Stiftung and SDSN 2020), including the United States (USOMB 2018) and its 100 largest cities (Prakash et al. 2017).

The UN SDG Good Health and Well-Being Target 3.4 proposes to reduce pre-mature mortality from NCDs by one-third by 2030. To monitor achievement of this longer-term health impact target, SDG Indicator #23 (SDSN n.d.b.) measures the probability of dying between the ages of 30 and 70 in each nation from any NCD (WHO n.d.q.).

In addition to these longer-term health impacts, school health programs could also improve longer-term education impacts. Multiple studies have shown that students with various chronic health conditions are absent more frequently and that these absences are associated with lower scores across many indica-tors of academic achievement (CDC 2017k). Evidence suggests that well-planned school health programs can help these students and their parents manage chronic health conditions, reduce absences, and improve academic performance

(Jacobsen et al. 2016; NACDD 2016c; TFAH and HSC 2015; Tollit et al. 2015). HP 2020 includes national objectives to improve longer-term education impacts, including decreasing school absenteeism among adolescents due to illness or injury and increasing the percentage of students who graduate from high school (USDHHS n.d.a.; n.d.n.).

Step Three: Epidemiological Assessment B to Improve Shorter-Term Genetic, Behavioral, and Environmental Impacts (Table 12.1, Phases 2B and 7B)

In Phase 2B, partners can conduct an **epidemiological assessment B** of shorter-term NCD risk behaviors and resulting metabolic/physiological conditions that are modifiable causes of longer-term NCDs. The prevalence of these risk behaviors is increasing rapidly, especially among adolescents in low- and middle-income countries (Patton 2012). Increasingly unhealthful diets and physical inactivity among the world's young people have led to a tenfold increase in the number of 5- to 19-year-olds who have obesity, from 11 million young people in 1975 to 124 million in 2016. In 2016, 6% of the world's girls and 8% of its boys had obesity (see figure 4.3 in chapter 4 for youth vs. adult trends in obesity from 1999 to 2016; NCD Risk Factor Collaboration 2017). In the United States, the percentage of young people who have obesity has tripled since the 1970s (Fryar et al. 2016). By 2015–2016, 19% of US 2- to 19-year olds had obesity (Hales et al. 2017); the prevalence does not appear to be abating (Skinner at al. 2018), and one projection suggests that 57% of US young people will have obesity by age 35 (Ward et al. 2017).

As referenced earlier, in 2013, the WHO established the WHO Global Action Plan for the Prevention and Control of Noncommunicable Diseases 2013–2020, which can enable schools to help attain four of its 25 global indicators: to reduce tobacco use, harmful alcohol use, physical inactivity, and overweight/obesity (WHO 2013; n.d.d.). In addition, in 2014, the WHO established the Commission on Ending Childhood Obesity, which published recommendations to help schools reduce these NCD risks (WHO n.d.b.; 2016b; n.d.a.). To help attain the UN SDG Good Health and Well-Being Target 3.4 for reducing premature mortality from NCDs, the WHO is monitoring and helping to attain two SDG indicators. That is, the WHO is working to reduce SDG Indicator #24—percent of population overweight and obese and SDG Indicator #30—current use of any tobacco product (SDSN n.d.b.). In the United States, HP 2020 includes national health objectives to reduce tobacco use, harmful alcohol use, physical inactivity, unhealthy diets, and obesity among young people (USDHHS n.d.k.; n.d.l.; n.d.o.; n.d.p.).

WHO also has developed a STEPwise Approach to Noncommunicable Disease Risk Factor Surveillance (STEPS) to help interested countries monitor NCD behavioral risks (e.g., diet) and related physical risks (e.g., weight/height ratios) and biochemical risks (e.g., cholesterol) (Riley et al. 2016; WHO n.d.o.).[10] As part of STEPS, the WHO Global School-based Student Health Survey (GSHS) has been implemented in 120 nations to provide population data about the prevalence of student risk behaviors, including student tobacco use, harmful alcohol use, physical inactivity, dietary behaviors, and obesity (CDC 2018d; WHO n.d.f.). Further, in collaboration with the WHO Regional Office for Europe, the Health Behavior in School-Aged Children Survey is conducted every four years to monitor similar student health risk behaviors in 48 countries across Europe and North America (HBSC International Coordinating Center n.d.; WHO/EURO n.d.). In addition, by 2007, more than 140 nations had implemented the WHO Global Youth Tobacco Survey to monitor tobacco use by students (CDC n.d.c.; WHO n.d.h.). In the United States, these shorter-term student health behavior impacts are monitored by the CDC's Youth Risk Behavior Surveillance System (YRBSS) (CDC 2018r) and other surveys (Holt et al. 2015). For example, in 2017, YRBSS data indicated that 9% of all US high school students were using cigarettes and 13% of all students were using an electronic vaping product (e.g., e-cigarettes, vape pipes, vaping pens) (Kann et al. 2018). Notably, e-cigarette vaping has emerged as a serious epidemic among school students (Farzal et al. 2019; WHO 2017a).

By addressing these shorter-term *health* impacts, school health programs also consequently might improve shorter-term *education* impacts such as student mood, classroom behavior, academic effort, and concentration (CDC 2014; 2017b). Students who are more physically active perform better in school (Álvarez-Bueno et al. 2017; CDC 2010; Howie and Pate 2012; IOM 2013a), as do students who have healthier dietary behaviors (Frisvold 2015; IOM 2007). Evidence suggests that students with obesity are more likely to perform poorly in school. They are absent more frequently, engage less in school, demonstrate less academic effort, have more behavioral problems, exhibit lower reading scores and grade point averages, and are more likely to repeat a grade (Carey et al. 2015; Halfon et al. 2013; Kolbe 2019; Ramaswamy et al. 2010). The UN Interagency Task Force on NCDs has described "What Ministries of Education Need to Know" about how collaborative efforts to prevent NCDs risks also can help improve education outcomes (WHO 2016a).

Step Four: Educational and Ecological Assessment to Improve School Health Program Processes (Table 12.1, Phases 3 and 6)

During the mid-1980s, the CDC developed a multicomponent school health framework based on the PRECEDE-PROCEED model. This school health framework included eight interactive process components to improve both health and education outcomes (Allensworth and Kolbe 1987; Kolbe 1986). In 2014, the

CDC and ASCD (a national nongovernmental education organization) jointly improved the eight-component model to develop a Whole School, Whole Community, Whole Child (WSCC) Framework that includes the ten integrated process components depicted in figure 12.1 (ASCD n.d.a.; n.d.b.; 2016; CDC 2018p; Lewallen 2015; NACDD 2017b).

These ten WSCC process components are listed in table 12.1 under Phase 3. The tenets and purposes of the WSCC Framework are to assure that all students are healthy, safe, supported by caring adults, effectively engaged in learning, challenged academically, and prepared to be successful in life (Lewallen et al. 2015). The CDC offers resources that can be used to help implement each of these components, including the CDC's online School Health Index and interactive Virtual Healthy School (CDC 2015b; 2018n; 2018o). National, state, and local

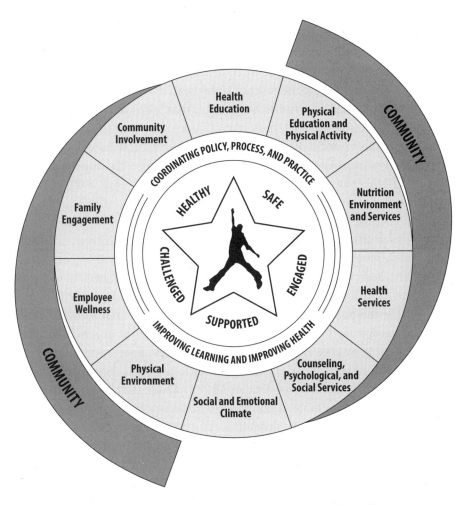

FIGURE 12.1. The Whole School, Whole Community, Whole Child (WSCC) Model: A Collaborative Approach to Learning and Health

data to monitor the provision of these school health component processes are generated by the CDC's School Health Policies and Practices Study (CDC 2017m) and by the CDC's School Health Profiles (CDC 2017n).

Although the WSCC has been widely implemented within the United States, many other nations use the WHO's Health Promoting School Framework (SHE Network n.d.; WHO n.d.i.; n.d.m.; n.d.n.; n.d.p.; 2017b; WHO/WPRO n.d.). The WHO Framework includes five core process components, including policy, skill-based health education, a supportive social and physical environment, community partnerships, and health services (Langford et al. 2017; Tang et al. 2009; Young 2005). Three international mechanisms have been developed to help monitor and evaluate the implementation of such school health program process components. The WHO has developed the Global School Health Policies and Practices Survey (WHO n.d.e.), the World Bank has developed indicators of school health policy and institutional development (World Bank n.d.; 2012), and the FRESH Partnership has developed school health program core and thematic indicators (UNESCO 2013; 2014).

Numerous evaluations have been conducted to assess the effectiveness of both single- and multicomponent school interventions to reduce various health risks. For example, several studies have found that, even in communities with high SARS-CoV-2 transmission, multicomponent school health programs—that include mask use, physical distancing, improved ventilation, hand hygiene, and appropriate isolation and quarantine protocols—reduced the spread of SARS-CoV-2 in schools that offered in-person learning (Dawson et al. 2021; Falk et al. 2021; Honein et al. 2021; Macartney et al. 2020). In addition, numerous systematic literature reviews have been published that aggregate and synthesize findings from such studies. For example, one synthesis of 139 intervention studies found that different combinations of school nutrition, physical activity, family engagement, and community involvement components produced at least moderate evidence of effectiveness in preventing childhood obesity (Wang et al. 2015). During the past two decades, such evaluation research syntheses have been increasingly used to identify effective evidence-based programs or practices (EBPs). At least 20 EBP Registries (EBPRs) disseminate information about the evidence of effectiveness of relevant health and education interventions (Burkhardt et al. 2015). Examples of these EBPRs include the Cochrane Database (Cochrane n.d.) and the Guide to Community Preventive Services (CPSTF n.d.b.). Those who plan school health programs can consult these EBPRs to identify school health EBPs (e.g., CHRR 2018; CPSTF n.d.a.).

Depending on how the ten school health component processes are interpreted, they variously can be categorized in the PRECEDE-PROCEED Model as processes that either: *predispose* students to engage in targeted behaviors, *reinforce* those behaviors, or *enable* those behaviors (Green et al. 2022). The ten component processes accordingly are categorized and outlined below as processes that variously may predispose, reinforce, or enable risk behaviors.

Predisposing Component Processes

1. *Health Education*—Can improve the health literacy of young people, including relevant cognitive and social skills that *predispose* young people throughout their lives to engage in healthier behaviors and collective actions that can improve their own health and the health of their families, communities, and nations (CDC 2017e; IOM 2004; Kickbusch et al. 2013; McDaid 2016; Nutbeam 2000; Sørensen et al. 2012; WHO/EMRO 2012). The Shanghai Declaration on Promoting Health in the 2030 Agenda for Sustainable Development recognized that the health literacy of citizens is essential to ensure a healthy society, and that health literacy is developed over a lifetime, "first and foremost through the school curriculum" (WHO 2016c; 2018c). In addition, to help schools achieve SDG #3 for Good Health and Well-Being, UNESCO has developed 15 Learning Objectives for SDG #3 (UNESCO 2016; 2017b; n.d.a.). Further, UNICEF is helping schools implement Life Skills-Based Health Education (UNICEF n.d.; WHO 2003). In the United States, the third goal of the US National Action Plan to Improve Health Literacy is to enable child care agencies, schools, and universities to provide effective health education (USDHHS 2010). The US HP 2020 includes objectives to increase the proportion of schools that provide health education and qualified staff to teach school health education (USDHHS n.d.e.; n.d.f.). The CDC offers a variety of resources to help schools implement effective health education (CDC 2015a; 2016c; 2017c).

2. *Social and Emotional Climate*—Can *predispose* students to engage in healthier behaviors (Carroll-Scott et al. 2015; Gilstad-Hayden et al. 2014), and teachers can create school climates that nurture such behaviors (CDC n.d.e.).

Reinforcing Component Processes

3. *Family Engagement*—Can help parents and families *reinforce* healthier student behaviors (AHK and PTA 2018; CDC 2018i; Cowgill et al. 2014; Gruber and Halderman 2009; Van Lippevelde et al. 2012).

4. *Community Involvement*—Can help community agencies establish partnerships with schools and families to *reinforce* healthier student behaviors (Blank 2015; Hoelscher et al. 2013; Park et al. 2017).

Enabling Component Processes

5. *Physical Environment*—Can *enable* students to avoid tobacco use. The US HP 2020 includes an objective to increase tobacco-free environments in all school facilities, properties, vehicles, and school events (USDHHS n.d.p.). Various resources are available to improve the effectiveness of school policies that prohibit tobacco use in schools (PHLC n.d.e.; RMC Health n.d.; Stanford Medicine n.d.; UNESCO 2017a), including school policies that prohibit the use of electronic nicotine delivery systems (FDA n.d.; PHLC n.d.f.; WHO 2017a).

6. *Nutrition Environment and Services*—Can *enable* students to eat healthier foods in schools. The HP 2020 includes objectives to increase the proportion of schools that offer nutritious foods and beverages for students (USDHHS n.d.k., n.d.a.). The World Food Program (WFP n.d.) and the World Bank (n.d.; 2012) help schools in many nations to provide food for students. A wide range of resources is available to help improve the school nutrition environment and services (Drake et al. 2016; CDC 2017m; 2018l; n.d.b.; USDA 2016; 2017a; 2017b; 2018).

7. *Physical Education and Physical Activity*—Can *enable* students to engage in healthier physical activity (IOM 2013b). The WHO has developed a Global Action Plan on Physical Activity 2018–2030, which includes whole-of-school approaches and indicators to improve physical activity in schools (WHO 2018a; n.d.k.). The US HP 2020 includes objectives to increase the proportion of schools that provide physical activity for students (USDHHS n.d.l.). The United States is implementing a National Physical Activity Plan that includes strategies and tactics to help schools improve physical activity (NPAPA n.d.). Numerous resources are available to help improve school physical education and physical activity (CDC 2017n; 2018m; 2021; PHLC n.d.a.; SHAPE n.d.).

8. *Health Services*—Can *enable* all students to prevent NCDs, and can especially *enable* the many students who have obesity (Hales et al. 2017), asthma (CDC 2017h), diabetes (CDC 2020a), and other chronic health conditions to improve their health and consequently their education performance (CDC 2017f; 2017g; NACDD 2015b; 2016b; NASN 2014; 2017). The HP 2020 includes a national objective to increase the proportion of schools that have an appropriate full-time registered school nurse-to-student ratio (USDHHS n.d.f.).

9. *Counseling, Psychological, and Social Services*—Can help *enable* students to prevent NCDs, and can help *enable* students with chronic health conditions to improve their health and consequently their education performance (Cook and Heyden 2018; CDC 2017j; Hamlet et al. 2011).

10. *Employee Wellness*—Each of the nine school health component processes developed for students also can be developed for school employees, especially as a means to *enable* school employees to improve their own health and productivity and as a means to reduce school employee health care costs from NCDs (AHG n.d.a.; Asay et al. 2016; CDC 2018g; 2018q; 2021c; Cigna Corporation 2011; Kaiser Permanente n.d.; NACDD 2019; Pennsylvania State University 2016).

The CDC (CDC 2017i; 2017l; 2018a; 2018e; 2018j; n.d.a.), the NACDD (n.d.b.), and the WHO (n.d.i.) offer a variety of websites and resources to help integrate each of the various component processes into the broader school health program.

Step Five: Policy, Administrative, and Implementation Assessment to Improve School Health Program Inputs (Table 12.1, Phases 4 and 5)

A wide range of national (i.e., federal), state, and local laws, policies, rules, and regulations (PHLC n.d.d.) can provide inputs to support one or more of the school health component processes outlined above. For example, the World Bank is working to improve educational outcomes, in part by improving and monitoring school health and school feeding policies and institutions (World Bank n.d.). The WHO has also established a WHO School Policy Framework (WHO 2008) to improve multiple school health components as part of the WHO Global Strategy on Diet, Physical Activity and Health (WHO n.d.g.).

In the United States, the CDC and other national organizations have identified numerous school policies to prevent NCDs and means to monitor and improve such policies (CDC n.d.d.; 2018h; Everett-Jones 2008; NACDD 2015c; Rudd Center 2013). Phase 4 in table 12.1 lists five broad United States national policies that provide various types of support for school programs to prevent NCDs. These five national policies include:

- The Every Student Succeeds Act provides support for education in each state, including various types of support for school health programs (NACDD n.d.a.; 2016a; Health Impact Project et al. 2017; HSC 2018; HSC and AHG 2017; USED n.d.b.; 2017).

- The Individuals with Disabilities Education Act provides support for special education services for students who have acute and chronic health conditions and learning problems (Lipkin and Okamoto 2015; USED n.d.c.).

- The Patient Protection and Affordable Care Act, amended by the Health Care and Education Reconciliation Act, provides support for some school health services and school counseling, psychological, and social services (CDC 2017d; Pudelski 2017; Vaughn et al. 2013).

- The Pro-Children Act supports the prohibition of tobacco use in school facilities (PHLC n.d.e.).
- The Healthy, Hunger-Free Kids Act provides support for schools to make nutritious food available, especially for children in low-income households (CDC 2018l; NACDD 2015a; PHLC n.d.b.; n.d.c.; USDA 2017a; 2017b).

In the United States, state policies drive school priorities, time, and funding. In 2019, the National Association of State Boards of Education (NASBE) reorganized its State Policy Database on School Health (NASBE n.d.b.) to monitor and describe each state's school health policies for each of the ten WSCC school health components, including school physical education and school nutrition. With these data, Child Trends (n.d.) created a website entitled *Using Policy to Create Healthy Schools: Resources to Support Policymakers and Advocates*, and described the extent to which each state's policies addressed each of the ten WSCC components (Chriqui et al. 2019). In addition, the National Cancer Institute has established a Classification of Laws Associated with School Students (CLASS) website to score and monitor state-level laws for school physical education and school nutrition (NCI n.d.).

Those who plan, implement, and evaluate school health programs as described above must comply with federal, and applicable state, laws created to assure the privacy of all individual education data and health data (ASTHO n.d.b.; USED n.d.d.).[11]

Step Six: Implement, Monitor, and Improve the Planned School Health Program (Table 12.1)

By identifying the relevant policy inputs in Phase 4 as described above, program planners thus complete the PRECEDE stage of the planning process—after which they can implement the program and then monitor and improve program effects through the PROCEED stage sequentially via Phases 5, 6, 7, and 8.

SUMMARY

Virtually every community in the world is afflicted by the combined health, education, and economic costs of NCDs. During the past four decades, researchers and practitioners across nations have developed many practical resources that local, state, national, and international health and education agencies collaboratively might use to:

- More effectively plan, implement, and evaluate school health programs that simultaneously can both prevent NCDs and improve education outcomes;

- Help integrate and amplify their respective efforts across jurisdictions; and

- Adapt, update, and improve the above-described school health program planning process and resources over time.

ACKNOWLEDGMENT

The authors are grateful for the work of their many school health colleagues around the world, referenced and unreferenced in this chapter. We apologize to many whose good work is not referenced in this admittedly limited chapter.

EXERCISES

Complete one or more of the following exercises.

1. Select a jurisdiction for which you might plan, implement, and evaluate efforts to help schools in that jurisdiction improve specific health and education impacts: e.g., to prevent NCDs, HIV, other STDs, teen pregnancy, or other health problems. Identify for that jurisdiction: (a) an agency or agencies that might convene potential stakeholder organizations; (b) individuals in the convening agency or agencies who might delegate time and resources to help develop and implement the plan; (c) potential stakeholder organizations that might be convened to participate in the plan; (d) a rough and tentative timeline to pursue the planning, implementation, and evaluation processes; and (e) a rough agenda and materials that can be used for the first meeting of stakeholder organizations to be convened.

2. For the first meeting of stakeholder organizations to be convened for the jurisdiction, prepare a relatively brief background document that outlines the draft purposes, participants, and processes to be pursued at the first and subsequent meetings of interested stakeholder organizations.

3. For the first and subsequent meetings of interested organizations, prepare a relatively brief draft background document that interested stakeholder organizations can use to help them complete each of the following school health planning phases: Phases 1 and 8, Phases 2A and 7A, Phases 2B and 7B, Phases 3 and 6, and Phases 4 and 5. In the draft background document, identify potential indicators and information resources that stakeholders can use to help them complete each phase.

Notes

1. The number of students in the world, its regions, and its nations during any recent year can be calculated by accessing the online UNESCO Institute for Statistics Database (UNESCO n.d.b.) From the iterative dropdown menus, select "Education," "Population," "School-age," "School-age population by level of education," "Primary education, both sexes," and "Secondary education, both sexes." For example, when accessed on October 23, 2018, the UNESCO Database suggested that in 2017, worldwide, 716,849,962 students attended primary school and 771,143,108 attended secondary school, for a total of 1,487,993,070 primary and secondary school students.

2. School health has been defined as a cross-disciplinary field of study and a fundamental strategy that can be used to improve both health and education outcomes. For a broader analysis of school health as a strategy to improve both public health and education, see Kolbe (2019).

3. One can often find and review the scope of each organization's efforts by electronically accessing the organization's home website and entering "school health" into the website search bar.

4. For the updated, searchable, bibliography of published applications of the PRECEDE-PROCEED model, go to http://www.lgreen.net.

5. Similar to the PRECEDE-PROCEED model, the WHO's 2018 Impact and Accountability Framework includes—from left to right—Inputs, Activities, Outputs, Outcomes, and Impacts. For more information, see WHO (2018d).

6. The ASCD is an international nongovernmental education organization (formerly known as the Association for Supervision and Curriculum Development). The International School Health Network (ISHN) is a network of practitioners, researchers, and organizations that work to improve human development. The ASCD and ISHN have called for the health system in each jurisdiction to work within the education system, including the education system's mandates and constraints, instead of assuming that the education system can simply adopt and address health system priorities. For more information, see ASCD (n.d.c.).

7. In past decades, research agencies invested in developing and assessing the effectiveness of school-based interventions to prevent NCDs. In future decades, research agencies could progressively develop and assess means to help large numbers of schools implement and sustain evidence-informed if not evidence-based (Kumah et al. 2019) interventions that can improve both public health and education. See, for example, Brownson et al. (2018), Chambers (2018), and Kolbe (2019).

8. The US CDI include 124 standardized indicators that offer comparable state-level and selected metropolitan-level data across the following 18 topic groups: alcohol; arthritis; asthma; cancer; cardiovascular disease; chronic kidney disease; chronic obstructive pulmonary disease; diabetes; immunization; nutrition, physical activity, and weight status; oral health; tobacco; overarching conditions; disability; mental health; older adults; reproductive health; and school health. See CDC (2018c; 2020) and Holt et al. (2015).

9. The 2030 Agenda for Sustainable Development was adopted by all UN member states in 2015 to achieve a better and more sustainable future for all people in each nation. Its 17 SDGs offer a shared blueprint for action by all countries through a global partnership to reduce poverty, improve health and education, reduce inequality, spur economic growth, and stem climate change. For more information, see UN (2015).

10. By 2015, 122 countries across all six WHO regions had implemented STEPS to monitor main NCD risk factors. See Riley et al. (2016) and WHO (n.d.o).

11. To ensure the privacy of student education records and student health records, respectively, the US Congress passed the Family Educational Rights and Privacy Act (FERPA) of 1974 and the Health Insurance Portability and Accountability Act (HIPAA) of 1996. The US Department of Education (USED n.d.d.) and the Association of State and Territorial

Health Officials (ASTHO n.d.b.) provide information about requirements to protect the privacy of data about students, including, for example, data about student educational achievement, health behaviors, and health conditions.

References

American Academy of Pediatrics (AAP). (n.d.) *Council on School Health (COSH)*. American Academy of Pediatrics. Retrieved April 21, 2021, from https://services.aap.org/en /community/aap-councils/council-on-school-health/

Action for Healthy Kids (AHK). (n.d.) *Action for Healthy Kids*. AHK. Retrieved July 15, 2018, from http://www.actionforhealthykids.org/

Action for Healthy Kids (AHK), & National Parent Teachers Association (PTA). (2018). *Parents for Healthy Kids*. AHK. https://parentsforhealthykids.org/

Allensworth, D.D., & Kolbe, L.J. (1987). The comprehensive school health program: Exploring an expanded concept. *Journal of School Health, 57*(10), 409–12.

Alliance for a Healthier Generation (AHG). (n.d.a.). *Staff Well-Being*. Clinton Foundation. Retrieved July 24, 2018, from https://www.healthiergeneration.org/take_action/schools /employee_wellness/

Alliance for A Healthier Generation (AHG). (n.d.b.). *Schools*. AHG. Retrieved July 15, 2018, from https://www.healthiergeneration.org/take_action/schools/

Álvarez-Bueno, C., Pesce, C., Cavero-Redondo, I., Sánchez-López, M., Garrido-Miguel, M., & Martínez-Vizcaíno, M. (2017). Academic achievement and physical activity: A meta-analysis. *Pediatrics, 140*(6), e20171498. https://doi.org/10.1542/peds.2017-1498

Arbeit, M.L., Johnson, C.C., Mott, D.S., Harsha, D.W., Nicklas, T.A., Webber, L.S., & Berenson, G.S. (1992). The Heart Smart cardiovascular school health promotion: Behavior correlates of risk factor change. *Preventive Medicine, 21*(1), 18–32. https://doi.org/10.1016/0091 -7435(92)90003-z

Asay, G., Roy, K., Lang, J., Payne, R., & Howard, D. (2016). Absenteeism and employer costs associated with chronic diseases and health risk factors in the US workforce. *Preventing Chronic Disease, 13*, 150503. http://dx.doi.org/10.5888/pcd13.150503

ASCD (formerly Association for Curriculum Supervision and Development). (n.d.a.). *ASCD Whole Child Initiative*. Retrieved July 21, 2018, from http://www.ascd.org/whole-child.aspx

ASCD (formerly Association for Curriculum Supervision and Development). (n.d.b.). *Learning and Health: Whole School, Whole Community, Whole Child*. Retrieved July 21, 2018, from http://www.ascd.org/programs/learning-and-health/wscc-model.aspx.

ASCD (formerly Association for Supervision and Curriculum Development) and International School Health Network (ISHN). (n.d.c.). *Statement on the Integration of Health and Education*. ASCD. Retrieved July 15, 2018, from http://www.ascd.org/ASCD/pdf/siteASCD /wholechild/Statement-for-the-Integration-of-Health-and-Education_English.pdf

ASCD (formerly Association for Curriculum Supervision and Development). (2016). *The Whole School, Whole Community, Whole Child Model: Ideas for Implementation*. ASCD. Retrieved July 21, 2018, from http://www.ascd.org/ASCD/pdf/siteASCD/wholechild /WSCC_Examples_Publication.pdf

American School Health Association (ASHA). (n.d.) *American School Health Association*. ASHA. Retrieved July 15, 2018, from http://www.ashaweb.org/

Association of State and Territorial Health Officials (ASTHO). (n.d.a.). *ASTHO Public Health and Schools Toolkit*. ASTHO. Retrieved July 15, 2018, from http://www.astho.org/Programs /Preparedness/Public-Health-Emergency-Law/Public-Health-and-Schools-Toolkit/Public -Health---Schools-Toolkit/

Association of State and Territorial Health Officials (ASTHO). (n.d.b.). *Public Health Access To Student Health Data: Authorities And Limitations In Sharing Information Between Schools And Public Health Agencies*. http://www.astho.org/Programs/Preparedness/Public-Health -Emergency-Law/Public-Health-and-Schools-Toolkit/Public-Health-Access-to-Student -Health-Data/

Bauer, U., Briss, P., Goodman, R., & Bowman, B. (2014). Prevention of chronic disease in the 21st century: elimination of the leading preventable causes of premature death and disability in the USA. *The Lancet, 384*(9937), 45–52. https://doi.org/10.1016/S0140-6736 (14)60648-6

Belansky, E.N., Cutforth, N., Chavez, R., Waters, E., & Bartlett-Horch, K. (2011). An adapted version of intervention mapping (AIM) is a tool for conducting community-based participatory research. *Health Promotion Practice, 12*(3), 440–55. https://doi.org/10.1177 /1524839909334620

Belansky, E.N., Cutforth, N., Chavez, R., Crane, L., Waters, E., & Marshall, J. (2013). Adapted intervention mapping: A strategic planning process for increasing physical activity and healthy eating opportunities in schools via environment and policy change. *Journal of School Health, 83*(3), 194–205. https://doi.org/10.1111/josh.12015

Berenson, G.S., Arbeit, M.L., Hunter, S.M., Johnson, C.C., & Nicklas, T.A. (1991). Cardiovascular health promotion for elementary school children: The Heart Smart Program. *Annals of the New York Academy of Sciences, 623*(1), 299–313. https://doi.org/10.1111/j.1749 -6632.1991.tb43739.x

Bertelsmann Stiftung and Sustainable Development Solutions Network (SDSN). (2020). *Sustainable Development Report 2020:The Sustainable Development Goals and COVID-19 (Includes the SDG Index and Dashboards).* SDSN. https://s3.amazonaws.com/sustainable development.report/2020/2020_sustainable_development_report.pdf

Blank, M. (2015). Building sustainable health and education partnerships: Stories from local communities. *Journal of School Health, 85*(11), 810–6. https://doi.org/10.1111/josh.12311

Brownson, R.C., Fielding, J.E., & Green, L.W. (2018). Building capacity for evidence-based public health: Reconciling the pulls of practice and the push of research. *Annual Review of Public Health, 39*, 27–53. https://doi.org/10.1146/annurev-publhealth-040617-014746

Bundy, D. (2011). *Rethinking School Health: A Key Component of Education for All.* World Bank. https://openknowledge.worldbank.org/handle/10986/2267

Bundy, D., Shaeffer, S., Jukes, M.C.H., Beegle, K., Gillespie, A., Drake, L., Lee, S.F., Hoffman, A.M., Jones, J., Mitchell, A., Barcelona, D., Camara, B., Golmar, C., Savoli, L., Sembene, M., Takeuchi, T., & Wright, C. (2006). School-based health and nutrition programs. In Jamison, D., Breman, J., Measham, A., Alleyne, G., Claeson, M., Evans, D., Jha, P., Mills, A., & Musgrove, P., *Disease Control Priorities in Developing Countries* (2nd ed., pp. 1091–108). World Bank.

Burkhardt, J.T., Schröter, D.C., Magura, S., Means, S.N., & Coryn, C.L.S. (2015). An overview of evidence-based program registers (EBPRs) for behavioral health. *Evaluation and Program Planning, 48*, 92–99. https://doi.org/10.1016/j.evalprogplan.2014.09.006

Bush, P.J., Zuckerman, A.E., Theiss, P.K., Taggart, V.S., Horowitz, C., Sheridan, M.J., & Walter, H.J. (1989). Cardiovascular risk factor prevention in black school children: Two-year results of the "Know Your Body" Program. *American Journal of Epidemiology, 129*(3), 466–82. https://doi.org/10.1093/oxfordjournals.aje.a115158

Buttorff, C., Ruder, T., & Bauman, M. (2017). *Multiple Chronic Conditions in the United States.* RAND Corporation.

Cameron, R., Manske, S., Brown, K.S., Jolin, M.A., Murnaghan, D., & Lovato, C. (2007). Integrating public health policy, practice, evaluation, surveillance, and research: The School Health Action Planning and Evaluation System. *American Journal of Public Health, 97*(4), 648–54. https://doi.org/10.2105/AJPH.2005.079665

Carey, F.R., Singh, G.K., Brown, H.S., & Wilkinson, A.V. (2015). Educational outcomes associated with childhood obesity in the United States: Cross-sectional results from the 2011–2012 National Survey of Children's Health. *International Journal of Behavioral Nutrition and Physical Activity, 12*(Suppl. 1), S3. https://doi.org/10.1186/1479-5868-12-S1-S3

Carroll-Scott, A., Gilstad-Hayden, K., Rosenthal, L., Eldahan, A., McCaslin, C., Peters, S.M., & Ickovics, J.R. (2015). Associations of neighborhood and school socioeconomic and social contexts with body mass index among urban preadolescent students. *American Journal of Public Health, 105*(12), 2496–502. https://doi.org/10.2105/AJPH.2015.302882

Centers for Disease Control and Prevention (CDC). (n.d.a.). *Collection of Online Resources & Inventory Database: Organized and Readily Accessible (CORIDOR).* CDC.

Centers for Disease Control and Prevention (CDC). (n.d.b.). *Comprehensive Framework for Addressing the School Nutrition Environment and Services.* CDC. Retrieved July 23, 2018, from https://www.cdc.gov/healthyschools/nutrition/pdf/School_Nutrition_Framework _508tagged.pdf

Centers for Disease Control and Prevention (CDC). (n.d.c.). *Global Tobacco Surveillance System Data (GTSSData): Global Youth Tobacco Survey (GYTS) — Overview.* CDC. Retrieved July 21, 2018, from https://nccd.cdc.gov/GTSSDataSurveyResources/Ancillary/Documentation .aspx?SUID=1&DOCT=1

Centers for Disease Control and Prevention (CDC). (n.d.d.). *School-Based Obesity Prevention Strategies for State Policymakers.* CDC. https://www.cdc.gov/healthyyouth/policy/pdf /obesity_prevention_strategies.pdf

Centers for Disease Control and Prevention (CDC). (n.d.e.). *Tips for Teachers: Promoting Healthy Eating and Physical Activity in the Classroom.* CDC. https://www.cdc.gov /healthyschools/npao/pdf/tips-for-teachers.pdf

Centers for Disease Control and Prevention (CDC). (2010). *The Association Between School Based Physical Activity, Including Physical Education, and Academic Performance.* CDC. https://www.cdc.gov/healthyyouth/health_and_academics/pdf/pa-pe_paper.pdf

Centers for Disease Control and Prevention (CDC). (2014). *Health and Academic Achievement.* CDC. https://www.cdc.gov/healthyyouth/health_and_academics/pdf/health-academic -achievement.pdf

Centers for Disease Control and Prevention (CDC). (2015a). *Characteristics of an Effective Health Education Curriculum.* CDC. https://www.cdc.gov/healthyschools/sher /characteristics/index.htm

Centers for Disease Control and Prevention (CDC). (2015b, September 15). *SHI Resources by Module [Component].* CDC. https://www.cdc.gov/healthyschools/shi/resources.htm

Centers for Disease Control and Prevention (CDC). (2016a, June 9). *Health in All Policies.* CDC. https://www.cdc.gov/policy/hiap/index.html

Centers for Disease Control and Prevention (CDC). (2016b, May 27). *Health-Related Quality of Life (HRQOL).* CDC. https://www.cdc.gov/hrqol/index.htm

Centers for Disease Control and Prevention (CDC). (2016c). *National Health Education Standards.* CDC. https://www.cdc.gov/healthyschools/sher/standards/index.htm

Centers for Disease Control and Prevention (CDC). (2017a, June 27). *Funded Non-Governmental Organizations for Healthy Schools.* CDC. https://www.cdc.gov/healthyschools/ngo.htm

Centers for Disease Control and Prevention (CDC). (2017b, October 28). *Health and Academics.* CDC. https://www.cdc.gov/healthyyouth/health_and_academics/

Centers for Disease Control and Prevention (CDC). (2017c). *Health Education Curriculum Analysis Tool (HECAT).* CDC. https://www.cdc.gov/healthyyouth/hecat/index.htm

Centers for Disease Control and Prevention (CDC). (2017d). *Health Insurance for Children: How Schools Can Help.* CDC. https://www.cdc.gov/healthyschools/chronic_conditions /pdfs/2017_04_13-FactSheet-InsuranceHowSchoolsCanHelp_CLEARED_508.pdf

Centers for Disease Control and Prevention (CDC). (2017e, July 26). *Health Literacy.* CDC. https://www.cdc.gov/healthliteracy/

Centers for Disease Control and Prevention (CDC). (2017f). *Managing Chronic Health Conditions in Schools: The Role of the School Nurse.* CDC. https://www.cdc.gov/healthyschools/ chronic_conditions/pdfs/2017_02_15-FactSheet-RoleOfSchoolNurses_FINAL_508.pdf

Centers for Disease Control and Prevention (CDC). (2017g, May 9). *Managing Chronic Conditions in Schools.* CDC. https://www.cdc.gov/healthyschools/chronicconditions.htm

Centers for Disease Control and Prevention (CDC). (2017h, February 10). *2015 National Health*

Interview Survey (NHIS) Data: Table 4.1—Current Asthma Prevalence Percents by Age, United States: National Health Interview Survey, 2015. CDC. https://www.cdc.gov/asthma/nhis/2015/table4-1.htm

Centers for Disease Control and Prevention (CDC). (2017i, December 20). *Out of School Time: Out of School Time Supports Student Health and Learning.* CDC. https://www.cdc.gov/healthyschools/ost.htm

Centers for Disease Control and Prevention (CDC). (2017j). *Research Brief: Addressing the Needs of Students with Chronic Health Conditions: Strategies for Schools.* CDC. https://www.cdc.gov/healthyschools/chronic_conditions/pdfs/2017_02_15-How-Schools-Can-Students-with-CHC_Final_508.pdf

Centers for Disease Control and Prevention (CDC). (2017k). *Research Brief: Chronic Health Conditions and Academic Achievement.* CDC. https://www.cdc.gov/healthyschools/chronic_conditions/pdfs/2017_02_15-CHC-and-Academic-Achievement_Final_508.pdf

Centers for Disease Control and Prevention (CDC). (2017l, September 5). *School Health Guidelines.* CDC. https://www.cdc.gov/healthyschools/npao/strategies.htm

Centers for Disease Control and Prevention (CDC). (2017m, September 18). *School Health Policies and Practices Study (SHPPS).* CDC. https://www.cdc.gov/healthyyouth/data/shpps/index.htm

Centers for Disease Control and Prevention (CDC). (2017n, November 2). *School Health Profiles.* CDC. https://www.cdc.gov/healthyyouth/data/profiles/index.htm

Centers for Disease Control And Prevention (CDC). (2018a, June 26). *Adolescent and School Health.* CDC. https://www.cdc.gov/healthyyouth/

Centers for Disease Control and Prevention (CDC). (2018b). *CDC Evaluation Documents, Workbooks, and Tools—Logic Models.* CDC. https://www.cdc.gov/eval/tools/logic_models/index.html

Centers for Disease Control and Prevention (CDC). (2018c). *Chronic Disease Indicators.* CDC. https://www.cdc.gov/cdi/index.html

Centers for Disease Control and Prevention (CDC). (2018d, January 9). *Global School-based Student Health Survey (GSHS).* CDC. https://www.cdc.gov/GSHS/

Centers for Disease Control And Prevention (CDC). (2018e, May 14). *CDC Healthy Schools.* CDC. https://www.cdc.gov/healthyschools/index.htm

Centers for Disease Control and Prevention (CDC). (2018f, October 18). *Funded School Health Partners: Improving Student Health and Academic Achievement through Nutrition, Physical Activity and the Management of Chronic Conditions in Schools (DP18-1801).* CDC. https://www.cdc.gov/healthyschools/fundedpartners.htm

Centers for Disease Control and Prevention (CDC). (2018g, February 14). *Local School Wellness Policies.* CDC. https://www.cdc.gov/healthyschools/npao/wellness.htm

Centers for Disease Control and Prevention (CDC). (2018h, June 21). *Overweight and Obesity: Early Care and Education (ECE).* CDC. https://www.cdc.gov/obesity/strategies/childcareece.html

Centers for Disease Control and Prevention (CDC). (2018i, March 9). *Parents for Healthy Schools.* CDC. https://www.cdc.gov/healthyschools/parentengagement/parentsforhealthyschools.htm

Centers for Disease Control and Prevention (CDC). (2018j, February 26). *Professional Training and Development.* CDC. https://www.cdc.gov/healthyschools/trainingtools.htm

Centers for Disease Control and Prevention (CDC). (2018k, February 27). *School Health Index.* CDC. https://www.cdc.gov/healthyschools/shi/index.htm

Centers for Disease Control and Prevention (CDC). (2018l, February 14). *School Nutrition.* CDC. https://www.cdc.gov/healthyschools/nutrition/schoolnutrition.htm

Centers for Disease Control and Prevention (CDC). (2018m, January 18). *School Physical Education and Physical Activity.* CDC. https://www.cdc.gov/healthyschools/physicalactivity/index.htm

Centers for Disease Control and Prevention (CDC). (2018n, March 12). *Virtual Healthy School Resource List by WSCC Components*. CDC. https://www.cdc.gov/healthyschools/vhs/resources.html

Centers for Disease Control and Prevention (CDC). (2018o, July 21). *Virtual Healthy School*. CDC. https://www.cdc.gov/healthyschools/vhs/index.html

Centers for Disease Control and Prevention (CDC). (2018p, May 4). *Whole School, Whole Community, Whole Child: A Collaborative Approach to Learning and Health*. CDC. https://www.cdc.gov/healthyschools/wscc/index.htm

Centers for Disease Control and Prevention (CDC). (2018q, June 26). *Workplace Health Promotion*. CDC. https://www.cdc.gov/workplacehealthpromotion/index.html

Centers for Disease Control and Prevention (CDC). (2018r, June 14). *Youth Risk Behavior Surveillance System (YRBSS)*. CDC. https://www.cdc.gov/healthyyouth/data/yrbs/index.htm

Centers for Disease Control and Prevention (CDC). (2020a). *National Diabetes Statistics Report, 2020 Estimates of Diabetes and Its Burden in the United States*. CDC. https://www.cdc.gov/diabetes/pdfs/data/statistics/national-diabetes-statistics-report.pdf

Centers for Disease Control and Prevention (CDC). (2020b). PLACES: Local Data for Better Health. CDC. https://www.cdc.gov/places/index.html

Centers for Disease Control and Prevention (CDC). (2021a). *About Chronic Diseases*. CDC. https://www.cdc.gov/chronicdisease/about/index.htm

Centers for Disease Control and Prevention (CDC). (2021b). *Physical Education and Physical Activity*. CDC. https://www.cdc.gov/healthyschools/physicalactivity/index.htm

Centers for Disease Control and Prevention (CDC). (2021c). *School Employee Wellness*. CDC. https://www.cdc.gov/healthyschools/employee_wellness.htm

Chambers, D. (2018). Commentary: Increasing the connectivity between implementation science and public health: Advancing methodology, evidence integration, and sustainability. *Annual Review of Public Health, 39*, 1–4. https://doi.org/10.1146/annurev-publhealth-110717-045850

Chaney, J., Hunt, B., & Schulz, J. (2000). An examination using the PRECEDE model framework to establish a comprehensive program to prevent school violence. *American Journal of Health Studies, 16*(4), 199–204.

Child Trends. (n.d.) *Using Policy to Create Healthy Schools: Resources to Support Policymakers and Advocates*. Child Trends. Retrieved October 17, 2019, from https://www.childtrends.org/publications/using-policy-to-create-healthy-schools

Chriqui, J., Stuart-Cassel, V., Piekarz-Porter, E., Temkin, D., Lao, K., Steed, H., Harper, K., Leider, J., & Gabriel, A. (2019). *Using State Policy to Create Healthy Schools Coverage of the Whole School, Whole Community, Whole Child Framework in State Statutes and Regulations School Year 2017-2018*. Child Trends. Retrieved October 17, 2019, from https://www.childtrends.org/wp-content/uploads/2019/01/WSCCStatePolicyReportSY2017-18_ChildTrends_January2019.pdf

Cigna Corporation. (2011). *A Guide to School Employees' Well-Being*. Cigna Corporation. https://www.cigna.com/assets/docs/employers-and-organizations/school-well-being-wellness-guide.pdf

Cochrane. (n.d.) *Cochrane Library*. Cochrane. https://www.cochranelibrary.com/

County Health Rankings and Roadmaps (CHRR). (n.d.a.). *County Health Rankings and Roadmaps*. University of Wisconsin Population Health Institute. Retrieved July 19, 2018, from http://www.countyhealthrankings.org/

County Health Rankings and Roadmaps (CHRR). (n.d.b.). *County Health Rankings and Roadmaps: Education*. University of Wisconsin Population Health Institute. Retrieved July 19, 2018, from https://www.countyhealthrankings.org/explore-health-rankings/measures-data-sources/county-health-rankings-model/health-factors/social-and-economic-factors/education

County Health Rankings and Roadmaps (CHRR). (n.d.c.). *County Health Rankings and Road-maps: Work Together*. CHRR. Retrieved July 15, 2018, from http://www.countyhealthrankings.org/take-action-improve-health/action-center/work-together

County Health Rankings and Roadmaps (CHRR). (2018, May 10). *County Health Rankings and Roadmaps: Multi-component school-based obesity prevention intervention*. CHRR. http://www.countyhealthrankings.org/take-action-to-improve-health/what-works-for-health/policies/multi-component-school-based-obesity-prevention-interventions

Community Preventive Services Task Force (CPSTF). (n.d.a.). *The Community Guide: In Action Story—Healthy Schools Equals Healthy Kids*. Retrieved July 21, 2018, from https://www.thecommunityguide.org/stories/healthy-schools-equal-healthy-kids

Community Preventive Services Task Force (CPSTF). (n.d.b.). *The Community Guide*. CDC. Retrieved July 21, 2018, from https://www.thecommunityguide.org/

Cook, A., & Heyden, L. (2018). Obesity prevention among Latino youth: School counselors' role in promoting healthy lifestyle. *Professional School Counseling Journal, 16*(1), 7–17. https://doi.org/10.5330/PSC.n.2012-16.7

Cowgill, B., Chung, P., Thompson, L., Elijah, J., Lamb, S., Garcia, V., & Bastani, R. (2014). Parents' views on engaging families of middle school students in obesity prevention and control in a multiethnic population. *Preventing Chronic Disease, 11*, E54. https://doi.org/10.5888/pcd11.130138

Dawson, P., Worrell, M.C., Malone, S., Tinker, S.C., Fritz, S., Maricque, B., Junaidi, S., Purnell, G., Lai, A.M., Neidich, J.A., Lee, J.S., Orscheln, R.C., Charney, R., Rebmann, T., Mooney, J., Yoon, N., Petit, M., Schmidt, S., Grabeel, J., . . . CDC COVID-19 Surge Laboratory Group (2021). Pilot Investigation of SARS-CoV-2 Secondary Transmission in Kindergarten Through Grade 12 Schools Implementing Mitigation Strategies — St. Louis County and City of Springfield, Missouri, December 2020. *MMWR Morbidity and Mortality Weekly Report, 70*(12), 449–55. http://doi.org/10.15585/mmwr.mm7012e4

Drake, L., Woolnough, A., Burbano, C., & Bundy, D. (2016). *Global School Feeding Sourcebook: Lessons from 14 Countries*. Imperial College Press. https://openknowledge.worldbank.org/handle/10986/24418

Everett-Jones, S. (Ed.). (2008). A CDC Review of School Laws and Policies Concerning Child and Adolescent Health. *Journal of School Health, 78*(2), 69–128. https://doi.org/10.1111/j.1746-1561.2007.00272_1.x

European Union (EU). (2018). *Eurostat Statistics Explained: Quality of Life Indicators—Measuring Quality of Life*. European Union.

Falk, A., Benda, A., Falk, P., Steffen, S., Wallace, Z., & Høeg, T.B. (2021). COVID-19 cases and transmission in 17 K-12 schools—Wood County, Wisconsin, August 31–November 29, 2020. *MMWR Morbidity and Mortality Weekly Report, 70*(4), 136–40. https://doi.org/10.15585/mmwr.mm7004e3

Farzal, Z., Perry, M.F., Yarbrough, W.G., & Kimple, A.J. (2019). The adolescent vaping epidemic in the United States—How it happened and where we go from here. *JAMA Otolaryngology–Head & Neck Surgery, 145*(10), 885–6. https://doi.org/10.1001/jamaoto.2019.2410

Food and Drug Administration (FDA). (n.d.) *Vaporizers, E-Cigarettes, and other Electronic Nicotine Delivery Systems (ENDS)*. FDA. https://www.fda.gov/tobaccoproducts/labeling/productsingredientscomponents/ucm456610.htm

FRESH Partnership. (n.d.) *FRESH Partnership (Focusing Resources on Effective School Health)*. https://www.fresh-partners.org/fresh-partnership.html

Frieden, T. (2010). A framework for public health action: The Health Impact Pyramid. *American Journal of Public Health, 100*(4), 590–5. https://doi.org/10.2105/AJPH.2009.185652

Frisvold, D. (2015). Nutrition and cognitive achievement: An evaluation of the School Breakfast Program. *Journal of Public Economics, 124*, 91–104. https://doi.org/10.1016/j.jpubeco.2014.12.003

Fryar, C., Carroll, M., & Ogden, C. (2016). Prevalence of overweight and obesity among children and adolescents: United States, 1963–1965 through 2011–2012. *Health E-Stats.* https://www.cdc.gov/nchs/data/hestat/obesity_child_11_12/obesity_child_11_12.htm

Gilstad-Hayden, K., Carroll-Scott, A., Rosenthal, L., Peters, S., McCaslin, C., & Ickovics, J. (2014). Positive school climate is associated with lower body mass index percentile among urban preadolescents. *Journal of School Health, 84*(8), 502–6. https://doi.org/10.1111/josh.12177

Green, L.W. (1974). Toward cost-benefit evaluations of health education: Some concepts, methods, and examples. *Health Education Monographs, 2*(Suppl. 1), 34–64. https://doi.org/10.1177/10901981740020S106

Green, L.W., Gielen, A., Kreuter, M.W., Ottoson, J.M., & Peterson, D. (Eds.) (2022). *Health Program Planning, Implementation, and Evaluation: Creating Behavioral, Environmental and Policy Change.* Johns Hopkins University Press.

Gruber, K., & Haldeman, L. (2009). Using the family to combat childhood and adult obesity. *Preventing Chronic Disease, 6*(3), A106.

Hales, C., Carroll, M., Fryar, C., & Ogden, C. (2017). Prevalence of obesity among adults and youth: United States, 2015–2016. *NCHS Data Brief, 288*, 1–8. https://www.cdc.gov/nchs/data/databriefs/db288.pdf

Halfon, N., Larson, K., & Slusser, W. (2013). Associations between obesity and comorbid mental health, developmental, and physical health conditions in a nationally representative sample of US children aged 10 to 17. *Academic Pediatrics, 13*(1), 6–13. https://doi.org/10.1016/j.acap.2012.10.007

Hamlet, H., Gergar, P., & Schaefer, B. (2011). Students living with chronic illness: The school counselor's role. *Professional School Counseling Journal, 14*(3), 202–10. https://doi.org/10.1177/2156759X1101400304

HBSC International Coordinating Center. (n.d.) *Health Behavior in School-Aged Children: World Health Organization Collaborative Cross-National Survey.* University of St Andrews, Child and Adolescent Health Research Unit. Retrieved July 21, 2018, from http://www.hbsc.org/

Health Impact Project, Robert Wood Johnson Foundation, & Pew Charitable Trusts. (2017). *The Every Student Succeeds Act Creates Opportunities to Improve Health and Education at Low-Performing Schools.* The Pew Charitable Trusts. http://www.pewtrusts.org/~/media/assets/2017/08/hip_the_every_student_succeeds_act_creates_opportunities_to_improve_health_and_education_at_low_performing_schools.pdf

Healthy Schools Campaign (HSC) & Alliance for a Healthier Generation (AHG). (2017). *State ESSA Plans to Support Student Health and Wellness: A Framework for Action* (3rd ed.). HSC. https://healthyschoolscampaign.org/wp-content/uploads/2017/03/ESSA-State-Framework.pdf

Healthy Schools Campaign (HSC). (2018). *State ESSA Plans to Support Student Health and Wellness: A Framework for Action.* HSC. https://healthyschoolscampaign.org/state-essa-framework/

Helliwell, J., Layard, R., & Sachs, J. (Eds.) (2018). *World Happiness Report 2018.* United Nations Sustainable Development Solutions Network. https://s3.amazonaws.com/happiness-report/2018/WHR_web.pdf

Hoelscher, D., Kirk, S., Ritchie, L., & Cunningham-Sabo, L., for the Academy Positions Committee. (2013). Position of the Academy of Nutrition and Dietetics: Interventions for the prevention and treatment of pediatric overweight and obesity. *Journal of the Academy of Nutrition and Dietetics, 113*(10), 1375–94. https://doi.org/10.1016/j.jand.2013.08.004

Holt, J., Huston, S., Heidari, K., Schwartz, R., Gollmar, C., Tran, A., Bryan, L., Liu, B., & Croft, J. (2015). Indicators for chronic disease surveillance—United States, 2013. *Morbidity and Mortality Weekly Report, 64*(RR01), 1–252. https://www.cdc.gov/mmwr/preview/mmwrhtml/rr6401a1.htm

Honein, M.A., Barrios, L.C., & Brooks, J.T. (2021). Data and policy to guide opening schools safely to limit the spread of SARS-CoV-2 infection. *JAMA, 325*(9), 823–4. https://doi .org/10.1001/jama.2021.0374

Howat, P., Jones, S., Hall, M., Cross, D., & Stevenson, M. (1997). The PRECEDE-PROCEED Model: Application to planning a child pedestrian injury prevention program. *Injury Prevention, 3*(4), 282–7. https://doi.org/10.1136/ip.3.4.282

Howie, E., & Pate, R. (2012). Physical activity and academic achievement in children: a historical perspective. *Journal of Sport and Health Science, 1*(3), 160–9. https://doi.org/10.1016 /j.jshs.2012.09.003

Institute of Medicine (IOM). (2004). *Health Literacy: A Prescription to End Confusion.* National Academies Press.

Institute of Medicine (IOM). (2007). Chapter 2—Nutrition Related Health Concerns, Dietary Intakes, and Eating Behaviors of Children and Adolescents. In *Nutrition Standards for Foods in Schools* (pp. 29–72). National Academies Press.

Institute of Medicine (IOM). (2013a). Chapter 4—Physical Activity, Fitness, And Physical Education: Effects On Academic Performance. In *Educating the Student Body: Taking Physical Activity and Physical Education to School* (pp. 161–96). National Academies Press.

Institute of Medicine (IOM). (2013b). *Educating The Student Body: Taking Physical Activity And Physical Education To School.* National Academies Press. https://www.nap.edu/catalog /18314/educating-the-student-body-taking-physical-activity-and-physical-education

International School Health Network (ISHN). (2018). *International School Health Network.* ISHN. Retrieved July 19, 2018, from http://www.internationalschoolhealth.org/about -ishn.html

Jacobsen, K., Meeder, L., & Voskuil, V., for the National Association of School Nurses (NASN). (2016). School nurses' role in combating chronic absenteeism. *NASN School Nurse, 31,* 179–85.

Kaiser-Permanente. (n.d.) *Thriving Schools—School Employee Well-Being.* Kaiser-Permanente. Retrieved July 24, 2018, from https://thrivingschools.kaiserpermanente.org/school -employees/

Kann, L., McManus, T., Harris, W., Shanklin, S., Flint, K., Queen, B., Lowry, R., Chyen, D., Whittle, L., Thornton, J., Lim, C., Bradford, D., Yamakawa, Y., Leon, M., Brener, N., & Ethier, K.A. (2018). Youth Risk Behavior Surveillance—United States, 2017. *Morbidity and Mortality Weekly Report, 67*(8), 1–114. http://dx.doi.org/10.15585/mmwr.ss6708a1

Kickbusch, I., Pelikan, J., Apfel, F., & Tsouros, A. (2013). *Health Literacy: The Solid Facts.* World Health Organization European Regional Office.

Kolbe, L. (1986). Increasing the impact of school health promotion programs: Emerging research perspectives. *Health Education Journal, 17*(5), 47–52.

Kolbe, L. (2015). On national strategies to improve both education and health—An open letter. *Journal of School Health, 85*(1), 1–7. https://doi.org/10.1111/josh.12223

Kolbe, L. (2019). School health as a strategy to improve both public health and education. *Annual Review of Public Health, 40,* 443–63. https://doi.org/10.1146/annurev-publhealth -040218-043727

Kolbe, L., Allensworth, D., Potts-Datema, W., & White, D. (2015). What have we learned from collaborative partnerships to concomitantly improve both education and health? *Journal of School Health, 85*(11), 766–74. https://doi.org/10.1111/josh.12312

Kolbe, L., Kann, L., Patterson, B., Wechsler, H., Osorio, J., & Collins, J. (2004). Enabling the nation's schools to help prevent heart disease, stroke, cancer, COPD, diabetes, and other serious health problems. *Public Health Reports, 119*(3), 286–302. https://doi.org/10.1016 /j.phr.2004.04.008

Kumah, E.A., McSherry, R., Bettany-Saltikov, J., Hamilton, S., Hogg, J., Whittaker, V., & van Schaik, P. (2019). PROTOCOL: Evidence-informed practice versus evidence-based practice educational interventions for improving knowledge, attitudes, understanding, and behavior toward the application of evidence into practice: A comprehensive systematic review of undergraduate students. *Campbell Systematic Reviews, 15*(1–2), e1015. https://doi.org/10.1002/cl2.1015

Langford, R., Bonell, C., Komro, K., Murphy, S., Magnus, D., Waters, E., Gibbs, L., & Campbell, R. (2017). The Health Promoting Schools Framework: Known unknowns and an agenda for future research. *Health Education and Behavior, 44*(3), 463–75. https://doi.org/10.1177/1090198116673800

Lewallen, T., Hunt, H., Potts-Datema, W., Zaza, S., & Giles, W. (2015). The Whole School, Whole Community, Whole Child Model: A new approach for improving educational attainment and healthy development for students. *Journal of School Health, 85*(11), 729–39. https://doi.org/10.1111/josh.12310

Lipkin, P., & Okamoto, J. for The American Academy Of Pediatrics Council On Children With Disabilities and Council on School Health. (2015). The Individuals With Disabilities Education Act (IDEA) for Children With Special Educational Needs. *Pediatrics, 136*(6), e1650–62. https://doi.org/10.1542/peds.2015-3409

Luepker, R.V., Perry, C.L., McKinlay, S.M., Nader, P.R., Parcel, G.S., Stone, E.J., Webber, L.S., Elder, J.P., Feldman, H.A., Johnson, C.C., Kelder, S.H., Wu, M., Nader, P., Elder, J., McKenzie, T., Bachman, K., Broyles, S., Busch, E., Danna, S., . . . Verter, J. (1996). Outcomes of a field trial to improve children's dietary patterns and physical activity: The Child and Adolescent Trial for Cardiovascular Health (CATCH). *Journal of the American Medical Association, 275*(10), 768–76. https://doi.org/10.1001/jama.1996.03530340032026

Macartney, K., Quinn, H.E., Pillsbury, A.J., Koirala, A., Deng, L., Winkler, N., Katelaris, A.L., O'Sullivan, M.V.N., Dalton, C., Wood, N., and the NSW COVID-19 Schools Study Team (2020). Transmission of SARS-CoV-2 in Australian educational settings: a prospective cohort study. *The Lancet Child and Adolescent Health, 4*(11), 807–16. https://doi.org/10.1016/S2352-4642(20)30251-0

Macnab, A., Stewart, D., & Gagnon, F. (2014). Health Promoting Schools: Initiatives in Africa. *Health Education Journal, 114*(4), 246–59. https://doi.org/10.1108/HE-11-2013-0057

Michael, S., Merlo, C., Basch, C., Wentzel, K., & Wechsler, H. (2015). Critical connections: Health and academics. *Journal of School Health, 85*(11), 740–58. https://doi.org/10.1111/josh.12309

McDaid, D. (2016). *Investing in Health Literacy: What Do We Know about the Co-Benefits to the Education Sector of Actions Targeted at Children and Young People?* World Health Organization European Regional Office.

National Association of Chronic Disease Directors (NACDD). (n.d.a.). *Resources Related to the Every Student Succeeds Act (ESSA).* NACDD.

National Association of Chronic Disease Directors (NACDD). (n.d.b.). *School Health.* NACDD. Retrieved July 15, 2018, from http://www.chronicdisease.org/page/SchoolHealth

National Association of Chronic Disease Directors (NACDD). (2009). *Partnering for Success: How Health Departments Work and How to Work with Health Departments.* NACDD. https://c.ymcdn.com/sites/chronicdisease.site-ym.com/resource/resmgr/school_health/cdchhdwbrochureweblogo.pdf

National Association of Chronic Disease Directors (NACDD). 2012. *Thinking Outside the Box: Building and Sustaining School Health Programs in State Health Agencies without Dedicated Funding.* NACDD. https://www.chronicdisease.org/resource/resmgr/school_health/sustainability_case_studies_.pdf

National Association of Chronic Disease Directors (NACDD). (2013). *Speaking Education's Language: A Guide for Public Health Professionals Working in the Education Sector.* NACDD. https://chronicdisease.org/resource/resmgr/school_health/nacdd_educationsector_guide_.pdf

National Association of Chronic Disease Directors (NACDD). (2015a). *Nevada: Improving School Nutrition, Strengthened by a State Wellness Policy.* NACDD. https://c.ymcdn.com

/sites/chronicdisease.site-ym.com/resource/resmgr/School_Health/Nevada_Case_study
_2015_-_Pub.pdf

National Association of Chronic Disease Directors (NACDD). (2015b). *State Health Department Leadership in Addressing Chronic Conditions in Schools: Case Studies from Massachusetts and Missouri.* NACDD. https://chronicdisease.org/resource/resmgr/school_health
/chronic_conditions_case_stud.pdf

National Association of Chronic Disease Directors (NACDD). (2015c). *State School Health
Policy Matrix 2.0.* NACDD. https://chronicdisease.org/resource/resmgr/school_health
/policy_matrix_ii_final.pdf

National Association of Chronic Disease Directors (NACDD). (2016a). *A Guide for Incorporating Health and Wellness into School Improvement Plans.* NACDD. https://chronicdisease
.org/resource/resmgr/school_health/nacdd_sip_guide_2016.pdf

National Association of Chronic Disease Directors (NACDD). (2016b). *Opportunities for School
and Hospital Partnership in the Management of Chronic Health Conditions.* NACDD.
https://chronicdisease.org/resource/resmgr/school_health/nacdd_school_and_hospital
_pa.pdf

National Association of Chronic Disease Directors (NACDD). (2016c). *School Attendance,
Chronic Health Conditions and Leveraging Data for Improvement: Recommendations for
State Education and Health Departments to Address Student Absenteeism.* NACDD. https://
chronicdisease.org/resource/resmgr/school_health/nacdd_school_attendance_and_.pdf

National Association of Chronic Disease Directors (NACDD). (2017a). *Local Health Department and School Partnerships: Working Together To Build Healthier Schools.* NACDD.
https://chronicdisease.org/resource/resmgr/school_health/nacdd_school_attendance
and.pdf

National Association of Chronic Disease Directors (NACDD). (2017b). *The WSCC Model:
A Guide to Implementation.* NACDD. https://chronicdisease.org/resource/resmgr/school
_health/nacdd_thewholeschool_final.pdf

National Association of Chronic Disease Directors (NACDD). (2019). *Healthy School, Healthy
Staff, Healthy Students: A Guide to Improving School Employee Wellness.* NACDD. https://
chronicdisease.org/resource/resmgr/school_health/school_employee_wellness/nacdd
_schoolemployeewellness.pdf

National Association of School Nurses (NASN). (2014). *Transition Planning for Students
with Healthcare Needs (Position Statement).* NASN. https://www.nasn.org/advocacy
/professional-practice-documents/position-statements/ps-transition

National Association of School Nurses (NASN). (2017). *Chronic Health Conditions (Students
with): The Role of the School Nurse (Position Statement).* NASN. https://www.nasn.org
/nasn/advocacy/professional-practice-documents/position-statements/ps-chronic
-health

National Association of State Boards of Education (NASBE). (n.d.a.). *Health and Wellness.*
NASBE. Retrieved July 15, 2018, from https://www.nasbe.org/policy-area/health-and
-wellness/

National Association of State Boards of Education (NASBE). (n.d.b.) *State Policy Database—
Health Policies.* Alexandria, VA: NASBE. Retrieved October 17, 2019, from https://state
policies.nasbe.org/

National Cancer Institute (NCI). (n.d.) *The Classification of Laws Associated with School
Students (CLASS).* NCI. https://class.cancer.gov/

National Physical Activity Plan Alliance (NPAPA). (n.d.) *National Physical Activity Plan—
Education.* http://www.physicalactivityplan.org/theplan/education.html

NCD Risk Factor Collaboration. (2017). Worldwide trends in body-mass index, underweight,
overweight, and obesity from 1975 to 2016: A pooled analysis of 2416 population-based
measurement studies in 128.9 million children, adolescents, and adults. *The Lancet,
390*(10113), 2627–42. https://doi.org/10.1016/S0140-6736(17)32129-3

Nutbeam, D. (2000). Health literacy as a public health goal: A challenge for contemporary health education and communication strategies into the 21st century. *Health Promotion International, 15*(3), 259–67. https://doi.org/10.1093/heapro/15.3.259

Organization for Economic Cooperation and Development (OECD). (n.d.) *Better Life Initiative: Measuring Well-Being and Progress.* OECD. Retrieved July 19, 2018, from http://www .oecd.org/statistics/better-life-initiative.htm

Organization for Economic Cooperation and Development (OECD). (2020). *How's Life? 2020: Measuring Well-Being.* OECD. http://www.oecd.org/statistics/how-s-life-23089679.htm,

Park, B., Cantrell, L., Hunt, H., Farris, R., Schumacher, P., & Bauer, U. (2017). State public health actions to prevent and control diabetes, heart disease, obesity and associated risk factors, and promote school health. *Preventing Chronic Disease, 14,* E127. http://dx.doi .org/10.5888/pcd14.160437

Partnership for Child Development (PCD). (n.d.). *Improving Educational Outcomes through Health and Nutrition.* Imperial College London Faculty of Medicine. Retrieved July 19, 2018, from https://www.imperial.ac.uk/partnership-for-child-development

Patton, G., Coffey, C., Cappa, C., Currie, D., Riley, L., Gore, F., Degenhardt, L., Richardson, D., Astone, N., Sangowawa, A., Mokdad, A., & Ferguson, J. (2012). Health of the world's adolescents: A synthesis of internationally comparable data. *The Lancet, 379*(9826), 1665–75. https://doi.org/10.1016/S0140-6736(12)60203-7

Pennsylvania State University & the Robert Wood Johnson Foundation. (2016). *Teacher Stress and Health: Effects on Teachers, Students, and Schools.* Pennsylvania State University. https://www.rwjf.org/content/dam/farm/reports/issue_briefs/2016/rwjf430428

Perry, C., Stone, E., Parcel, G., Ellison, R., Nader, P., Webber, L., & Luepker, R. (1990). School-based cardiovascular health promotion: The Child and Adolescent Trial for Cardiovascular Health (CATCH). *Journal of School Health, 60*(8), 406–13. https://doi.org/10.1111 /j.1746-1561.1990.tb05960.x

Prakash, M., Teksoz, K., Espey, J., Sachs, J., Shank, M., & Schmidt-Traub, G. (2017). 2017 US Cities Sustainable Development Goals Index: Achieving a Sustainable Urban America. 2017. UNSDN. https://sdgindex.org/reports/2017-u.s.-cities-sdg-index/

Public Health Law Center (PHLC). (n.d.a.). *Physical Activity in Schools.* Mitchell Hamline School of Law. Retrieved July 24, 2018, from http://www.publichealthlawcenter.org/topics/active -living/physical-activity-schools

Public Health Law Center (PHLC). *Food in Schools.* (n.d.b.). Mitchell Hamline School of Law. Retrieved July 24, 2018, from http://www.publichealthlawcenter.org/topics/healthy -eating/food-schools

Public Health Law Center (PHLC). (n.d.c.). *Out of School Time.* Mitchell Hamline School of Law. Retrieved July 24, 2018, from http://www.publichealthlawcenter.org/topics/healthy -eating/out-of-school-time

Public Health Law Center (PHLC). (n.d.d.). *Laws, Policies and Regulations: Key Terms and Concepts.* Mitchell Hamline School of Law. Retrieved July 24, 2018, from http://www .publichealthlawcenter.org/sites/default/files/resources/tclc-fs-laws-policies-regs -commonterms-2015.pdf

Public Health Law Center (PHLC). (n.d.e.). *Schools.* Mitchell Hamline School of Law. Retrieved July 23, 2018, from http://www.publichealthlawcenter.org/topics/tobacco-control/smoke -free-tobacco-free-places/schools

Public Health Law Center (PHLC). (n.d.f.). *Public Health Concerns About Youth and Young Adult Use of JUUL.* Mitchell Hamline School of Law. http://www.publichealthlawcenter .org/blogs/2018-02-19/public-health-concerns-about-youth-young-adult-use-juul

Pudelski, S. (2017). *Cutting Medicaid: A Prescription to Hurt the Neediest Kids.* AASA (formerly American Association of School Administrators). http://aasa.org/uploadedFiles/Policy _and_Advocacy/Resources/medicaid.pdf

Ramaswamy, R., Mirochna, M., & Perlmuter, L. (2010). The negative association of BMI with classroom effort in elementary school children. *Journal of Child Health Care, 14*(2), 161–9. https://doi.org/10.1177/1367493509359222

Rasberry, C., Tiu, G., Kann, L., McManus, T., Michael, S., Merlo, C., Lee, S., Bohm, M., Annor, F., & Ethier, K. (2017). Health-related behaviors and academic achievement among high school students, 2015. *Morbidity and Mortality Weekly Report, 66*(35), 921–7. https://doi .org/10.15585/mmwr.mm6635a1

Resnicow, K., Cohn, L., Reinhardt, J., Cross, D., Futterman, R., Kirschner, E., Wynder, E., & Allegrante, J. (1992). Three-Year Evaluation of the Know Your Body Program in Inner-City Schoolchildren. *Health Education Quarterly, 19*(4), 463–80. https://doi.org/10.1177/1090 19819201900410

Resnicow, K., Cross, D., & Wynder, E. (1993). The Know Your Body program: A review of evaluation studies. *Bulletin of the New York Academy of Medicine, 70*(3), 188–207.

Riley, L., Guthold, R., Cowan, M., Savin, S., Bhatti, L., Armstrong, T., & Bonita, R. (2016). The World Health Organization STEPwise Approach to Noncommunicable Disease Risk-Factor Surveillance: Methods, challenges, and opportunities. *American Journal of Public Health, 106*(1), 74–78. https://doi.org/10.2105/AJPH.2015.302962

RMC Health. (n.d.) *Tobacco-Free Schools Policy Checklist Toolkit*. RMC Health. Retrieved July 23, 2018, from http://rmc.org/what-we-do/substance-abuse-prevention-education /tobacco-free-policy-checklist/

Rudd Center (Rudd Center for Food Policy and Obesity). (2013). *Wellness School Assessment Tool 3.0*. University of Connecticut. Retrieved April 22, 2021, from http://wellsat.org/

Robert Wood Johnson Foundation (RWJF). (n.d.) *RWJF–School Health Resources*. RWJF. Retrieved July 15, 2018, from https://www.rwjf.org/en/search-results.html?u=&k=school +health

Save the Children. (n.d.) *School Health and Nutrition*. Save the Children. Retrieved July 19, 2018, from https://www.savethechildren.org/us/what-we-do/global-programs/education /school-health-and-nutrition

Schools for Health in Europe Network (SHE). (n.d.) *Schools for Health in Europe*. University College South Denmark. Retrieved July 21, 2018, from http://www.schools-for-health.eu /she-network

Skinner, A., Ravanbakht, S., Skelton, J., Perrin, E., & Armstrong, S. (2018). Prevalence of obesity and severe obesity in US children, 1999–2016. *Pediatrics, 141*(3), e20173459. https:// doi.org/10.1542/peds.2017-3459

Social Progress Imperative (SPI). (n.d.) *Social Progress Index*. SPI. Retrieved July 19, 2018, from http://www.socialprogressimperative.org/

Society of Health and Physical Educators America (SHAPE). (n.d.) *SHAPE America*. SHAPE America. Retrieved July 23, 2018, from https://www.shapeamerica.org/

Sørensen, K., Van den Broucke, S., Fullam, J., Doyle, G., Pelikan, J., Slonska, Z., Brand, H. and (HLS-EU) Consortium Health Literacy Project European. (2012). Health literacy and public health: A systematic review and integration of definitions and models. *BMC Public Health, 12*(80). https://doi.org/10.1186/1471-2458-12-80

Stanford Medicine. (n.d.) *Tobacco Prevention Toolkit–School Policies*. Stanford Medicine. Retrieved April 22, 2021, from https://med.stanford.edu/tobaccopreventiontoolkit-old /parents-and-school-policy.html

Stone, E., Perry, C., & Luepker, R. (1989). Synthesis of cardiovascular behavioral research for youth health promotion. *Health Education Quarterly, 16*(2), 155–69. https://doi.org /10.1177/109019818901600202

Sustainable Development Solutions Network (SDSN). (n.d.a.). *Indicators and a Monitoring Framework* . UN. Retrieved July 20, 2018, from http://indicators.report/indicators/

Sustainable Development Solutions Network (SDSN). (n.d.b.). *Indicators and a Monitoring Framework–Target 3.4 Indicators*. UN. Retrieved July 20, 2018, from http://indicators. report/targets/3-4/

Tang, K.C., Nutbeam, D., Aldinger, C., St. Leger, L., Bundy, D., Hoffman, A.M., Yankah, E., McCall, D., Bujis, G., Arnaout, S., Morales, S., Robinson, F., Torranin, C, Drake, L., Abolfotouh, M., Whitman, C.V., Meresman, S., Odete, C., Joukhadar, A.H., . . . Heckert, K. (2009). Schools for health, education and development: A call for action. *Health Promotion International, 24*(1), 68–77. https://doi.org/10.1093/heapro/dan037

Taylor, M., Coovadia, H., Kvalsvig, J., Jinabhai, C., & Reddy, P. (1999). Helminth Control as an entry point for Health-Promoting Schools In Kwazulu-Natal. *South African Medical Journal, 89*(3), 273–9.

Tollit, M., Sawyer, S., Ratnapalan, S., & Barnett, T. (2015). Education support services for improving school engagement and academic performance of children and adolescents with a chronic health condition. *Cochrane Database of Systematic Reviews.* https://www .cochranelibrary.com/cdsr/doi/10.1002/14651858.CD011538/full

Trust for America's Heath (TFAH) and Healthy Schools Campaign (HSC). (2015). *Brief on Chronic Absenteeism and School Health.* http://www.attendanceworks.org/wordpress /wp-content/uploads/2011/03/Chronic-Absenteeism-and-School-Health-Brief-1.pdf

United Nations (UN). (n.d.a.). *SDG Knowledge Platform.* United Nations. Retrieved July 19, 2018, from https://sustainabledevelopment.un.org/

United Nations (UN). (n.d.b.). *Sustainable Development Goal Indicators.* United Nations. Retrieved July 20, 2018, from https://unstats.un.org/sdgs/

United Nations (UN). (2015). *Transforming Our World: The 2030 Agenda for Sustainable Development.* United Nations. https://sustainabledevelopment.un.org/post2015 /transformingourworld/publication

United Nations (UN). (2020). *The Sustainable Development Goals Report 2020.* United Nations. https://unstats.un.org/sdgs/report/2020/

United Nations Development Program (UNDP). (n.d.). *Human Development Reports.* UNDP. Retrieved July 19, 2018, from http://hdr.undp.org/en

United Nations Educational, Scientific, and Cultural Organization (UNESCO). (n.d.a.). *Education for Health and Well-Being.* UNESCO. Retrieved July 19, 2018, from https:// en.unesco.org/themes/health-education

United Nations Educational, Scientific, and Cultural Organization (UNESCO), Institute for Statistics (UIS). (n.d.b.). *Welcome to UIS.Stat.* UNESCO. Retrieved July 15, 2018, from http://data.uis.unesco.org/

United Nations Educational, Scientific, and Cultural Organization (UNESCO). (2013). *Monitoring and Evaluation Guidance for School Health Programs: Eight Core Indicators to Support FRESH (Focusing Resources on Effective School Health).* UNESCO. http:// hivhealthclearinghouse.unesco.org/sites/default/files/resources/FRESH_M%26E_CORE _INDICATORS.pdf

United Nations Educational, Scientific, and Cultural Organization (UNESCO). (2014). *Monitoring And Evaluation Guidance For School Health Programs: Thematic Indicators Supporting FRESH (Focusing Resources on Effective School Health).* UNESCO. http:// hivhealthclearinghouse.unesco.org/sites/default/files/resources/FRESH_M%26E _THEMATIC_INDICATORS.pdf

United Nations Educational, Scientific, and Cultural Organization (UNESCO). (2016). *UNESCO Strategy on Education for Better Health and Well-Being: Contributing to the Sustainable Development Goals.* UNESCO. http://unesdoc.unesco.org/images/0024 /002464/246453e.pdf

United Nations Educational, Scientific and Cultural Organization (UNESCO), United Nations Office on Drugs and Crime, & World Health Organization. (2017a). *Good Policy and Practice in Health Education: Booklet 10—Education Sector Responses to the Use of Alcohol, Tobacco and Drugs.* UNESCO. https://cdn.who.int/media/docs/default-source/substance -use/247509eng.pdf?sfvrsn=51329e52_2&download=true

United Nations Educational, Scientific, and Cultural Organization (UNESCO). (2017b).

Learning Objectives for SDG #3—Good Health and Well-Being. In *Education for Sustainable Development Goals: Learning Objectives, 16–17.* UNESCO. http://unesdoc.unesco.org /images/0024/002474/247444e.pdf

United Nations International Children's Emergency Fund (UNICEF). (n.d.) *Life Skills and Citizenship Education.* UNICEF. Retrieved April 22, 2020, from https://www.unicef.org /mena/life-skills-and-citizenship-education

US Department of Agriculture (USDA) Food and Nutrition Service (FNS). (2016, October 19). *About Team Nutrition.* USDA/FNS. https://www.fns.usda.gov/tn/about-team-nutrition

US Department of Agriculture (USDA) Food and Nutrition Service (FNS). (2017a, October 5). *School Breakfast Program: Healthy, Hunger-Free Kids Act.* USDA/FNS. https://www.fns .usda.gov/school-meals/healthy-hunger-free-kids-act

US Department of Agriculture (USDA) Food and Nutrition Service (FNS). (2017b). *Team Nutrition: Local School Wellness Policy.* USDA/FNS. Retrieved November 6, 2017, from https://www.fns.usda.gov/tn/local-school-wellness-policy

US Department of Agriculture (USDA) Food and Nutrition Service (FNS). (2018, March 5). *Child Nutrition Programs.* USDA/FNS. https://www.fns.usda.gov/school-meals/child -nutrition-programs

US Department of Education (USED), & National Center for Education Statistics 2017. (n.d.a.). *Back to School Statistics for 2017.* USED. Retrieved July 15, 2018, from https://nces.ed.gov /fastfacts/display.asp?id=372

US Department of Education (USED). (n.d.b.). *Every Student Succeeds Act (ESSA).* USED. Retrieved July 24, 2018, from https://www.ed.gov/esea

US Department of Education (USED). (n.d.c.). *Individuals with Disabilities Education Act.* USED. Retrieved July 24, 2018, from https://sites.ed.gov/idea/

US Department of Education (USED). (n.d.d.). *Student Privacy 101: Student Privacy at the US Department of Education.* USED. Retrieved July 24, 2018, from https://studentprivacy .ed.gov/

US Department of Education (USED). (2017, November 8). *ESSA State Plan Submission.* USED. https://www2.ed.gov/admins/lead/account/stateplan17/statesubmission.html

US Department of Health and Human Services (USDHHS). (n.d.a.). *Adolescent Health.* USDHHS. https://www.healthypeople.gov/2020/topics-objectives/topic/Adolescent -Health/objectives

US Department of Health and Human Services (USDHHS). (n.d.b.). *Healthy People 2020: Cancer Objectives Website.* USDHHS. https://www.healthypeople.gov/2020/topics -objectives/topic/cancer/objectives

US Department of Health and Human Services (USDHHS). (n.d.c.). *Development of the National Health Promotion and Disease Prevention Objectives for the Nation for 2030.* USDHHS. Retrieved July 19, 2018, from https://www.healthypeople.gov/2020/About -Healthy-People/Development-Healthy-People-2030

US Department of Health and Human Services (USDHHS). (n.d.d.). *Diabetes.* USDHHS. https://www.healthypeople.gov/2020/topics-objectives/topic/diabetes/objectives

US Department of Health and Human Services (USDHHS). (n.d.e.). *Early and Middle Childhood Objectives.* USDHHS. Retrieved July 22, 2018, from https://www.healthypeople.gov /2020/topics-objectives/topic/early-and-middle-childhood

US Department of Health and Human Services (USDHHS). (n.d.f.). *Educational and Community-Based Programs.* USDHHS. Retrieved July 22, 2018, from https://www. healthypeople.gov/2020/topics-objectives/topic/educational-and-community-based -programs/objectives

US Department of Health and Human Services (USDHHS). (n.d.g.). *Foundation Health Measures.* USDHHS. Retrieved July 19, 2018, from https://www.healthypeople.gov/2020 /About-Healthy-People/Foundation-Health-Measures

US Department of Health and Human Services (USDHHS). (n.d.h.). *Framework—The Vision, Mission, and Goals of Healthy People 2020*. USDHHS. Retrieved July 19, 2018, from https://www.healthypeople.gov/sites/default/files/HP2020Framework.pdf

US Department of Health and Human Services (USDHHS). (n.d.i.). *Health-Related Quality of Life and Well-Being*. USDHHS. Retrieved July 19, 2018, from https://www.healthypeople.gov/2020/topics-objectives/topic/health-related-quality-of-life-well-being

US Department of Health and Human Services (USDHHS). (n.d.j.). *Heart Disease and Stroke*. USDHHS. https://www.healthypeople.gov/2020/topics-objectives/topic/heart-disease-and-stroke/objectives

US Department of Health and Human Services (USDHHS). (n.d.k.). *Nutrition and Weight Status*. USDHHS. Retrieved July 20, 2018, from https://www.healthypeople.gov/2020/topics-objectives/topic/nutrition-and-weight-status/objectives

US Department of Health and Human Services (USDHHS). (n.d.l.). *Physical Activity*. USDHHS. Retrieved July 20, 2018, from https://www.healthypeople.gov/2020/topics-/topic/physical-activity/

US Department of Health and Human Services (USDHHS). (n.d.m.). *Respiratory Diseases*. USDHHS. https://www.healthypeople.gov/2020/topics-/topic/respiratory-diseases/

US Department of Health and Human Services (USDHHS). (n.d.n.). *Social Determinants of Health*. USDHHS. https://www.healthypeople.gov/2020/topics-/topic/social-determinants-of-health/

US Department of Health and Human Services (USDHHS). (n.d.o.). *Substance Abuse*. USDHHS. Retrieved July 20, 2018, from https://www.healthypeople.gov/2020/topics-/topic/substance-abuse/

US Department of Health and Human Services (USDHHS). (n.d.p.). *Tobacco Use*. USDHHS. Retrieved July 20, 2018, from https://www.healthypeople.gov/2020/topics-/topic/tobacco-use/

US Department of Health and Human Services (USDHHS). (2010). *National Action Plan to Improve Health Literacy*. USDHHS. https://health.gov/communication/hlactionplan/pdf/Health_Literacy_Action_Plan.pdf

US Office of Management and Budget (USOMB), Office of Information and Regulatory Affairs. (2018). US National Statistics for the U.N. Sustainable Development Goals. USOMB. https://sdg.data.gov/

Van Lippevelde, W., Verloigne, M., De Bourdeaudhuij, I., Brug, J., Bjelland, M., Lien, N., & Maes, L. (2012). Does parental involvement make a difference in school-based nutrition and physical activity interventions? A systematic review of randomized controlled trials. *International Journal of Public Health, 57*(4), 673–8. https://doi.org/10.1007/s00038-012-0335-3

Vaughn, B., Princiotta, D., Barry, M., Fish, H., & Schmitz, H. (2013). *Schools and the Affordable Care Act*. American Institutes for Research. https://safesupportivelearning.ed.gov/sites/default/files/1953_Schools%20Affordable%20Care%20Brief_d3%20lvr.pdf

Walter, H. (1989). Primary prevention of chronic disease among children: The school-based "Know Your Body" intervention trials. *Health Education Quarterly, 16*(2), 201–14. https://doi.org/10.1177/109019818901600205

Wang, Y., Cai, L., Wu, Y., Wilson, R., Weston, C., Fawole, O., Bleich, S., Cheskin, L.J., Showell, N.N., Lau, B.D., Chiu, D.T., Zhang, A., & Segal, J. (2015). What childhood obesity prevention programmes work? A systematic review and meta-analysis. *Obesity Reviews, 16*(7), 547–65. https://doi.org/10.1111/obr.12277

Ward, Z., Long, M., Resch, S., Giles, C., Cradock, A., & Gortmaker, S. (2017). Simulation of growth trajectories of childhood obesity into adulthood. *New England Journal of Medicine, 377*, 2145–53. https://doi.org/10.1056/NEJMoa1703860

WK Kellogg Foundation (WKKF). (2004). *Logic Model Development Guide: Using Logic Models to Bring Together Planning, Evaluation, and Action*. WK Kellogg Foundation.

World Bank. (n.d.) *Systems Approach for Better Education Results (SABER): School Health and School Feeding.* http://saber.worldbank.org/index.cfm?indx=8&pd=9&sub=0

World Bank. (2012). What Matters Most for School Health and School Feeding: A Framework Paper. In *Systems Approach for Better Education Results (SABER): Working Paper Series 3,* 1–88. World Bank. http://wbgfiles.worldbank.org/documents/hdn/ed/saber/supporting _doc/Background/SHN/Framework_SABER-School_Health.pdf

World Food Program (WFP). (n.d.) *School feeding.* WFP. Retrieved July 19, 2018, from http:// www1.wfp.org/school-meals

World Health Organization (WHO). (n.d.a.). Building a Healthy School Environment. In *Policy Briefs: Preventing Chronic Diseases, 2–3.* WHO. Retrieved July 21, 2018, from http://www .who.int/chp/advocacy/policy.brief_EN_web.pdf

World Health Organization (WHO). (n.d.b.). *Commission on Ending Childhood Obesity.* WHO. Retrieved July 20, 2018, from http://www.who.int/end-childhood-obesity/en/

World Health Organization (WHO). (n.d.c.). *Global Coordination Mechanism on the Prevention and Control of NCDs.* WHO. Retrieved October 17, 2019, from https://www.who.int /activities/gcm

World Health Organization (WHO). (n.d.d.). *The Global Health Observatory— Noncommunicable diseases: Risk factors.* WHO. Retrieved July 15, 2018, from http://www.who.int/gho /ncd/risk_factors/en/

World Health Organization (WHO). (n.d.e.). *Global School Health Policies and Practices Survey.* WHO. https://www.who.int/teams/noncommunicable-diseases/surveillance/systems -tools/global-school-health-policies-and-practices-survey

World Health Organization (WHO). (n.d.f.). *Global School-based Student Health Survey (GSHS).* WHO. Retrieved July 19, 2018, from http://www.who.int/ncds/surveillance/gshs/en/

World Health Organization (WHO). (n.d.g.). *Global Strategy on Diet, Physical Activity and Health.* WHO. Retrieved July 24, 2018, from https://www.who.int/dietphysicalactivity /background/en/

World Health Organization (WHO). (n.d.h.). *Global Youth Tobacco Survey (GYTS).* WHO. Retrieved July 20, 2018, from http://www.who.int/tobacco/surveillance/gyts/en/

World Health Organization (WHO). (n.d.i.) *Health Promoting Schools.* WHO. Retrieved April 20, 2021, from https://www.who.int/health-topics/health-promoting-schools#tab=tab_1

World Health Organization (WHO). (n.d.j.). *Knowledge Action Portal on NCDs.* Geneva, Switzerland: WHO. Retrieved October 17, 2019, from https://www.knowledge-action -portal.com/

World Health Organization (WHO). (n.d.k.). *Global Action Plan on Physical Activity 2018-2030: More Active People for a Healthier World.* WHO. http://apps.who.int/iris/bitstream/handle /10665/272722/9789241514187-eng.pdf

World Health Organization (WHO). (n.d.l.). *NCD Global Monitoring Framework.* WHO. Retrieved July 19, 2018, from http://www.who.int/nmh/global_monitoring_framework/en/

World Health Organization (WHO). (n.d.m.). *School and Youth Health: What Is a Health Promoting School?* WHO. http://www.who.int/school_youth_health/gshi/hps/en/

World Health Organization (WHO). (n.d.n.). *School and Youth Health.* Geneva, Switzerland: WHO. Retrieved July 15, 2018, from https://www.who.int/school_youth_health/gshi/en/

World Health Organization (WHO). (n.d.o.). *STEPwise Approach to Noncommunicable Disease Risk Factor Surveillance (STEPS).* WHO. Retrieved July 20, 2018, from http://www.who.int /ncds/surveillance/steps/riskfactor/en/

World Health Organization (WHO). (n.d.p.). *WHO Information Series on School Health.* WHO. Retrieved July 21, 2018, from http://www.who.int/school_youth_health/resources /information_series/en/

World Health Organization (WHO). (n.d.q.). *World Health Statistics Data Visualizations Dashboard: SDG Target 3.4—Noncommunicable Diseases and Mental Health.* WHO. Retrieved July 20, 2018, from http://www.who.int/gho/data/node.sdg.3-4

World Health Organization (WHO). (2003). *Skills for Health: Skills-based Health Education Including Life Skills: An Important Component of a Child-Friendly/Health-Promoting School.* WHO. http://www.who.int/iris/handle/10665/42818

World Health Organization (WHO). (2008). *School Policy Framework: Implementation of the WHO Global Strategy on Diet, Physical Activity and Health.* WHO. http://apps.who.int/iris/bitstream/10665/43923/1/9789241596862_eng.pdf

World Health Organization (WHO). (2011). Education: Shared Interests in Well-Being and Development. In *Social Determinants of Health Sectoral Briefing Series, 1–27.* WHO. http://www.who.int/iris/handle/10665/44737

World Health Organization (WHO). (2013). *Global Action Plan For The Prevention And Control Of Noncommunicable Diseases 2013–2020.* WHO. http://apps.who.int/iris/bitstream/handle/10665/94384/9789241506236_eng.pdf?sequence=1

World Health Organization (WHO). (2014a). *Global Status Report on Noncommunicable Diseases 2014.* WHO. http://apps.who.int/iris/bitstream/handle/10665/148114/9789241564854_eng.pdf?sequence=1

World Health Organization (WHO). (2014b). *Health in All Policies: Framework for Country Action.* WHO. http://www.who.int/healthpromotion/frameworkforcountryaction/en/

World Health Organization (WHO). (2014c). *Noncommunicable Diseases Country Profiles 2014.* WHO. http://apps.who.int/iris/bitstream/handle/10665/128038/9789241507509_eng.pdf?sequence=1

World Health Organization (WHO). (2014d). *WHO Tools to Prevent and Control Noncommunicable Diseases.* WHO. http://www.who.int/nmh/ncd-tools/en/

World Health Organization (WHO). (2015). *Health in All Policies Training Manual.* WHO. http://www.who.int/social_determinants/publications/9789241507981/en/

World Health Organization (WHO) for the UN Interagency Task Force on NCDs. (2016a). *Noncommunicable Diseases: What Ministries of Education Need to Know.* WHO. http://apps.who.int/iris/handle/10665/250231

World Health Organization (WHO). (2016b). *Report of the Commission on Ending Childhood Obesity.* WHO. http://apps.who.int/iris/bitstream/handle/10665/204176/9789241510066_eng.pdf?sequence=1

World Health Organization (WHO). (2016c). *Shanghai Declaration on Promoting Health in the 2030 Agenda for Sustainable Development.* WHO. http://www.who.int/healthpromotion/conferences/9gchp/shanghai-declaration.pdf?ua=1

World Health Organization (WHO). (2017a). *Electronic Nicotine Delivery Systems and Electronic Non-Nicotine Delivery Systems (ENDS/ENNDS).* WHO. http://www.who.int/tobacco/communications/statements/eletronic-cigarettes-january-2017/en/

World Health Organization (WHO). (2017b). *Health Promoting Schools: An Effective Approach to Early Action on Noncommunicable Disease Risk Factors.* WHO. http://apps.who.int/iris/bitstream/handle/10665/255625/WHO-NMH-PND-17.3-eng.pdf?sequence=1

World Health Organization (WHO). (2018a). *Global Action Plan on Physical Activity 2018–2030: More Active People for a Healthier World.* WHO. http://apps.who.int/iris/bitstream/handle/10665/272722/9789241514187-eng.pdf?ua=1

World Health Organization (WHO). (2018b). *Noncommunicable diseases country profiles 2018.* WHO. https://www.who.int/nmh/publications/ncd-profiles-2018/en/

World Health Organization (WHO). (2018c). *Promoting Health: Guide to National Implementation of the Shanghai Declaration.* WHO. http://apps.who.int/iris/bitstream/handle/10665/260172/WHO-NMH-PND-18.2-eng.pdf?sequence=1

WHO (World Health Organization). (2018d). Translating GPW 13 into action: The New Framework for Impact and Accountability for the Program Budget, Monitoring, and Performance Assessment. In *Thirteenth General Program of Work [GPW 13] 2019–2023,* 43–46. WHO. http://apps.who.int/gb/ebwha/pdf_files/WHA71/A71_4-en.pdf?ua=1

World Health Organization Regional Office for the Eastern Mediterranean (WHO/EMRO). (2010). *A Practical Guide to Developing and Implementing School Policy on Diet and Physical Activity*. WHO/EMRO. http://applications.emro.who.int/dsaf/dsa1038.pdf?ua=1 http://www.emro.who.int/health-education/publications/school-health.html

World Health Organization Eastern Mediterranean Regional Office (WHO/EMRO). (2012). *Health Education: Theoretical Concepts, Effective Strategies and Core Competencies*. WHO/EMRO. http://applications.emro.who.int/dsaf/EMRPUB_2012_EN_1362.pdf?ua=1

World Health Organization Regional Office for Europe (WHO/EURO). (n.d.) *Health Behavior in School-Aged Children*. WHO/EURO. Retrieved July 21, 2018, from http://www.euro.who.int/en/health-topics/Life-stages/child-and-adolescent-health/health-behaviour-in-school-aged-children-hbsc

World Health Organization Western Pacific Regional Office (WHO/WPRO). (n.d.) *Health Promoting Schools: Experiences from the Western Pacific Region*. WHO/WPRO. Retrieved April 22, 2021, from https://www.who.int/publications/i/item/9789290617884

Young, I. (2005). Health promotion in schools: A historical perspective. *Global Health Promotion, 12*(3–4), 112–7. https://doi.org/10.1177/10253823050120030103

CHAPTER 13

Applications in Health Care Settings

•

John P. Allegrante and Janey C. Peterson

Learning Objectives

After completing the chapter, the reader will be able to:

- Identify challenges and opportunities in the contemporary health care setting for using PRECEDE-PROCEED to improve the management of chronic diseases and infectious conditions.
- Discuss the characteristics of the patient-centered, outcomes-oriented approach to health care and identify at least three key factors that can be exploited by health care providers to address issues of health behavior.
- Provide specific examples of the application of PRECEDE-PROCEED as an effective planning framework for patient education in health care.
- Describe the applications of the PRECEDE-PROCEED model to planning, implementation, and evaluation in the development of (a) a community awareness campaign designed to improve mental health literacy and encourage early help-seeking for mental health problems, and (b) an educational program designed to improve self-care behaviors, health outcomes, and quality of life in people with rheumatoid arthritis.

INTRODUCTION

The original PRECEDE model dates back to the early 1970s, when Lawrence Green and his colleagues and students in public health at Johns Hopkins University developed and tested, in a series of controlled clinical and population trials, the seminal model for planning and evaluation to address the predisposing, enabling, and reinforcing factors in health-related behavior (Green et al. 1975; Green 1977; Levine et al. 1979; Morisky et al. 1978).[1] The Johns Hopkins University School of Medicine was the first in the United States to adopt and apply scientific methods in medical education. Green, like his innovative predecessors in medicine and public health at Hopkins, was interested in bringing rigorous scientific methods to the practice of public health education. He realized that planning health education programs lacked methodologic rigor, was often conducted without clear and measurable goals, and was rarely grounded in the kind of diagnostic orientation found in clinical medicine (Green 1977; Kreuter and Green 1978). Thus, he sought to develop a diagnostic approach to health education planning—an analogue to diagnosis in medicine—that could have applications in clinical care, but also in broader community health settings.

In doing so, Green effectively put the science and practice of health education and its focus on improving population health on a footing similar to that of how medical providers traditionally approached the diagnosis and treatment of individual patients in the clinical setting. He later collaborated with Marshall Kreuter to expand the model to include policy, regulatory, and organizational diagnoses in varied other settings in what is now the widely adopted PRECEDE-PROCEED planning framework for addressing the behavioral and environmental changes necessary to promote population health (Green and Kreuter 2005). Since then, nowhere has the evidence been more compelling for the utility and efficacy of the model than in the health care setting.[2] As has been demonstrated in schools, worksites, and other community settings in the previous chapters, disease prevention and health promotion program planning in health care—hospitals, clinics, pharmacies, and primary care settings (including dental, nursing, and physical therapy practices)—can be strengthened by the educational and ecological approach of PRECEDE-PROCEED. Meta-analyses and systematic reviews of the professional and continuing education literature in the health care setting also have a long history of applying PRECEDE to examine the factors influencing behavioral and organizational change among physicians and other providers in health care settings (Davis et al. 1992; 1995; Oxman et al. 1995; Tamblyn and Battista 1993).

This chapter will show how PRECEDE-PROCEED has been applied effectively over more than four decades to patient populations in the health care setting. Part one briefly reviews the contemporary challenges and opportunities practitioners and researchers face in the management of chronic diseases and infectious conditions in the context of dynamic change in health care delivery systems; in addition, it highlights the changes in health care provider practice that are required by patient-centered care and the focus on improving health outcomes and quality of life. Part two summarizes the many applications of PRECEDE-PROCEED in the health care setting. In part three, we present two case studies that describe the application and utility of the model in planning, implementing, and evaluating health promotion and disease prevention in the health care setting. Finally, we conclude with a brief comment about the value of the model in achieving disease prevention, health promotion, and self-care priorities in the health care setting and beyond.

CHALLENGES AND OPPORTUNITIES IN THE MANAGEMENT OF CHRONIC AND INFECTIOUS CONDITIONS IN THE HEALTH CARE SETTING

Central to the work of health care is the evolving role of the provider in the context of evidence-based and outcomes-oriented medicine (Brownson et al. 2017; Glasgow et al. 2006; Green et al. 2009; Green and Ottoson 2004; Gurses et al. 2010). Part of the evolution of provider roles is the recognition of some limitations of "evidence-based" medicine when it is applied too mechanically. Evidence-based medicine needs to take into consideration that, in the quest for internal validity, highly controlled randomized trials often add layers of artificial circumstances to what would be the usual or prevailing circumstances of local practice. The rote implementation of evidence-based practices without an assessment and educational diagnosis of the local realities can miss the mark of what the patients and local circumstances may require. In this context, another aspect of the evolution has been a mounting pressure to implement evidence-based medicine "with fidelity," despite the dubious fit in many circumstances and for many patients where deviation from the "evidence" or guideline would be clinically justifiable, and indeed essential for appropriate fit. Gurses and colleagues (2010) have illustrated this dilemma by conceptualizing the system, provider, and guideline characteristics that influence clinician uptake and implementation of evidence-based guidelines in health care practice, as shown in figure 13.1.

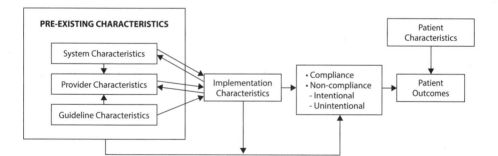

FIGURE 13.1. An interdisciplinary conceptual framework of clinicians' compliance with evidence-based guidelines. *Source:* Gurses, A.P., Marstellar, J.A., Ant Ozok, A., Xiao, Y., Owens, S., & Pronovost, P.J. (2010). Using an interdisciplinary approach to identify factors that affect clinician's compliance with evidence-based guidelines. *Critical Care Medicine, 38*(Suppl. 8), S282–91. https://doi.org/10.1097/CCM.0b013e3181e69e02

What physicians, nurses, therapists, and other health care providers—and their patients—must do to improve chronic disease management is key to achieving the goals of treatment and improving health outcomes. Health care providers need to emphasize the active and informed engagement of patient decision-making and control from the earliest stages of diagnosis to the post-medical or postsurgical course of self-monitoring and maintenance of recommended lifestyle and environmental changes.

While the emphasis on patient engagement may be recognized by providers, much of the traditional provider-centered practice model has focused on clinical proficiency during the clinical encounter—conducting a physical examination, asking questions, taking a history, developing a diagnosis, and implementing a treatment plan to address a chronic disease. But traditional practice sometimes presents several problems that can lead to poor quality of care and poor health outcomes. For example, patients often resist medical advice; education about disease is not optimally delivered (e.g., not tailored to the patient's health literacy or readiness for change), and therefore not uniformly correlated with changes in patient or caregiver behavior; and patient motivation to comply with medical advice is frequently variable. Moreover, from the perspective of clinical practice, acute care tends to take precedence over preventive care in the practice of physicians and other health care providers, insofar as acute cases are urgent and call directly on the provider's clinical acumen, skills, and resources. However, while the control and cultural authority inherent in the traditional model of provider-centered practice has, historically, proven effective for acute care, such a model of health care is no longer sufficient for facilitating the long-term management of chronic diseases and other conditions for which skills in coping, communication, control (Daltroy and Liang 1993), and patient behavioral self-management (Bodenheimer et al. 2002; Grady and Gough 2014; Holman and Lorig 2000; Peterson et al. 2014) are critical to achieving optimal treatment outcomes and improvements in quality of life.

Considerable clinical and epidemiologic evidence has emerged for the impact of patient education and behavioral self-management on health outcomes in chronic disease and infectious conditions. Although the scope of this chapter does not permit a full review of the literature—nor will it permit attention to the challenges of preventing and treating the emergent COVID-19 (SARS-CoV-2) pandemic of 2020-21 (e.g., see Allegrante et al. 2020; Fauci et al. 2020; Gates 2020)—we encourage the reader to consult the following for representative examples of the history and contemporary reviews of this evidence: Allegrante (2018); Allegrante et al. (1993); Allegrante et al. (2019); Allegrante and Marks (2003); Grady and Gough (2014); Lorig et al. (1999; 2001); Marks et al. (2005a; 2005b); McGinnis (1993). The large body of work that has been conducted over several decades to demonstrate the relationship between educational intervention, changes in health behavior, and health outcomes suggests that physicians and other health care providers must assume the role of applied behavioral scientist to foster better patient coping, communication, and control.

THE CHALLENGES

Health care expenditures in the United States continue to outpace inflation and now account for approximately 18% of the nation's GDP, with costs exceeding $2.6 trillion (figure 13.2).[3] Much of the economic burden comes from chronic diseases and conditions—heart disease, stroke, cancer, type 2 diabetes, obesity, and arthritis. According to the CDC, these are among the most common, costly, and preventable of all health problems, and are the leading causes of mortality and disability. Moreover, addressing patterns of health behavior that lead to chronic diseases—estimated to account for 50% of all deaths in the United States—may constitute the single most critical opportunity to improve health and quality of life (Green et al. 2015; Schroeder 2007).[4] Thus, the challenge of addressing chronic diseases and conditions will require that the United States make progress in meeting the *Healthy People 2030* goal to improve health care (Office of Disease Prevention and Health Promotion n.d.a.). One means by which this can be accomplished is through effective planning for health education.

The failure to manage chronic diseases has long been recognized as a significant driver of rising health care costs and poor health outcomes. This is because managing complex medical conditions increasingly involves long-term adherence to a preventive or therapeutic regimen that typically involves lifestyle behavioral changes. Such changes are likely to include altering patterns of diet and physical activity, taking medications as prescribed, and scheduling and keeping

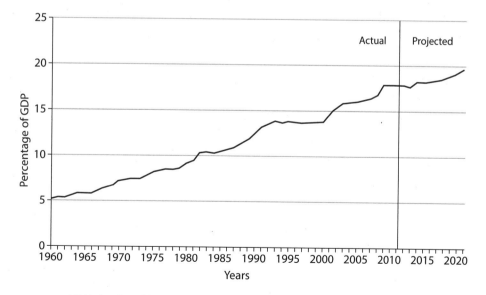

FIGURE 13.2. US National Health Expenditures as a Share of GDP, 1960–2021. *Source:* Centers for Medicare and Medicaid Services.

regular medical appointments. Thus, health care providers need to emphasize the active and informed engagement of patient decision-making and control from the start of the therapeutic relationship, beginning with primary prevention and consideration of socioeconomic and environmental circumstances of the patient. This, in turn, sets the stage for early diagnosis, to postmedical or postsurgical self-monitoring and maintenance of behavioral and environmental changes.

To accomplish effective patient engagement, providers must go beyond performing the customary clinical skills necessary to conduct a health history and examination and arrive at a diagnosis; they must become adept at applying the methods of applied behavioral science to a range of other tasks. For example, providers must be skilled at listening to what patients say about their preferences and the utilities they ascribe to competing prevention or treatment approaches in response to their diagnosis and recommended available treatments. Providers must also calibrate patient expectations of realistic treatment outcomes, as well as clearly communicate the potential unintended consequences of any treatment. Employing peer coaches and patient navigators to discuss with patients how they view anticipated problems of coping with the medical care system, compliance, and barriers to treatment adherence all become critical to effective clinical practice and improvement of health outcomes. Providers need to do all these things by engaging their patients in a partnership that fosters trust and rapport and builds patient confidence in the treatment and treatment team, as well as in themselves. Finally, patient-centered care, fostering patient empowerment, and ensuring patients' rights—and the relationship of these to health outcomes—have continued to be important considerations in the present context of managed care. Each aims to engage consumers more effectively in greater self-care and in a government-sponsored health care setting that increasingly seeks to serve a population less dependent on the medical system while reducing costs. Numerous specific applications of PRECEDE in perceived control and empowerment in relating patient or community needs and capacities to those of health professionals have been published (e.g., Allison 1991; Hill 1996; Jenny 1993).

THE OPPORTUNITIES

A patient-centered, outcomes-oriented approach to health care calls for several departures from the traditional medical model that has dominated health care planning for over a century, a process that can be facilitated by applying the PRECEDE-PROCEED model. First, clinical providers must recognize the opportunities and potential effectiveness they can have in improving patient outcomes. Second, a break from the traditional medical approach of concentrating health care diagnosis and planning on the individual patient must be accompanied by a broader focus on family and population health and the social determinants of health. In addition to its capacity to be applied at the individual level, the added value of PRECEDE-PROCEED can be achieved in health care settings where an epidemiologic approach to population-based health needs can be applied to large numbers of people in the community. Finally, the educational and ecological approach that characterizes PRECEDE-PROCEED requires a third departure from the traditional medical model as practiced in most health care settings: a greater emphasis on self-care and patient-centered autonomy and responsibility for planning and controlling the health care regimen is required. This aligns with the first phase of patient or population participation and engagement when applying the PRECEDE-PROCEED model.

An impressive body of literature suggests that health care providers, working in partnership with trained peer counselors or patient navigators, can play a major role in strengthening the motivation and capabilities of patients to change specific health-related behaviors such as stopping smoking and other tobacco use, getting more physical activity, and changing diet and nutrition.[5] In addition, taking medicine and monitoring biologic functions such as blood pressure or blood glucose levels are behaviors that patients may have to learn, adopt, and maintain in order to successfully manage a disease condition.

By working in tandem with patients to address the often complex, durable, and deeply-rooted cultural, social, and psychological issues related to health behavior, providers can promote trust and respect, enhance the reach of behavioral interventions, and increase program participation and retention in both clinical and community settings.[6] This role should not be regarded as trivial or dispensable; without support and encouragement from the physician, nurse, therapist, or trained lay peer coach, many patients will fail to adopt or to maintain the process of change, and some of the critical community efforts to influence the broader social determinants of health will go unrealized. There is a substantial literature examining the opportunity to initiate, support, and reinforce complex lifestyle and behavioral changes from within the health care arena (e.g., Glanz 1999; Paluck et al. 2003; Pellmar et al. 2002; Williams et al. 2000).

The role for health care providers envisioned here exploits several key factors:

- the *credibility* and *cultural authority* of the health care provider in directing treatment, while at the same time recognizing the autonomy and responsibility of the engaged and empowered patient;
- the *access to patients at teachable moments* when they are particularly receptive to advice and guidance, especially at times of heightened concern about symptoms, susceptibility, and potential severity of disease (Becker 1978; Janz and Becker 1984; Rosenstock 1974);[7]

- an emerging *culture of health*[8] in which the health consciousness of the public has enlarged the inherent interest of patients in seeking not only the counsel of health care providers but also wider, Internet-based and crowd-sourced health information that can support decision-making and help them change health-directed behavior, cope with lifestyle issues, or address environmental factors that may threaten their health;
- the increased *readiness and capacity of physicians*[9] and *other clinical providers*[10] and their interest in health promotion and health-related behavioral change; and
- the *contributions of trained peer coaches* who themselves have valuable personal experience with the chronic condition of interest to the patient and who are particularly effective in delivering health-related information, especially to minority, low socioeconomic, and other hard-to-reach groups (Sokol and Fisher 2016).

PRECEDE-PROCEED represents a practical and scientifically credible logic model designed to enhance practitioners' preparation, practice environment, personal health beliefs and habits, and their understanding of and familiarity with the evidence base for effective disease prevention and health promotion interventions. In addition, it is designed to strengthen their capacity and skills to formulate, coordinate, and oversee an interdisciplinary health care team that can effectively counsel patients and assist them in navigating myriad behavioral self-management tasks.

PRECEDE-PROCEED IN HEALTH CARE

Although several models and frameworks have been developed to guide health planning and evaluation for different settings (Bartholomew-Eldridge et al. 2011; Czajkowski et al. 2015; Glasgow et al. 1999; Peterson et al. 2013),[11] the application of PRECEDE-PROCEED has proved itself to be an effective guiding framework with which to study or intervene on a wide range of problems and across settings. The PRECEDE-PROCEED model has been applied to the individual level of clinical decision-making in health care and broader community settings in the United States and globally. Many of these efforts have focused on chronic diseases and infectious conditions with high incidence or prevalence—including recent efforts to understand perceptions of COVID-19 related to prevention, coping, and testing (Bateman et al. 2021)—and where nonadherence to medical recommendations and failure to implement preventive health services results in poor outcomes and high costs to society. Others have implemented PRECEDE-PROCEED to plan broader population health improvement efforts being led by the health care team and that reach beyond the clinic and into the community.

Numerous more recent applications of PRECEDE-PROCEED highlight the planning, implementation, and evaluation of patient education. These include nutrition education (Buta et al. 2011); smoking- and vaping cessation (Aldiabat and Le Navenec 2013); health-related self-care, self-help, or self-management programs (Dizaji et al. 2014); and telehealth for managing chronic conditions (Salisbury et al. 2015). For decades, applications have spanned disease conditions where patient behavioral changes and adherence to prescribed medication are critical to the management of such diseases and conditions: arthritis and musculoskeletal conditions (Allegrante et al. 1993; Kovar et al. 1992; Marks and Allegrante 2001; Nadrian et al. 2011; Sullivan et al. 1998; Sezgin and Esin 2018), asthma (Bailey et al. 1987; Chiang et al. 2004), diabetes (Gary et al. 2003; 2009), hypertension (Levine et al. 1979; Morisky et al. 1990), infectious conditions like tuberculosis (Khortwong and Kaewkungwal 2013; Morisky et al. 1990), and mental health (Mo and Mak 2008; Wright 2006; Yeo et al. 2006). Recent work has also demonstrated the utility of PRECEDE-PROCEED in studies investigating a wide range of issues that are relevant to disease prevention and health promotion planning in specific health care processes, such as improving the implementation of health care information technology (Kukafka et al. 2003); assessing barriers to communication in community pharmacies (Paluck et al. 2003); addressing facilitators of and barriers to patient influenza vaccination from the physician's perspective (Zimmerman et al. 2004); identifying personal and structural factors that influence timely follow-up of abnormal mammograms among multicultural women (Arnsberger et al. 2006); addressing barriers to psychosocial care in oncology patients (Schofield et al. 2006); improving hand hygiene practices of health care personnel in the prevention of health care-based infections (Aboumatar et al. 2012); developing chronic disease interventions by nurses (Phillips et al. 2012); designing and evaluating oral health strategies for adults with intellectual and developmental disabilities (Binkley and Johnson 2013); understanding the quality of life among drug users (Matin et al. 2014); and developing pediatric interventions in the primary care setting to reduce antibiotic use (Lucas et al. 2017). Additional published applications of the model are available online[12] and have been cited in numerous Cochrane Database of Systematic Reviews.[13]

CASE STUDY 1: IMPROVING MENTAL HEALTH LITERACY

A practical and feasible application of PRECEDE-PROCEED that is relevant to health care is The Compass Strategy (Makrides et al. 1997; Wright et al. 2006).[14] Conducted in Australia in the early 2000s, The Compass Strategy is a theory-driven application of the model to the planning, implementation, and evaluation of a community awareness campaign designed to improve mental health literacy and encourage early help-seeking among young people. The program developers and investigators used focus group interviews, telephone surveys, and data from a prior preliminary study to conduct assessments for each of the PRECEDE-PROCEED phases. The PRECEDE-PROCEED model concepts as applied in the program are shown in figure 13.3.

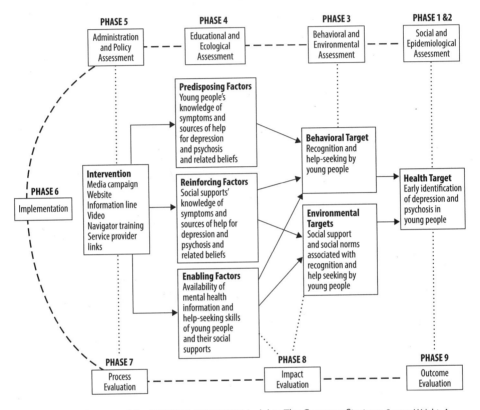

FIGURE 13.3. Application of the PRECEDE-PROCEED Model to The Compass Strategy. *Source:* Wright, A., McGorry, P.D., Harris, M.G., Jorm, A.F., & Pennell, K. (2006). Development and evaluation of a youth mental health community awareness campaign—The Compass Strategy. *BMC Public Health, 6,* 215. https://doi.org/10.1186/1471-2458-6-215

Social and Epidemiological Assessment (Phases 1 and 2)

Globally, the burden of mental health disorders is significant. A wide range of disorders require mental health treatment, as shown in box 13.1. In Australia, at the time of the study, mental disorders accounted for 55% of the total injury and disease burden in youth aged 15 to 24 years. Improved surveillance and treatment were believed to have the potential to substantially reduce disease burden and to improve health-related quality of life. Thus, in this study, the health target was the early identification and treatment of depression and psychosis in young people.

BOX 13.1

From the Clinic to the Community—Focus on Mental Health

According to the National Institute of Mental Health, mental illness is defined as a mental, behavioral, or emotional disorder that can vary in impact, ranging from no impairment to mild, moderate, and even severe impairment. Each year, mental illness affects approximately one in five adults in the United States (18.3%, or 44.7 million in 2016), and one in 25 adults experience a serious mental illness that substantially interferes with or limits one or more major life activities. Globally, anxiety disorders and depression are the most prevalent mental illnesses.

Mental illness that requires treatment includes a wide range of disorders, including:

- Anxiety disorders
- Attention deficit hyperactivity disorder (ADHD, ADD)
- Autism spectrum disorders (ASD)
- Bipolar disorder (manic-depressive illness)
- Borderline personality disorder
- Depression
- Disruptive mood dysregulation disorder
- Eating disorders
- Obsessive-compulsive disorder (OCD)
- Post-traumatic stress disorder (PTSD)
- Schizophrenia
- Seasonal affective disorder

In addition, the use of alcohol and other substances and experiencing traumatic events can contribute to mental health problems that often require treatment.

In 2016, young adults aged 18–25 years had the highest prevalence of any mental illness (22.1%) compared to adults aged 26–49 years (21.1%) and aged 50 and older (14.5%). Untreated and unresolved mental health problems can, in some cases, lead to suicide, which in 2016 was the second leading cause of death among young people between the ages of 10 and 24, and those adults between the ages of 25 and 34.

Public attitudes toward mental illness and efforts to treat people with mental illness have undergone dramatic changes during the last 50 years. While those with mental illness were once committed to institutional care and treated in isolation, scientific and clinical advancements in safe and effective treatments—including psychopharmacologic medication, psychotherapy, and complementary and alternative medicine—have made it possible for many people with mental health problems to live productive lives and function in the community without hospitalization.

Mental health is determined by a range of socioeconomic, biological, and environmental factors. Raising community awareness and promoting efforts to improve mental health literacy and encourage early help-seeking are critical in both the prevention and treatment of mental illness.

Sources: National Institute of Mental Health: https://www.nimh.nih.gov/health/statistics/mental-illness.shtml; https://www.nimh.nih.gov/health/statistics/suicide.shtml. World Health Organization: http://www.who.int/en/news-room/fact-sheets/detail/mental-disorders.

Behavioral and Environmental Assessment (Phase 3)

Previous population health interventions had demonstrated some success in increasing the recognition of mood disorders and taking action to seek help; thus, these behavioral targets were considered by the investigators to be potentially changeable. Because the recognition of depression and psychosis is the first step in the process of effective help-seeking, this study focused on increasing help-seeking behavior to obtain appropriate treatment.

Among the principal social-environmental factors associated with recognition and help-seeking were social support, social norms of expected behaviors and responses to mental health problems, a social network, and stigma associated with mental illness. Health care environmental factors, including the accessibility and availability of services and the quality of treatment by treating providers, were also considered to be important. However, the assessment concluded that fostering social norms and providing social support for recognition of symptoms and help-seeking would be priority environmental targets, again because strategies that had previously targeted these factors had shown some success.

Educational and Ecological Assessment (Phase 4)

The educational and ecological assessment in this study focused on the need for early identification and receipt of treatment for mental health problems.

Predisposing factors. Respondents possessed limited knowledge and awareness of the signs, symptoms, and potential seriousness of depression or psychosis and available treatments. In addition, respondents held beliefs that suggested they were not susceptible to these disorders or that they would be stigmatized if they sought help.

Reinforcing factors. Respondents identified family and friends, followed by teachers, counselors, and lay leaders (such as the clergy) as being among the principal sources of reinforcing factors, indicating that these individuals were most trusted to provide positive feedback and social support for seeking help.

Enabling factors. Respondents noted that the lack of available information about mental health problems and appropriate sources of help constituted barriers to effective help-seeking. They also reported that opportunities to develop specific help-seeking skills could further enable symptom recognition and seeking help.

Administrative and Policy Assessment (Phase 5)

The analysis of policies, resources, and circumstances in an organizational setting that either hinder or facilitate the development of a health promotion program showed that funding would be a key issue in supporting the program. A new Australian government mental health policy focusing on early intervention and mental health promotion facilitated the funding of the project. Funding, however, would be contingent on the capacity of the community and the service system to cooperate in undertaking such a mental health initiative. This is where interorganizational collaborations and coalitions, as proposed in chapter 8, can prove instrumental in leveraging the mutual interests and combined efforts of organizations.

Implementation (Phase 6)

The development and implementation of the intervention was shaped by the predisposing, reinforcing, and enabling factors that were identified in the educational and ecological assessment phase. The Process Model of Social Marketing Program Development (Lebvre and Rochlin 1996) was the theoretical framework used to guide strategy development, audience segmentation, key messages, and channels of communication. Once the proposed intervention was designed and the investigators obtained informed consent, it was pilot-tested, refined, and implemented, as discussed in chapter 9.

Process, Impact, and Outcome Evaluation (Phases 7–9)

An evaluation committee was organized to conduct the evaluation, the primary goal of which was to monitor program implementation and effectiveness in increasing help-seeking behavior and early identification of depression and psychosis. The process evaluation sought to determine whether the program was being implemented as planned and operated effectively; an impact evaluation focused on a wide range of post-campaign predisposing, reinforcing, and enabling variables; and the outcome evaluation was oriented toward assessing service utilization, duration of untreated mental illness, and number of contacts in the pathways to care. The evaluation trial included a cross-sectional telephone survey of mental health literacy among randomly selected independent samples of 600 young people aged 12–25 years from the region where the program was implemented and another 600 from a comparison region. The survey was undertaken before and after 14 months of the campaign; results indicated that the Compass Strategy proved to be effective. This effectiveness was in large part attributed to the PRECEDE-PROCEED model, which the investigators believed facilitated refinement of the campaign targets through the population assessment processes, the use of evidence-based campaign strategies, and the capacity to refine the campaign elements in response to regular reviews of process evaluation findings.

CASE STUDY 2: DEVELOPING EDUCATION TO IMPROVE SELF-CARE BEHAVIORS AND HEALTH OUTCOMES FOR PEOPLE WITH RHEUMATOID ARTHRITIS

A second case study of the application of PRECEDE-PROCEED further illustrates the value of the model, especially in the formative development and evaluation of educational and behavioral programs in the health care setting. This case comes from a study of the development of an education program designed to improve functioning and promote quality of life for patients with rheumatoid arthritis (RA) in Iran (Nadrian et al. 2011).

RA is the most common of inflammatory arthritis-related diseases. Patients with RA experience a broad spectrum of symptoms and disease impact, including fatigue, pain, and functional limitations that have significant impact on their health-related quality of life. Thus, in addition to medication, the clinical treatment and management of RA involves self-care behaviors that can help patients to manage the disease and their activities of daily living. In this study, the PRECEDE-PROCEED model was used by the developers as a conceptual framework with which to develop a patient education program to help patients engage in self-care behaviors that would enable and support them to better manage their disease.

First, the developers used the model to guide a comprehensive review of the literature of RA. The review included the signs and symptoms of RA, the functional challenges that people who have RA commonly encounter, and the effects of the disease on patient quality of life. In addition, the program developers sought to review what was known about previous educational programs and their design, to better understand the missed opportunities for improving health outcomes and the quality of life of patients living with the disease.

Next, in order to inform the development of the education program, the developers conducted a needs assessment of the intended patient population. This involved a cross-sectional survey of outpatients with RA who were residing in Yazd, a city located in the center of Iran. The survey questionnaire included questions about each of the predisposing, enabling, and reinforcing factors identified in the PRECEDE-PROCEED educational and ecological assessment (Phase 4) component of the model. Patients included in the survey responded to questions about their perceptions regarding those predisposing, enabling, and reinforcing factors they deemed relevant to managing their RA and symptoms.

The survey results showed that patients were most concerned with the impact low physical functioning due to chronic pain had on their quality of life. Given that one of the significant and potentially modifiable behavioral factors influencing pain and functional limitations was found to be patient self-care behaviors, the Rheumatoid Arthritis Patient Education Program (RAPEP) focused on fostering better self-care. Thus, the program sought to improve patients' knowledge, attitude, self-efficacy, enabling factors, and social support associated with better self-care behavior. A summary of the predisposing, enabling, and reinforcing factors related to self-care behavioral, health, and quality of life outcomes in RA patients is shown in figure 13.4.

Although the impact of RAPEP was not evaluated as part of the program development effort, the formative processes that used concepts and methods from the PRECEDE-PROCEED model to develop the educational program proved useful as a comprehensive conceptual framework. The study also demonstrated that, depending on setting and resources, using even only selected elements of the model for purposes of planning—in this case, only focusing on the educational and ecological factors of interest in relation to health and quality of life outcomes—can nevertheless provide program developers with important insights into patient preferences and priorities and how they can be leveraged and addressed in fostering behavioral change.

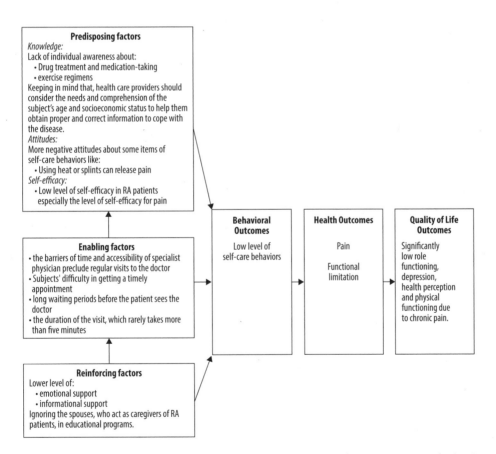

FIGURE 13.4. A summary of predisposing, enabling, and reinforcing factors (expressed as barriers) related to self-care behavioral outcomes, health outcomes, and quality of life outcomes in RA patients. *Source:* Nadrian, H., Morowatisharifabad, M.A., & Bahmanpour, K. (2011). Development of a rheumatoid arthritis education program using the PRECEDE-PROCEED Model. *Health Promotion Perspectives, 1*(2), 118–9. https://doi.org/10.5681/hpp .2011.013. Reprinted with permission.

CONCLUSION

The institutional culture and environment of health care settings, as well as the professional behavior of health care providers, continue to evolve in response to changing societal needs and the economic and other priorities of clinical health care related to the prevention, treatment, and management of chronic diseases. Considering the range and pervasiveness of influences beyond the biomedical on lifestyle, behavior, and health-related environments, perhaps society should ask itself whether the investment in disease prevention, health promotion, and a broader population health agenda is a more plausible alternative to that of clinical medicine in addressing such priorities.

This is a reasonable question because there is now impressive evidence demonstrating that lifestyle and behavior are influenced by a broad range of determinants—cultural, psychological, social, occupational, recreational, economic, structural, and political. The exposure of people to these influences indelibly shapes the attitudes, beliefs, and values that consciously drive their personal choices of health-directed behavior, such as seeking an immunization, a physical examination, or a low-fat food, or complying with prescribed medication. These purposeful actions are usually time-limited and reasonably responsive to clinical or office-based health care intervention. Nevertheless, one's history of exposure to social, structural, and other environmental conditions also shapes one's lifestyle and opportunities. Resultant enduring patterns of unconscious health-related behavior that can harm health and lead to chronic conditions include such behaviors as consumption of high-fat foods, physical inactivity, excessive stress, aggression or risk-taking, and harmful use of alcohol, tobacco, and drugs (Fisher et al. 2011). Because such behaviors and patterns of living are now known to be deeply rooted in one's personal development, experiences, social relationships, and environmental exposures, they resist intervention in such time-limited medical encounters typical of the health care setting.

The PRECEDE-PROCEED concepts, processes, and methods can be used to effectively address these influences and patterns, and have demonstrated universally broad utility across a wide range of populations and practice settings in doing so. Its hallmarks of flexibility and scalability, evidence-based process and evaluability, commitment to the principle of participation, and provision of a process for the appropriate adaptation of evidence-based practices to population and setting-specific circumstances make PRECEDE-PROCEED especially well-suited as a planning framework for health care settings. The model implicitly recognizes that the culture, environment, and professional behavior of health care providers—physicians, nurse practitioners, therapists, and others—must evolve and adapt to patient and community population needs if they are to support primary and secondary disease prevention, health promotion, and self-care priorities that are now well-established features of cost-effective health care. In the context of the health care setting, the PRECEDE-PROCEED model lends itself to a protocol for the triage and stepped care of patients as well as the continuing education of health care professionals and the broader community beyond the clinic. PRECEDE-PROCEED acknowledges that complex behavioral changes, the social determinants of health, and environmental influences all must be taken into consideration and addressed at both the individual clinical and population levels.

EXERCISES

1. For any given clinical health care practice setting, identify and describe the distribution of chronic diseases or infectious conditions presented by patients and prioritize them for health education planning.

2. For the highest-priority chronic disease or infectious condition, identify what the literature on the clinical epidemiology of the disease suggests are the potentially modifiable behaviors of interest for behavioral self-management in this population of patients, and write a behavioral objective for the highest priority behavior.

3. Develop an inventory of the predisposing, enabling, and reinforcing factors for the highest-priority behavior, identify the priorities for each factor, and describe the educational objectives, intervention methods, and health outcomes of interest for evaluation to facilitate patient behavioral self-management of the disease or condition.

4. Develop a parallel set of objectives, intervention strategies, and health outcomes of interest for evaluation to facilitate health care provider behavior and the organizational or system changes necessary to facilitate patient behavioral self-management of the disease or condition.

Notes

1. We thank Lawrence W. Green, Andrea C. Gielen, and Marshall Kreuter for the opportunity to contribute to this edition of PRECEDE-PROCEED and for the insightful comments, additions, and edits they contributed to drafts of this chapter. Special thanks to Elana Einstein-Sim for her assistance in manuscript preparation.

   In addition to these seminal research reports that provide the early scientific basis for PRECEDE, bibliographies containing numerous other demonstrations of PRECEDE in the health care and other settings can be found in the most recent edition previous to this volume (Green and Kreuter 2005), as well as earlier editions.

2. Because the literature is so voluminous for the health care setting, we refer the reader to a few of the classic or most representative earlier contributions, including those citations

contained in several seminal meta-analyses of the early literature (e.g., Dolan-Mullen et al. 1994; Mullen and Green 1985; Mullen et al. 1985; 1992; 1997). Evidence of effectiveness of behavioral intervention in health care, moreover, increasingly can be found in several sources of practice-based evidence, including participatory research and practice-based research networks, systematic reviews, and systems science (see Green and Allegrante 2020).

3. See the Centers for Medicare and Medicaid Services *National Health Expenditure Data* at https://www.cms.gov/Research-Statistics-Data-and-Systems/Statistics-Trends-and-Reports/NationalHealthExpendData/index.html. For a discussion of currently projected health care costs and their determinants, see Cuckler et al. (2018) at https://www.healthaffairs.org/doi/abs/10.1377/hlthaff.2017.1655.

4. See the CDC *Chronic Disease Overview* at https://www.cdc.gov/chronicdisease/about/index.htm and, in addition, the WHO *Global Status Report on Noncommunicable Diseases 2014* at http://www.who.int/nmh/publications/ncd-status-report-2014/en/. This documents the international comparative data on the prevalence of chronic conditions globally and shows that, while health systems and capacity differ across the European, Canadian, and Australasian countries, 40 million deaths—70% of all deaths—are attributable to chronic diseases. See the WHO *Noncommunicable Diseases* at http://www.who.int/topics/noncommunicable_diseases/en/.

5. The broad and central role of behavior in the prevention and treatment of disease and improvement of quality of life must be acknowledged. Considerable evidence now demonstrates the importance of behavior in adherence and other aspects of medical treatment in achieving health outcomes. For more expansive discussions, see Fisher (2008); Fisher et al. (2018); Glasgow et al. (2004); Green et al. (2015); McGinnis and Foege (1993); Nigg et al. (2002); and chapter 1 of this volume.

6. The RE-AIM framework conceptualizes and addresses the issues of reach, effectiveness, adoption, implementation, and maintenance in the translation of research in disease prevention and health promotion into action in a broad range of population health settings, including health care. For representative reading, see Gaglio et al. (2013); Glasgow and Estabrooks (2018); Glasgow et al. (1999); and Harden et al. (2019).

7. The Health Belief Model is a historically important social-psychological theoretical framework that conceptualized the role in health-related behavior of perceptions and beliefs, specifically those of symptoms of the disease or condition in question, susceptibility to it, the belief that one can have it and not know it, and potential severity of the disease. There are numerous published examples of the application of the Health Belief Model (see Janz and Becker 1984); however, at least one published meta-analysis of 16 studies of the Health Belief Model with adults showed equivocal predictive validity (see Harrison et al. 1992). For a recent example of how the Health Belief Model has been used to explain patient involvement in patient safety in the health care setting, see Bishop et al. (2015).

8. The Robert Wood Johnson Foundation's concept of "The Culture of Health" has emerged in recognition of health being greatly influenced by complex factors, such as where we live, work, play, and worship, and the strength of our families and communities. See https://www.rwjf.org/en/how-we-work/building-a-culture-of-health.html. The RWJF formulation of "The Culture of Health" builds on the earlier work and original conceptual framework of the WHO Commission on the Social Determinants of Health (see http://www.who.int/social_determinants/thecommission/finalreport/en/), which has also informed the present focus on social determinants in *Healthy People 2030* (see Office of Disease Prevention and Health Promotion n.d.b. and Green and Allegrante 2011). In addition, for work examining patient perceptions and public interest in and satisfaction with physician and nurse initiatives in disease prevention and health promotion, see Hughes (2003); Kottke et al. (1997); and Litaker et al. (2003).

9. The interest by physicians in disease prevention and health promotion has grown over the last three decades. For example, see McGinnis and Hamburg (1988); Mann and Putnam (1989; 1990); Mann et al. (1997); and Moser et al. (1991). For studies applying PRECEDE-PROCEED to the assessment of physician attitudes, barriers, and practices in clinical health promotion, see Battista et al. (1986); Burglehaus et al. (1997); Costanza (1992); Donovan (1991); Downey et al. (1989); Duke et al. (2000); Green (1987); Green et al. (1988); Herbert (1999); Heywood et al. (1996); Hiddink et al. (1995; 1997a; 1997b; 1997c; 1999); Langille et al. (1997); Love et al. (1996); Makrides et al. (1997); Mann and Putnam (1989; 1990); Singer et al. (1991); Solomon et al. (1998); Taylor et al. (1994); Thamer et al. (1998); Walsh and McPhee (1992); and Weinberger et al. (1982).

10. Much of what has been demonstrated concerning physicians, who control or at least influence the professional practices of most other health care providers in clinical settings, applies also to other providers. For applications of PRECEDE-PROCEED in assessing or influencing the health promotion practices of other health providers, see the following: *for nurses* (Berland et al. 1995; Cretain 1989; Han et al. 1996; Laitakari et al. 1997; Macrina et al. 1996; Pormehr and Shojaezadeh 2019; Shamian and Edgar 1987); *for dentists* (Canto et al. 2001; Frazier and Horowitz 1990); *for dietitians* (Miilunpalo et al. 1995; Smith et al. 1998); *for health education specialists* (Candeias 1991; Glanz and Oldenburg 1997); *for pharmacists* (Paluck et al. 2003); *for physical therapists and rehabilitation professionals* (Laitakari and Miilunpalo 1998; Laitakari et al. 1997); *and for other allied health professionals* (Bennett 1977; Goldenhar et al. 2001).

11. For related frameworks for planning and evaluation, see the Center for Community Health and Development at the University of Kansas Community Tool Box (https://ctb .ku.edu/en); Institute of Medicine Community Health Improvement Process (https:// www.nap.edu/read/5298/chapter/6); National Association of County & City Health Officials Assessment Protocol for Excellence in Public Health (http://archived.naccho .org/topics/infrastructure/APEXPH/index.cfm); Planned Approach to Community Health (PATCH) (http://www.lgreen.net/patch.pdf); and other available tool boxes for planning (https://www.cdc.gov/stltpublichealth/cha/assessment.html). Many of these models and frameworks have built upon, expanded, or elaborated on one or more aspects of PRECEDE-PROCEED in various settings.

12. An online searchable bibliography of over 1,200 published applications of PRECEDE-PROCEED, including those for the healthcare setting, is available at http://lgreen.net /bibliog.htm. The reader will find a link to the online abstract and a link to the full text of the article for all open-access publications.

13. Selected reviews contained in the Cochrane Database of Systematic Reviews comprise the evidence base for effective behavioral interventions for several medical conditions that are relevant here. The reader is encouraged to consult the following: *arthritis* (Fransen et al. 2015; Hurley et al. 2018); *asthma* (Peytremann-Bridevaux et al. 2015); *chronic pain* (Eccleston et al. 2017; Geneen et al. 2017); *diabetes* (Boels et al. 2017; Duke et al. 2009; Renders et al. 2000; Vermeire et al. 2005); *hypertension* (Glynn et al. 2010; Schroeder et al. 2004); *infectious conditions* (Lutge et al. 2015; M'Imunya et al. 2012; van der Heijden et al. 2017); and multimorbidity (Smith et al. 2016).

14. For an example of how PRECEDE-PROCEED was applied as a practice model in an effort to guide physicians in more effectively educating and counselling their patients about health issues, and specifically coronary heart disease prevention, see Makrides et al. 1997.

References

Aboumatar, H., Ristaino, P., Davis, R.O., Thompson, C.B,. Maragakis, L., Cosgrove, S., Rosenstein, B., & Perl, T.M. (2012). Infection prevention promotion program based on the PRECEDE Model: Improving hand hygiene behaviors among healthcare personnel. *Infection Control and Hospital Epidemiology, 33*(2), 144–51. https://doi.org/10.1086/663707

Aldiabat, K.M., & Le Navenec, C.-L. (2013). Developing smoking cessation program for older Canadian people: An application of Precede-Proceed Model. *American Journal of Nursing Science, 2*(3), 33–9. https://doi.org/10.11648/j.ajns.20130203.13

Allegrante, J.P. (2018). Advancing the science of behavioral self-management of chronic disease: The arc of a research trajectory. *Health Education and Behavior, 45*(1), 6–13. https://doi.org/10.1177/1090198117749010

Allegrante, J.P., Auld, M.E., & Natarajan, S. (2020). Preventing COVID-19 and its sequela: "There Is No Magic Bullet . . . It's Just Behaviors." *American Journal of Preventive Medicine, 59*(2), 288–292. https://doi.org/10.1016/j.amepre.2020.05.004

Allegrante, J.P., Kovar, P.A., MacKenzie, C.R., Peterson, M.G.E., & Gutin, B. (1993). A walking education program for patients with osteoarthritis of the knee: Theory and intervention strategies. *Health Education Quarterly, 20*(1), 63–81. https://doi.org/10.1177/109019819302000107

Allegrante, J.P., & Marks, R. (2003). Self-efficacy in management of osteoarthritis. *Rheumatic Diseases Clinics of North America, 29*(4), 747–68.

Allegrante, J.P., Wells, M.T., & Peterson, J.C. (2019). Interventions to support behavioral self-management of chronic diseases. *Annual Review of Public Health, 40*, 127–46. https://doi.org/10.1146/annurev-publhealth-040218-044008

Allison, K.R. (1991). Theoretical issues concerning the relationship between perceived control and preventive health behaviour. *Health Education Research, 6*(2), 141–51. https://doi.org/10.1093/her/6.2.141

Arnsberger, P., Fox, P., Ryder, P., Nussey, B., Zhang, X., & Otero-Sabogal, R. (2006). Timely follow-up among multicultural women with abnormal mammograms. *American Journal of Health Behavior, 30*(1), 51–61.

Bailey, W.C., Richards, J.M. Jr., Manzella, B.A., Windsor, R.A., Brooks, C.M., & Soong, S.J. (1987). Promoting self-management in adults with asthma: An overview of the UAB program. *Health Education Quarterly, 14*(3), 345–55. https://doi.org/10.1177/109019818701400308

Bartholomew-Eldridge, L.K., Markham, C.M., Ruiter, R.A.C., Fernández, M.E., Kok, G., Parcel, G.S. (2011). *Planning Health Promotion Programs: An Intervention Mapping Approach* (4th ed.).Wiley.

Bateman, L.B., Schoenberger, Y.M., Hansen, B., Osborne, T.N., Okoro, G.C., Speights, K.M., & Fouad, M.N. (2021). Confronting COVID-19 in under-resourced, African American neighborhoods: a qualitative study examining community member and stakeholders' perceptions. *Ethnicity & Health, 26*(1), 49–67. https://doi.org/10.1080/13557858.2021.1873250

Battista, R.N., Williams, J.I., & MacFarlane, L.A. (1986). Determinants of primary medical practice in adult cancer prevention. *Medical Care, 24*(3), 216–24. https://doi.org/10.1097/00005650-198603000-00004

Becker, M.H. (Ed.) (1978). The Health Belief Model and personal health behavior. *Health Education Monographs, 2*(4), 324–73.

Bennett, B.E. (1977). A model for teaching health education skills to primary care practitioners. *International Journal of Health Promotion and Education, 20*(4), 232–9.

Berland, A., Whyte, N.B., Maxwell, L. (1995). Hospital nurses and health promotion. *Canadian Journal of Nursing Research, 27*(4), 13–31.

Binkley, C.J., & Johnson, K.W. (2013). Application of the PRECEDE-PROCEED planning model in designing an oral health strategy. *Journal of Theory and Practice of Dental Public Health, 1*(3), 1–18.

Bishop, A.C., Baker, G.R., Boyle, T.A., & MacKinnon, N.J. (2015). Using the Health Belief Model to explain patient involvement in patient safety. *Health Expectations, 18*(6), 3019–33. https://doi.org/10.1111/hex.12286

Bodenheimer, T., Lorig, K., Holman, H., & Grumbach, K. (2002). Patient self-management of chronic disease in primary care. *Journal of the American Medical Association, 288*(19), 2469–75. https://doi.org/10.1001/jama.288.19.2469

Boels, A.M., Vos, R.C., Metzendorf, M.-I., & Rutten, G.E.H.M. (2017). Diabetes self-management education and support delivered by mobile health (m-health) interventions for adults with type 2 diabetes mellitus. *Cochrane Database of Systematic Reviews, 11*, CD012869. https://doi.org/10.1002/14651858.CD012869

Brownson, R.C., Fielding, J.E., & Green, L.W. (2017). Building capacity for evidence-based public health: Reconciling the pulls of practice and the push of research. *Annual Review of Public Health, 39*, 27–53. https://doi.org/10.1146/annurev-publhealth-040617-014746

Burglehaus, M.J., Smith, L.A., Sheps, S.B., & Green, L.W. (1997). Physicians and breast-feeding: Beliefs, knowledge, self-efficacy and counseling practices. *Canadian Journal of Public Health, 88*(6), 383–87. https://doi.org/10.1007/BF03403911

Buta, B., Brewer, L., Hamlin, D.L., Palmer, M.W., Bowie, J., & Gielen, A. (2011). An innovative faith-based healthy eating program: From class assignment to real-world application of PRECEDE/PROCEED. *Health Promotion Practice, 12*(6), 867–75. https://doi.org/10.1177/1524839910370424

Candeias, N.M. (1991). Evaluating the quality of health education programmes: Some comments on methods and implementation. *Journal of Hygiene, 10*(2), 40–5.

Canto, M.T., Drury, T.F., & Horowitz, A.M. (2001). Maryland dentists' knowledge of oral cancer risk factors and diagnostic procedures. *Health Promotion Practice, 2*(3), 255–62. https://doi.org/10.1177/152483990100200309

Chiang, L.C., Huang, J.L., Yeh, K.W., & Lu, C.M. (2004). Effects of a self-management asthma educational program in Taiwan based on PRECEDE-PROCEED model for parents with asthmatic children. *Journal of Asthma, 41*(2), 205–15. https://doi.org/10.1081/jas-120026078

Costanza, M.E., Stoddard, A.M., Zapka, J.G., Gaw, V.P., & Barth, R. (1992). Physician compliance with mammography guidelines: Barriers and enhancers. *Journal of the American Board of Family Practice, 5*(2), 143–52.

Cretain, G.K. (1989). Motivational factors in breast self-examination. Implications for nurses. *Cancer Nursing, 12*(4), 250–6.

Cuckler, G.A., Sisko, A.M., Poisal, J.A., Keehan, S.P., Smith, S.D., Madison, A.J., Wolfe, C.J., & Hardesty, J.C. (2018). National health expenditure projections, 2017–26: Despite uncertainty, fundamentals primarily drive spending growth. *Health Affairs, 37*(3), 482–92. https://doi.org/10.1377/hlthaff.2017.1655

Czajkowski, S.M., Powell, L.H., Adler, N., Naar-King, S., Reynolds, K.D., Hunter, C.M., Laraia, B., Olster, D.H., Perna, F.M., Peterson, J.C., Epel, E., Boyington, J.E., & Charlson, M.E. (2015). From ideas to efficacy: The ORBIT model for developing behavioral treatments for chronic diseases. *Health Psychology, 34*(10), 971–82. https://doi.org/10.1037/hea0000161

Daltroy, L.H., & Liang, M.H. (1993). Arthritis education: Opportunities and state of the art. *Health Education Quarterly, 20*(1), 3–16. https://doi.org/10.1177/109019819302000103

Davis, D.A., Thomson, M.A., Oxman, A.D., & Haynes, R.B. (1992). Evidence for the effectiveness of CME: A review of 50 randomized controlled trials. *Journal of the American Medical Association, 268*(9), 1111–7.

Davis, D.A., Thomson, M.A., Oxman, A.D., & Haynes, R.B. (1995). Changing physician performance: A systematic review of the effect of continuing medical education strategies. *Journal of the American Medical Association, 274*(9), 700–5.

Dizaji, M.B., Taghdisi, M.H., Solhi, M., Hoseini, S.M., Shafieyan, Z., Qorbani, M., Mansourian, M., Charkazi, A., & Rezapoor, A. (2014). Effects of education based on PRECEDE model on self-care behaviors and control in patients with type 2 diabetes in 2012. *Journal of Diabetes and Metabolic Disorders, 13*, 72. https://doi.org/10.1186/2251-6581-13-72

Dolan-Mullen, P.D., Ramirez, G., & Groff, J.Y. (1994). A meta-analysis of randomized trials of prenatal smoking cessation interventions. *American Journal of Obstetrics and Gynecology, 171*(5), 1328–34. https://doi.org/10.1016/0002-9378(94)90156-2

Donovan, C.L. (1991). Factors predisposing, enabling and reinforcing routine screening of patients for preventing fetal alcohol syndrome: A survey of New Jersey physicians. *Journal of Drug Education, 21*(1), 35–42. https://doi.org/10.2190/BT5C-3UHU-C9WA-7JE9

Downey, A.M., Cresanta, J.L., & Berenson, G.S. (1989). Cardiovascular health promotion in children: "Heart Smart" and the changing role of physicians. *American Journal of Preventive Medicine, 5*(5), 279–95.

Duke, S.A.S., Colagiuri, S., & Colagiuri, R. (2009). Individual patient education for people with type 2 diabetes mellitus. *Cochrane Database of Systematic Reviews, 1*, CD005268. https://doi.org/10.1002/14651858.CD005268.pub2

Duke, S.S., McGraw, S.A., Avis, N.E., & Sherman, A. (2000). A focus group study of DES daughters: Implications for health care providers. *Psycho-Oncology, 9*(5), 439–44. https://doi.org/10.1002/1099-1611(200009/10)9:5<439::aid-pon470>3.0.co;2-l

Eccleston, C., Fisher, E., Thomas, K.H., Derry, S., Stannard, C., Knaggs, R., & Moore, R.A. (2017). Interventions for the reduction of prescribed opioid use in chronic non-cancer pain. *Cochrane Database of Systematic Reviews, 11*, CD010323. https://doi.org/10.1002/14651858.CD010323.pub3

Fauci, A.S., Lane, H.C., & Redfield, R.R. (2020). Covid-19 – Navigating the Uncharted. *New England Journal of Medicine, 382*(13), 1268–9. https://doi.org/10.1056/NEJMe2002387

Fisher, E.B., Cameron, L.D., Christensen, A.J., Ehlert, U., Guo, Y., Oldenburg, B., & Snoek, F.J. (Eds.) (2018). *Principles and Concepts of Behavioral Medicine: A Global Handbook*. Springer Publishing.

Fisher, E.B., Fitzgibbon, M.L., Glasgow, R.E., Haire-Joshu, D., Hayman, L.L., Kaplan, R.M., Nanney, M.S., & Ockene, J.S. (2011). Behavior matters. *American Journal of Preventive Medicine, 40*(5), e15–e30. https://doi.org/10.1016/j.amepre.2010.12.031

Fisher, E.B. (2008). The Importance of Context in Understanding Behavior and Promoting Health. *Annals of Behavioral Medicine, 35*(1), 3–18. https://doi.org/10.1007/s12160-007-9001-z

Fransen, M., McConnell, S., Harmer, A.R., Van der Esch, M., Simic, M., & Bennell, K.L. (2015). Exercise for osteoarthritis of the knee. *Cochrane Database of Systematic Reviews, 1*, CD004376. https://doi.org/10.1002/14651858.CD004376.pub3

Frazier, P.J., & Horowitz, A.M. (1990). Oral health education and promotion in maternal and child health: A position paper. *Journal of Public Health Dentistry, 50*(special no. 6), 390–5. https://doi.org/10.1111/j.1752-7325.1990.tb02154.x

Gaglio, B., Shoup, J.A., & Glasgow, R.E. (2013). The RE-AIM framework: A systematic review of use over time. *American Journal of Public Health, 103*(6), e38–46. https://doi.org/10.2105/AJPH.2013.301299

Gary, T.L., Batts-Turner, M., Yeh, H.C., Hills-Briggs, F., Bone, L.R., Wang, N.Y., Levine, D.M., Powe, N.R., Saudek, C.D., Hill, M.N., McGuire, M., & Brancati, F.L. (2009). The effects of a nurse case manager and a community health worker team on diabetic control, emergency department visits, and hospitalizations among urban African Americans with type 2 diabetes mellitus, A randomized controlled trial. *Archives of Internal Medicine, 169*(19), 1788–94. https://doi.org/10.1001/archinternmed.2009.338

Gary, T.L., Bone, L.R., Hill, M.N., Levine, D.M., McGuire, M., Saudek, C., & Brancati, F.L. (2003). Randomized controlled trial of the effects of nurse case manager and community health worker interventions on risk factors for diabetes-related complications in urban African Americans. *Preventive Medicine, 37*(1), 23–32. https://doi.org/10.1016/s0091-7435(03)00040-9

Gates, B. (2020). Responding to Covid-19 – A Once-in-a-Century Pandemic? *New England Journal of Medicine, 382*(18), 1677–9. https://doi.org/10.1056/NEJMp2003762

Geneen, L.J., Moore, R.A., Clarke, C., Martin, D., Colvin, L.A., & Smith, B.H. (2017). Physical activity and exercise for chronic pain in adults: An overview of Cochrane reviews. *Cochrane Database of Systematic Reviews, 4*, CD011279. https://doi.org/10.1002/14651858.CD011279.pub2

Glanz, K., & Oldenburg, B. (1997). Relevance of health behavior research to health promotion and health education. In Gochman, D.S. (Ed.), *Handbook of Health Behavior Research IV: Relevance for Professional and Issue for the Future* (pp. 143–61). Plenum Press.

Glanz, K. (1999). Progress in dietary behavior change. *American Journal of Health Promotion, 14*(2), 112–7. https://doi.org/10.4278/0890-1171-14.2.112

Glasgow, & R.E., Estabrooks, P.A. (2018). Pragmatic applications of RE-AIM for health care initiatives in community and clinical settings. *Preventing Chronic Disease, 15*, E02. https://doi.org/10.5888/pcd15.170271

Glasgow, R.E., Green, L.W., Klesges, L.M., Abrams, D.B., Fisher, E.B., Goldstein, M.G., Hayman, L.L., Ockene, J.K., & Orleans, C.T. (2006). External validity: We need to do more. *Annals of Behavioral Medicine, 31*(2), 105–8. https://doi.org/10.1207/s15324796abm3102_1

Glasgow, R.E., Klesges, L.M., Dzewaltowski, D.A., Bull, S.S., & Estabrooks, P. (2004). The future of health behavior change research: What is needed to improve translation of research into health promotion practice? *Annals of Behavioral Medicine, 27*(1), 3–12. https://doi.org/10.1207/s15324796abm2701_2

Glasgow, R.E., Vogt, T.M., & Boles, S.M. (1999). Evaluating the public health impact of health promotion interventions: The RE-AIM framework. *American Journal of Public Health, 89*(9), 1322–7. https://doi.org/10.2105/ajph.89.9.1322

Glynn, L.G., Murphy, A.W., Smith, S.M., Schroeder, K., & Fahey, T. (2010). Interventions used to improve control of blood pressure in patients with hypertension. *Cochrane Database of Systematic Reviews, 3*, CD005182. https://doi.org/10.1002/14651858.CD005182.pub4

Goldenhar, L.M., LaMontagne, A.D., Katz, T., Heaney, C., & Landsbergis, P. (2001). The intervention research process in occupational safety and health: An overview from the National Occupational Research Agenda Intervention Effectiveness Research Team. *Journal of Occupational and Environmental Medicine, 43*(7), 616–22. https://doi.org/10.1097/00043764-200107000-00008

Grady, P.A., & Gough, L.L. (2014). Self-management: A comprehensive approach to management of chronic conditions. *American Journal of Public Health, 104*(8), e25–31. https://doi.org/10.2105/AJPH.2014.302041

Green, L.W. (1977). Evaluation and measurement: Some dilemmas for health education. *American Journal of Public Health, 67*(2), 155–61. https://doi.org/10.2105/ajph.67.2.155

Green, L.W. (1987). How physicians can improve patients' participation and maintenance in self-care. *Western Journal of Medicine, 147*(3), 346–49.

Green, L.W., & Allegrante, J.P. (2011). Healthy People 1980-2020: Raising the ante decennially or just the name from public health education to health promotion to social determinants? *Health Education and Behavior, 38*(6), 558–62. https://doi.org/10.1177/1090198111429153

Green, L.W., & Allegrante, J.P. (2020). Practice-based evidence and the need for more diverse methods and sources in epidemiology, public health and health promotion. *American Journal of Health Promotion, 34*(8), 946–948. https://doi.org/10.1177/0890117120960580b

Green, L.W., Eriksen, M.P., & Schor, E.L. (1988). Preventive practices by physicians: Behavioral determinants and potential interventions. *American Journal of Preventive Medicine, 4*(Suppl. 4), 101–7.

Green, L.W., Glasgow, R.E., Atkins, D., & Stange, K. (2009). Making evidence from research more relevant, useful, and actionable in policy, program planning, and practice: Slips "twixt cup and lip." *American Journal of Preventive Medicine, 37*(6 Suppl. 1), S187–91. https://doi.org/10.1016/j.amepre.2009.08.017

Green, L.W., Hiatt, R.A., & Hoeft, K.S. (2015). Behavioural determinants of health and disease. In Detels, R., Gulliford, M., Karim, Q.A., & Tan, K.C. (Eds.), *Oxford Textbook of Public Health* (6th ed., pp. 218–33). Oxford University Press.

Green, L.W., & Kreuter, M.W. (2005). *Health Program Planning: An Educational and Ecological Approach* (4th ed.). McGraw Hill.

Green, L.W., Levine, D.M., & Deeds, S. (1975). Clinical trials of health education for hypertensive outpatients: Design and baseline data. *Preventive Medicine, 4*(4), 417–25. https://doi.org/10.1016/0091-7435(75)90030-4

Green, L.W., & Ottoson, J.M. (2004). From efficacy to effectiveness to community and back: Evidence-based practice vs. practice-based evidence. In Green, L., Hiss, R., & Glasgow, R. (Eds.), *From Clinical Trials to Community: The Science of Translating Diabetes and Obesity Research* (pp. 15–18). National Institutes of Health.

Gurses, A.P., Marstellar, J.A., Ant Ozok, A., Xiao, Y., Owens, S., & Pronovost, P.J. (2010). Using an interdisciplinary approach to identify factors that affect clinician's compliance with evidence-based guidelines. *Critical Care Medicine, 38*(Suppl. 8), S282–91. https://doi.org/10.1097/CCM.0b013e3181e69e02

Han, Y., Ciofu Baumann, L., & Cimprich, B. (1996). Factors influencing registered nurses teaching breast self-examination to female clients. *Cancer Nursing, 19*(3), 197–203. https://doi.org/10.1097/00002820-199606000-00006

Harden, S.M., Smith, M.L., Ory, M.G., Smith-Ray, R.L., Estabrooks, P.A., & Glasgow, R.E. (2019). RE-AIM in clinical, community, and corporate settings: Perspectives, strategies, and recommendations to enhance public health impact. *Frontiers in Public Health, 6*(71), 1–10. https://doi.org/10.3389/fpubh.2018.00071

Harrison, J.A., Mullen, P.D., & Green, L.W. (1992). A meta-analysis of studies of the Health Belief Model with adults. *Health Education Research, 7*(1), 107–16. https://doi.org/10.1093/her/7.1.107

Herbert, C.P. (1999). Editorial: Should physicians assess lifestyle risk factors routinely? *Canadian Medical Association Journal, 160*(13), 1849–50.

Heywood, A., Firman, D., Sanson-Fisher, R., & Mudge, P. (1996). Correlates of physician counseling associated with obesity and smoking. *Preventive Medicine, 25*(3), 268–76. https://doi.org/10.1006/pmed.1996.0056

Hiddink, G.J., Hautvast, J.G., van Woerkum, C.M., Fieren, C.J., & van't Hof, M.A. (1995). Nutrition guidance by primary-care physicians: Perceived barriers and low involvement. *European Journal of Clinical Nutrition, 49*(11), 842–51.

Hiddink, G.J., Hautvast, J.G., van Woerkum, C.M., Fieren, C.J., & van't Hof, M.A. (1997a). Consumers' expectations about nutrition guidance: The importance of primary care physicians. *American Journal of Clinical Nutrition, 65*(Suppl. 6), 1974S–95S. https://doi.org/10.1093/ajcn/65.6.1974S

Hiddink, G.J., Hautvast, J.G., van Woerkum, C.M., Fieren, C.J., & van't Hof, M.A. (1997b). Information sources and strategies of nutrition Guidance used by primary care physicians. *American Journal of Clinical Nutrition, 65*(Suppl. 6), 1996S–2003S. https://doi.org/10.1093/ajcn/65.6.1996S

Hiddink, G.J., Hautvast, J.G., van Woerkum, C.M., Fieren, C.J., & van't Hof, M.A. (1997c). Driving forces for and barriers to nutrition guidance practices of Dutch primary care physicians. *Journal of Nutrition Education and Behavior, 29*(1), 36–41.

Hiddink, G.J., Hautvast, J.G., van Woerkum, C.M., Fieren, C.J., & van't Hof, M.A. (1999). Cross-sectional and longitudinal analyses of nutrition guidance by primary care physicians. *European Journal of Clinical Nutrition, 53*(Suppl. 2), S35–43. https://doi.org/10.1038/sj.ejcn.1600800

Hill, A.J. (1996). Predictors of regular physical activity in participants of a Canadian health promotion program. *Canadian Journal of Nursing Research, 28*(1), 119–41.

Holman, H., & Lorig, K. (2000). Patients as partners in managing chronic disease. Partnership is a prerequisite for effective and efficient health care. *The BMJ, 320*(7234), 526–7. https://doi.org/10.1136/bmj.320.7234.526

Hughes, S. (2003). The use of non-face-to-face communication to enhance preventive strategies. *Journal of Cardiovascular Nursing, 18*(4), 267–73. https://doi.org/10.1097/00005082-200309000-00005

Hurley, M., Dickson, K., Hallett, R., Grant, R., Haurari, H., Walsh, N., Stanfield, C., & Oliver, S. (2018). Exercise interventions and patient beliefs for people with hip, knee or hip and knee osteoarthritis: A mixed methods review. *Cochrane Database of Systematic Reviews, 4,* CD010842. https://doi.org/10.1002/14651858.CD010842.pub2

Janz, N.K., & Becker, M.H. (1984). The Health Belief Model: A decade later. *Health Education Quarterly, 11*(1), 1–47. https://doi.org/10.1177/109019818401100101

Jenny, J. (1993). A future perspective on patient/health education in Canada. *Journal of Advanced Nursing, 18*(9), 1408–14. https://doi.org/10.1046/j.1365-2648.1993.18091408.x

Khortwong, P., & Kaewkungwal, J. (2013). Thai health education program for improving TB migrant's compliance. *Journal of the Medical Association of Thailand, 96*(3), 365–73.

Kottke, T.E., Solberg, L.I., Brekke, M.L., & Marquez, M. (1997). Will patient satisfaction set the preventive services implementation agenda? *American Journal of Preventive Medicine, 13*(4), 309–16.

Kovar, P.A., Allegrante, J.P., MacKenzie, C.R., Peterson, M.G.E., Gutin, B., & Charlson, M.E. (1992). Supervised fitness walking in patients with osteoarthritis of the knee: A randomized, controlled trial. *Annals of Internal Medicine, 116*(7), 529–34. https://doi.org/10.7326/0003-4819-116-7-529

Kreuter, M.W., & Green, L.W. (1978). Evaluation of school health education: Identifying purpose, keeping perspective. *Journal of School Health, 48*(4), 228–35. https://doi.org/10.1111/j.1746-1561.1978.tb03798.x

Kukafka, R., Johnson, S.B., Linfante, A., & Allegrante, J.P. (2003). Grounding a new information technology implementation framework in behavioral sciences: A systematic analysis of the literature on IT use. *Journal of Biomedical Informatics, 36*(3), 218–27. https://doi.org/10.1016/j.jbi.2003.09.002

Laitakari, J., Miilunpalo, S., & Vuori, I. (1997). The process and methods of health counseling by primary health care personnel in Finland: A national survey. *Patient Education and Counseling, 30*(1), 61–70. https://doi.org/10.1016/s0738-3991(96)00956-1

Laitakari, J., & Miilunpalo, S. (1998). How can physical activity be changed—Basic concepts and general principles in the promotion of health-related physical activity. *Patient Education and Counseling, 33*(Suppl. 1), S47–59. https://doi.org/10.1016/s0738-3991(98)00009-3

Langille, D.B., Mann, K.V., & Gailiunas, P.N. (1997). Primary care physicians' perceptions of adolescent pregnancy and STD prevention practices in a Nova Scotia county. *American Journal of Preventive Medicine, 13*(4), 324–30.

Lebvre, R.C., & Rochlin, L. (1996). Social marketing. In Glanz, K., Lewis, F.M., & Rimer, B.K. (Eds.), *Health Behavior and Health Education Theory, Research and Practice* (2nd ed.). Jossey-Bass.

Levine, D.M., Green, L.W., Deeds, S.G., Chwalow, A.J., Russell, R.P., & Finlay, J. (1979). Health education for hypertensive patients. *Journal of the American Medical Association, 241*(16), 1700–03. https://doi.org/10.1001/jama.1979.03290420026019

Litaker, D., Mion, L., Planavsky, L., Kippes, C., Mehta, N., & Frolkis, J. (2003). Physician-nurse practitioner teams in chronic disease management: The impact on costs, clinical effectiveness, and patients' perception of care. *Journal of Interprofessional Care, 17*(3), 223–37. https://doi.org/10.1080/1356182031000122852

Lorig, K.R., Ritter, P., Stewart, A.L., Sobel, D.S., Brown, B.W., Bandura, A., Gonzalez, V.M., Laurent, D.D., & Holman, H.R. (2001). Chronic disease self-management program: 2-year health status and health care utilization outcomes. *Medical Care, 39*(11), 1217–23. https://doi.org/10.1097/00005650-200111000-00008

Lorig, K.R., Sobel, D.S., Stewart, A.L., Brown, B.W., Bandura, A., Gonzalez, V.M., Laurent, D.D., & Holman, H.R. (1999). Evidence suggesting that a chronic disease self-management program can improve health status while reducing hospitalization: A randomized trial. *Medical Care, 37*(1), 5–14. https://doi.org/10.1097/00005650-199901000-00003

Love, M.B., Davoli, G.W., & Thurman, Q.C. (1996). Normative beliefs of health behavior professionals regarding the psychosocial and environmental factors that influence health behavior change related to smoking cessation, regular exercise, and weight loss. *American Journal of Health Promotion, 10*(5), 371–9. https://doi.org/10.4278/0890-1171-10.5.371

Lucas, P.J., Ingram, J., Redmond, N.M., Cabral, C., Turnbull, S.L., & Hay, A.D. (2017). Development of an intervention to reduce antibiotic use for childhood coughs in UK primary care using critical synthesis of multi-method research. *BMC Medical Research Methodology, 17*(1), 175. https://doi.org/10.1186/s12874-017-0455-9

Lutge, E.E., Wiysonge, C.S., Knight, S.E., Sinclair, D., & Volmink, J. (2015). Incentives and enablers to improve adherence in tuberculosis. *Cochrane Database of Systematic Reviews, 9*, CD007952. https://doi.org/10.1002/14651858.CD007952.pub3

M'Imunya, J.M., Kredo, T., & Volmink, J. (2012). Patient education and counselling for promoting adherence to treatment for tuberculosis. *Cochrane Database of Systematic Reviews, 5*, CD006591. https://doi.org/10.1002/14651858.CD006591.pub2

Macrina, D., Macrina, N., Horvath, C., Gallaspy, J., & Fine, P.R. (1996). An educational intervention to increase use of the Glasgow Coma Scale by emergency department personnel. *International Journal of Trauma Nursing, 2*(1), 7–12. https://doi.org/10.1016/s1075-4210 (96)80038-1

Makrides, L., Veinot, P.L., Richard, J., & Allen, M.J. (1997). Primary care physicians and coronary heart disease prevention: A practice model. *Patient Education and Counseling, 32*(3), 207–17. https://doi.org/10.1016/s0738-3991(97)00031-1

Mann, K.V., Lindsay, E.A., Putnam, R.W., & Davis, D.A. (1997). Increasing physician involvement in cholesterol-lowering practices: The role of knowledge, attitudes and perceptions. *Advances in Health Sciences Education: Theory and Practice, 2*(3), 237–53. https://doi.org/10.1023/A:1009736628545

Mann, K.V., & Putnam, R.W. (1989). Physicians' perceptions of their role in cardiovascular risk reduction. *Preventive Medicine, 18*(1), 45–58. https://doi.org/10.1016/0091-7435(89)90053-4

Mann, K.V., & Putnam, R.W. (1990). Barriers to prevention: Physician perceptions of ideal versus actual practices in reducing cardiovascular risk. *Canadian Family Physician, 36*, 665–70.

Marks, R., Allegrante, J.P., & Lorig, K. (2005a). A review and synthesis of research evidence for self-efficacy-enhancing interventions for reducing chronic disability: Implications for health education practice (Part I). *Health Promotion Practice, 6*(1), 37–43. https://doi .org/10.1177/1524839904266790

Marks, R., Allegrante, J.P., & Lorig, K. (2005b). A review and synthesis of research evidence for self-efficacy-enhancing interventions for reducing chronic disability: Implications for health education practice (Part II). *Health Promotion Practice, 6*(2), 148–56. https:// doi.org/10.1177/1524839904266792

Marks, R., & Allegrante, J.P. (2001). Nonoperative management of osteoarthritis. *Critical Reviews in Physical and Rehabilitation Medicine, 13*(2), 131–58. https://doi.org/10.1615 /CritRevPhysRehabilMed.v13.i2-3.30

Matin, B.K., Jalilian, F., Alavije, M.M., Ashtarian, H., Mahboubi, M., & Afsar, A. (2014). Using the PRECEDE model in understanding determinants of quality of life among Iranian male addicts. *Global Journal of Health Science, 6*(6), 19–27. https://doi.org/10.5539/gjhs .v6n6p19

McGinnis, J.M., & Foege, W.H. (1993). Actual causes of death in the United States. *Journal of the American Medical Association, 270*(18), 2207–12.

McGinnis, J.M., & Hamburg, M.A. (1988). Opportunities for health promotion and disease prevention in the clinical setting. *Western Journal of Medicine, 149*(4), 468–74.

McGinnis, J.M. (1993). The role of patient education in achieving national health objectives. *Patient Education and Counseling, 21*(1–2), 1–3. https://doi.org/10.1016/0738-3991 (93)90054-Z

Miilunpalo, S., Laitakari, J., & Vuolo, I. (1995). Strengths and weaknesses in health counseling in Finnish primary health care. *Patient Education and Counseling, 25*(3), 317–28. https://doi.org/10.1016/0738-3991(95)00804-9

Mo, P.K., & Mak, W.W. (2008). Application of the PRECEDE model to understanding mental health promoting behaviors in Hong Kong. *Health Education Quarterly, 35*(4), 574–87. https://doi.org/10.1177/1090198108317409

Morisky, D.E., Levine, D.M., Green, L.W., Shapiro, S., Russell, R.P., & Smith, C.R. (1978). Five-year blood-pressure control and mortality following health education for hypertensive patients. *American Journal of Public Health, 73*(2), 153–62. https://doi.org/10.2105/ajph.73.2.153

Morisky, D.E., Malotte, C.K., Choi, P., Davidson, P., Rigler, S., Sugland, B., & Langer, M. (1990). A patient education program to improve adherence rates with antituberculosis drug regimens. *Health Education Quarterly, 17*(3), 253–66. https://doi.org/10.1177/109019819001700303

Moser, R., McCance, K.L., & Smith, K.R. (1991). Results of a national survey of physicians' knowledge and application of prevention capabilities. *American Journal of Preventive Medicine, 7*(6), 384–90.

Mullen, P.D., Green, L.W., & Persinger, G. (1985). Clinical trials of patient education for chronic conditions: A comparative meta-analysis of intervention types. *Preventive Medicine, 14*(6), 753–81. https://doi.org/10.1016/0091-7435(85)90070-2

Mullen, P.D., & Green, L.W. (1985). Meta-analysis points way toward more effective medication teaching. *Promoting Health, 6*(6), 6–8.

Mullen, P.D., Mains, D.A., & Velez, R. (1992). A meta-analysis of controlled trials of cardiac patient education. *Patient Education and Counseling, 19*(2), 143–62. https://doi.org/10.1016/0738-3991(92)90194-n

Mullen, P.D., Simons-Morton, D.G., Ramírez, G., Frankowski, R.F., Green, L.W., & Mains, D.A. (1997). A meta-analysis of trials evaluating patient education and counseling for three groups of preventive health behaviors. *Patient Education and Counseling, 32*(3), 157–73. https://doi.org/10.1016/s0738-3991(97)00037-2

Nadrian, H., Morowatisharifabad, M.A., & Bahmanpour, K. (2011). Development of a rheumatoid arthritis education program using the PRECEDE-PROCEED Model. *Health Promotion Perspectives, 1*(2), 118–29. https://doi.org/10.5681/hpp.2011.013

Nigg, C.R., Allegrante, J.P., & Ory, M. (2002). Theory-comparison and multiple-behavior research: Common themes advancing health behavior research. *Health Education Research, 17*(5), 670–9. https://doi.org/10.1093/her/17.5.670

Office of Disease Prevention and Health Promotion. (n.d.a.). Health care. *Healthy People 2030*. US Department of Health and Human Services. https://health.gov/healthypeople/objectives-and-data/browse-objectives/health-care

Office of Disease Prevention and Health Promotion. (n.d.b.). Social determinants of health. *Healthy People 2030*. US Department of Health and Human Services. https://health.gov/healthypeople/objectives-and-data/social-determinants-health

Oxman, A.D., Thomson, M.A., Davis, D.A., & Haynes, R.B. (1995). No magic bullets: A systematic review of 102 trials of interventions to improve professional practice. *Canadian Medical Association Journal, 153*(10), 1423–31.

Paluck, E.C., Green, L.W., Frankish, C.J., Fielding, D.W., & Haverkamp, B. (2003). Assessment of communication barriers in community pharmacies. *Evaluation and the Health Professions, 26*(4), 380–403. https://doi.org/10.1177/0163278703258104

Pellmar, T.C., Brandt, E.N. Jr., & Baird, M.A. (2002). Health and behavior: The interplay of biological, behavioral, and social influences: Summary of an Institute of Medicine report. *American Journal of Health Promotion, 16*(4), 206–19. https://doi.org/10.4278/0890-1171-16.4.206

Peterson, J.C., Czajkowski, S., Charlson, M.E., Link, A.R., Wells, M.T., Issen, A.M., Mancuso,

C.A., Allegrante, J.P., Boutin-Foster, C., Ogedegbe, G., & Jobe, J.B. (2013). Translating basic behavioral and social science research to clinical application: The EVOLVE mixed methods approach. *Journal of Consulting and Clinical Psychology, 81*(2), 217–30. https://doi.org/10.1037/a0029909

Peterson, J.C., Link, A.R., Jobe, J.B., Winston, G.J., Klimasiewfksi, E., & Allegrante, J.P. (2014). Developing self-management education in coronary artery disease. *Heart and Lung, 43*(2), 133–9. https://doi.org/10.1016/j.hrtlng.2013.11.006

Peytremann-Bridevaux, I., Arditi, C., Gex, G., Bridevaux, P.O., & Burnand, B. (2015). Chronic disease management programmes for adults with asthma. *Cochrane Database of Systematic Reviews, 5*, CD007988. https://doi.org/10.1002/14651858.CD007988.pub2

Phillips, J.L., Rolley, J.X., & Davidson, P.M. (2012). Developing targeted health service interventions using the PRECEDE-PROCEED model: Two Australian case studies. *Nursing Research and Practice, 2012*, 279431. https://doi.org/10.1155/2012/279431

Pormehr, A., & Shojaezadeh, D. (2019). The effects of educational intervention for anxiety reduction on nursing staffs based on PRECEDE-PROCEED Model. *Health Education and Health Promotion, 7*(3), 119–123. http://journals.modares.ac.ir/article-5-31840-en.html

Renders, C.M., Valk, G.D., Griffin, S.J., Wagner, E., van Eijk, J.T, & Assendelft, W.J.J. (2000). Interventions to improve the management of diabetes mellitus in primary care, outpatient and community settings. *Cochrane Database of Systematic Reviews, 4*, CD001481. https://doi.org/10.1002/14651858.CD001481

Rosenstock, I.M. (1974). Historical origins of the Health Belief Model. *Health Education Monographs 2*(4), 328–35. https://doi.org/10.1177/109019817400200403

Salisbury, C., Thomas, C., O'Cathain, A., Rogers, A., Pope, C., Yardley, L., Hollinghurst, S., Fahey, T., Lewis, G., Large, S., Edwards, L., Rowsell, A., Segar, J., Brownsell, S., & Montgomery, A.A. (2015). TElehealth in CHronic disease: Mixed-methods study to develop the TECH conceptual model for intervention design and evaluation. *BMJ Open, 5*(2), e006448. https://doi.org/10.1136/bmjopen-2014-006448

Schofield, P., Carey, M., Bonevski, B., & Sanson-Fisher, R. (2006). Barriers to the provision of evidence-based psychosocial care in oncology. *Psycho-Oncology, 15*(10), 863–72. https://doi.org/10.1002/pon.1017

Schroeder, K., Fahey, T., & Ebrahim, S. (2004). Interventions for improving adherence to treatment in patients with high blood pressure in ambulatory settings. *Cochrane Database of Systematic Reviews, 3*, CD004804. https://doi.org/10.1002/14651858.CD004804

Schroeder, S.A. (2007). We can do better—Improving the health of the American people. *New England Journal of Medicine, 357*(12), 1221–28. https://doi.org/10.1056/NEJMsa073350

Sezgin, D., & Esin, M.N. (2018). Effects of a PRECEDE-PROCEED model based ergonomic risk management programme to reduce musculoskeletal symptoms of ICU nurses. *Intensive and Critical Care Nursing, 47*, 89–97. https://doi.org/10.1016/j.iccn.2018.02.007

Shamian, J., & Edgar, L. (1987). Nurses as agents for change in teaching breast self-examination. *Public Health Nursing, 4*(1), 29–34. https://doi.org/10.1111/j.1525-1446.1987.tb00508.x

Singer, J., Lindsay, E.A., & Wilson, D.M. (1991). Promoting physical activity in primary care: Overcoming the barriers. *Canadian Family Physician, 37*, 2167–73.

Smith, P.H., Danis, M., & Helmick, L. (1998). Changing the health care response to battered women: A health education approach. *Family and Community Health, 20*(4), 1–18.

Smith, S.M., Wallace, E., O'Dowd, T., & Fortin, M. (2016). Interventions for improving outcomes in patients with multimorbidity in primary care and community settings. *Cochrane Database of Systematic Reviews, 3*, CD006560. https://doi.org/10.1002/14651858.CD006560.pub3

Sokol, R., & Fisher, E. (2016). Peer support for the hardly reached: A systematic review. *American Journal of Public Health, 106*(7), e1–8. https://doi.org/10.2105/AJPH.2016.303180

Solomon, D.H., Hashimoto, H., Daltroy, L., & Liang, M.H. (1998). Techniques to improve physicians' use of diagnostic tests. *Journal of the American Medical Association, 280*(23), 2020–7. https://doi.org/10.1001/jama.280.23.2020

Sullivan, T., Allegrante, J.P., Peterson, M.G., Kovar, P.A., & MacKenzie, C.R. (1998). One-year followup of patients with osteoarthritis of the knee who participated in a program of supervised fitness walking and supportive patient education. *Arthritis Care and Research, 11*(4), 228–33. https://doi.org/10.1002/art.1790110403

Tamblyn, R., & Battista, R. (1993). Changing clinical practice: Which interventions work? *Journal of Continuing Education in the Health Professions, 13*(4), 273–88. https://doi.org/10.1002/chp.4750130403

Taylor, V.M., Taplin, S.H., Urban, N., Mahloch, J., & Majer, K.A. (1994). Medical community involvement in a breast cancer screening promotional project. *Public Health Reports, 109*(4), 491–9.

Thamer, M., Ray, N.F., Henderson, S.C., Rinehart, C.S., Sherman, C.R., & Ferguson, J.H. (1998). Influence of the NIH Consensus Conference on Heliobacter pylori on physician prescribing among a Medicaid population. *Medical Care, 36*(5), 646–60. https://doi.org/10.1097/00005650-199805000-00005

van der Heijden, I., Abrahams, N., & Sinclair, D. (2017). Psychosocial group interventions to improve psychological well-being in adults living with HIV. *Cochrane Database of Systematic Reviews, 3*, CD010806. https://doi.org/10.1002/14651858.CD010806.pub2

Vermeire, E.I.J.J., Wens, J., Van Royen, P., Biot, Y., Hearnshaw, H., & Lindenmeyer, A. (2005). Interventions for improving adherence to treatment recommendations in people with type 2 diabetes mellitus. *Cochrane Database of Systematic Reviews, 2*, CD003638. https://doi.org/10.1002/14651858.CD003638.pub2

Walsh, J.M., & McPhee, S.J. (1992). A systems model of clinical preventive care, An analysis of factors influencing patient and physician. *Health Education Quarterly, 19*(2), 157–75. https://doi.org/10.1177/109019819201900202

Weinberger, M., Mazzuca, S.A., Cohen, S.J., & McDonald, C.J. (1982). Physicians' ratings of information sources about their preventive medicine decisions. *Preventive Medicine, 11*(6), 717–23. https://doi.org/10.1016/0091-7435(82)90034-2

Williams, J.M., Chinnis, A.C., & Gutman, D. (2000). Health promotion practices of emergency physicians. *American Journal of Emergency Medicine, 18*(1), 17–21. https://doi.org/10.1016/s0735-6757(00)90041-x

Wright, A., McGorry, P.D., Harris, M.G., Jorm, A.F., & Pennell, K. (2006). Development and evaluation of a youth mental health community awareness campaign–The Compass Strategy. *BMC Public Health, 6*, 215. https://doi.org/10.1186/1471-2458-6-215

Yeo, Y., Berzins, S., & Addington, D. (2006). Development of an early psychosis public education program using the PRECEDE PROCEED model. *Health Education Research, 22*(5), 639–47. https://doi.org/10.1093/her/cyl126

Zimmerman, R.K., Nowalk, M.P., Bardella, I.J., Fine, M.J., Janosky, J.E., Santibanez, T.A., Wilson, S.A., & Raymund, M. (2004). Physician and practice factors related to influenza vaccination among the elderly. *American Journal of Preventive Medicine, 26*(1), 1–10. https://doi.org/10.1016/j.amepre.2003.09.020

CHAPTER 14

Applications in Communication Technology

·

Robert S. Gold

Learning Objectives

After completing the chapter, the reader will be able to:

- Identify the contexts within which technology can play a role in applications of PRECEDE-PROCEED.
- Discuss how principles of user-centered design, co-design, and participatory design align with hallmarks of the PRECEDE-PROCEED model.
- Describe how PRECEDE-PROCEED elements have been used to develop a classification scheme to analyze health-related apps.

INTRODUCTION

In the decade between the fourth edition (Green and Kreuter 2005) and the publication of this book, the published applications of its framework have continued to grow. The record shows that the PRECEDE-PROCEED model is both robust and extensible to a wide variety of issues. More than 1,400 such applications in research and practice have been published, but with increasing use of health communications and **wearable technologies** in that time. In this chapter, we examine how PRECEDE-PROCEED has been used:

- To assist with applications of the PRECEDE-PROCEED model using current and emerging technologies that can assist in the comprehensive application of the model in any of its intended uses, not only by professional program planners, implementers, and evaluators, but by others designing more efficient and accessible communications to predispose, enable, and reinforce health-related behaviors.

- To develop technology-based/technology-related interventions or applications, including apps, websites, and social media interventions. As a planning-to-evaluation model, PRECEDE-PROCEED has been used to structure the full cycle of such development, from design through to development, implementation, and evaluation of interventions using smartphone apps, websites, other activity-monitoring devices, and various social media interventions.
- To assess the appropriateness of an intervention or examine gaps in the current pool of existing applications, taking a look at how the model has been used or can be used to evaluate technology-based interventions, even when the model was not used to develop those interventions.

The model allows emerging technologies for intervention design and delivery to be incorporated into various combinations of the planning, implementation, and evaluation aspects of health promotion. At the same time, emerging technologies provide new and effective ways to learn and to apply the model, along with its component assessments or phases of application, more efficiently.

Designing community or organization-wide interventions requires attention to several specific complexities:

- The array of social and health problems and issues, each with its own multiple and interacting determinants.
- The heterogeneous nature of human populations, each segment of the population with its unique culture, tradition, politics, demographic composition, and socioeconomic conditions.
- The increasingly sophisticated and demanding target audiences for assessments and interventions.
- The need to reconcile and integrate scientific evidence from afar with idiosyncratic data and preferences from the local situation.
- The number of skills and areas of expertise necessary to plan and implement interventions effectively and to evaluate their myriad outcomes.

Encompassing the entirety of the model for its most comprehensive and effective application requires participatory, collaborative, multidisciplinary efforts. Few individuals alone have the breadth of skills that can span the variety of assessments it calls for. In our work, as we discovered each new complexity, we began looking for ways that new information technologies could help us cope with them. Technology offers new ways to process large volumes of discursive information, to collaborate, and to receive technical assistance for complete implementation of the processes embodied in PRECEDE-PROCEED. Further, those involved in the design, development/adaptation, deployment, and evaluation of communications technologies such as computer-assisted instruction (CAI) can use the PRECEDE-PROCEED model as a framework. Accordingly, this chapter is divided into four sections:

- The contexts within which technology can play a role in applications of PRECEDE-PROCEED.

- Two case studies on the use of PRECEDE-PROCEED to develop technology-based/technology-related interventions.

- Two case studies on the use of PRECEDE-PROCEED to create a taxonomy used to classify mHealth applications.

- A case study illustrating how a PRECEDE-PROCEED study was facilitated by the use of technology during COVID-19 social distancing research restrictions and showed how access to technology, and how effective its use was, played roles as social determinants of health in underserved communities.

THE CONTEXTS WITHIN WHICH TECHNOLOGY CAN PLAY A ROLE IN APPLYING PRECEDE-PROCEED

Public health informatics has been defined as the systematic application of information and computer science and technology to public health practice, research, and learning (Yasnoff et al. 2000). More specifically, public health informatics "assures that the right technologies are used to improve timely [and often personalized] delivery of quality data and assists data-driven decision making" (Public Health Informatics Institute 2018). Examples include access to and the application of information on populations and the determinants of their health. It also involves the effective communication, interoperability, synthesis, and guided application of this growing information.

Health-related data have grown at an exponential rate for years, and that rate continues to climb. New technologies and strategies such as the Internet of Things (IoT) will only serve to increase that rate as more and more devices get connected to each other and to physiological, psychological, geographic, and sociometric sources of data. Our capacity to understand and apply data collection and communication innovations of this kind will enhance the effective applications of PRECEDE-PROCEED.

A sample of communication technologies we can now deploy and use is provided in table 14.1. The assets of those technologies can be summarized as follows: (1) mobile first; (2) socially connected, using distributed wearables (e.g., devices, patches, smart clothing, ingestibles, tattoos, etc.) with the ability to communicate (e.g., through Bluetooth or radio waves); (3) understanding the Internet of "health-related" things, such as connected devices, electronic monitors, the proliferation of data, appliances such as refrigerators, and electronic health records (EHRs)/personal health records (PHRs); (4) able to use the massive amounts of data with different structures that can be linked or unlinked (newly available big data tools); and (5) ubiquitous 24-7 access through broadband and the cloud. We can access existing data, collect real-time data, connect them together along with the data from smart city monitors (e.g., monitoring air quality, noise levels, traffic, you name it) and all your interconnected personal and health data, and have the big data analytics to be able to use these data in meaningful, productive, and healthful ways. This is surely a "nirvana" for public health practitioners, policy makers, planners, epidemiologists, evaluators, researchers, and their populations of interest.

TABLE 14.1. Select new technologies since 2005, in chronological order

Facebook	February 2004
HIPAA Security Rule enforced	2009
Google Maps	2005
Usability concerns for end users	2005
Web 2.0	2005; asynchronous JavaScript and XML made it possible
YouTube	First video, "Me at the zoo," published April 23, 2005
Hadoop	Open-source big data solution, 2006
Twitter	Launched March 2006
Nike+iPod	Activity tracker announced May 23, 2006
Nintendo's Wii	Launched November 2006
First time in the United States that more text messages were sent in a year than phone calls made	2007
Cloud computing	2007
Open APIs	Facebook, Google 2007
Amazon Kindle	First released November 2007
Netflix	2007
iPhone	Introduced June 29, 2007
iPhone App Store	2008
Software as a Strategy (SaaS)	Unveiled November 2008
Big data computing	December 2008 (Bryant, Katz, and Lazowska 2008)
Business intelligence highly prized	January 2009 (Gartner 2009)
First GPS-based asthma inhaler	Prototyped in 2009 (Ngo 2009)
Crowd-sourced funding	April 28, 2009
Google Maps Navigation	October 28, 2009

TABLE 14.1. (*continued*)

iPad and other tablets	2010
Instagram	Launched 2010
Android software	2010
Snapchat	Launched 2011
Fitbit Flex	First Fitbit released May 2013
Robot agility	2013–2014
Creation of Office of National Health Information Coordinator created, EHR system adoption supported through the American Recovery and Reinvestment Act, and concept of Meaningful Use created	2014
Augmented reality devices	Google Glass debuted 2014
Mobile devices #1 in Internet access	2014
Connecting Health and Care for the Nation: A Shared Nationwide Interoperability Roadmap	2015
3D-printed tracheal repair	January 2015
Apple Smartwatch	First available for purchase April 24, 2015
Drone product delivery	Amazon trial in summer 2016
90% of world's data produced in last two years	2016
Smart tattoos to monitor blood glucose and sun exposure	MIT and Harvard developing in 2017

These technologies can both facilitate a fuller application of PRECEDE-PROCEED to complex problems and guide the further development of intervention technologies. An overview of select new technology developments since the previous edition of this book in 2005 is provided in table 14.1.

Applications and contributions of new technologies remain to be exploited, but since 2010, many more have shown signs of taking root in the everyday working life of health professionals. Here are some examples of how your applications of these technologies help overcome the barriers to good planning and communication.

1. Technology provides new opportunities for the delivery of public health programs and services by reaching out to current target audiences in new ways, both asynchronously (e.g., email, computer-facilitated instruction) and synchronously (e.g., text messaging, chat and discussion rooms, social media), and providing on-demand access to information (e.g., World Wide Web-based information sources).

2. Technology allows for person-to-person, person-to-group, or group-to-group communication over short or vast distances, in many cases eliminating long-distance telephone costs and increasing the rate at which

information can be transferred to a larger number of people. This has been demonstrated most universally with the application of Zoom technology during the shutdown of travel and gatherings during the COVID-19 pandemic.

3. Technology-based applications for real-time assessment, monitoring, and message tailoring enable the ultimate application of individualized attention in the delivery of public health programs.

4. With the increasing speed and memory capacity of computers, growing accessible libraries of knowledge are becoming ever more available to the practitioner or consumer, with ever more complex and efficient search strategies.

TWO CASE REPORTS ON THE USE OF PRECEDE-PROCEED TO DEVELOP TECHNOLOGY-BASED/TECHNOLOGY-RELATED INTERVENTIONS

The terms "user-centered design" (Abujara et al. 2018; Collins et al. 2018), "co-design" (Desmond et al. 2018; Rawson et al. 2018) and "participatory design" (Hobson et al. 2018) have been in the language of technology developers for many years. For those unaware of the terms:

• User-centered design "can enable identification of high-priority information and the communication needs and expectations of [end] users while considering the generalizability and consistency of design within and across portals. Tailored designs based on patient and care partner literacy levels should provide innovative opportunities to advance patient education, such as using computer adaptive technology" (Collins et al. 2018, 208)

• Co-design "is the most appropriate means to realize empowerment and equality in service delivery, in research production and indeed in the consumer/provider partnership" (Desmond et al. 2018, 4).

• In participatory design, those likely to be affected by a new intervention or service have the right to define what that outcome is (or should be) and participatory design helps influence the design by offering end user experience, perspectives, and preferences (De Vito Dabbs et al. 2009).

Figure 14.1, referring to people-centered design (Sanders 2008), illustrates these combined concepts best in a single sentence. Users of the results of this process (whether technology or community-based participatory research) are seen as partners—that is, they are active co-creators (Sanders 2008).

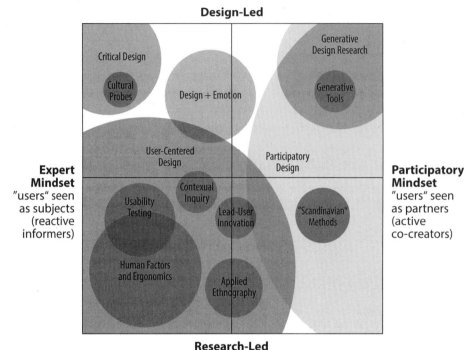

FIGURE 14.1. People-centered innovation overlaid on a map of design research. *Source:* Sanders (2008).

These strategies are *de rigueur* in technology design today because technology development and deployment should be designed in partnership with and for the intended end users. This is critical because, above all else, PRECEDE-PROCEED has been built on participatory engagement from the beginning. When fully applied from Phase 1, end users are involved. Even if a planner begins with constraints and does not begin at Phase 1, participatory engagement is essential at the earliest opportunity. As a result, adding user engagement as defined by participatory design is a natural outgrowth of the model. Let's take a look at how this happens in practice, and the benefits brought by the model's components.

CASE STUDY: DEVELOPMENT AND EVALUATION OF A YOUTH MENTAL HEALTH COMMUNITY AWARENESS CAMPAIGN—THE COMPASS STRATEGY

Wright and colleagues (2006) were concerned about the best strategies to detect mental disorders in adolescents and young adults, so they could be identified earlier to mitigate their long-term consequences (see figure 13.3 in chapter 13 and continue reading here about the technological applications of that study). They showed that until that time, there had been no systematic and effective outreach on mental health literacy specific to these young people that applied the rigorous standards becoming common in population health models considered "best practices." To address this, they set out to use the PRECEDE-PROCEED model to develop, implement, and evaluate a community awareness campaign designed to improve mental health literacy and early help-seeking amongst young people. They used focus groups, service provider consultations, and cross-sectional telephone surveys to gather their input data.

Epidemiological and Social Assessment. Wright and colleagues note specifically that since 55% of the total in-country (Australia) injury and disease burden is accounted for by mental disorders among 15- to 24-year-olds, they did not pursue further problem definition as part of the social assessment.

> " . . . an outstanding issue that usually occurs as part of the social assessment process is engagement of the target population and/or key organizational partners, which is vital to the long-term success and relevance of an intervention. This sub-assessment required the identification of the key stakeholders likely to have an investment in the mental health of young people, the young people and families themselves who have been affected or may be in the future, and those organizations and services which take responsibility for the treatment of these young people." (Wright et al. 2006, 3)

Behavioral Assessment. Based on focus groups and background research, the Australian researchers identified four steps essential to the early identification of high-risk youth: (1) recognition of the problem; (2) seeking help; (3) delivery of appropriate treatment; and, (4) compliance with treatment regimen. The latter two steps were not considered essential in their intervention, though they did partner with appropriate organizations to address them.

Environmental Assessment. Again, through their focus group data, telephone survey data, and previous research, the researchers focused on factors in the social and physical environments linked causally to their priority behavioral targets: social support for help-seeking and social norms of expected behaviors were considered the highest priorities for this project. These would qualify in most adolescent behavioral risk projects as the appropriate focus for intervention on the social environment. In projects with a broad base of civic support, additional attention is often warranted toward social and institutional (e.g., school) policies affecting the formal norms of behavior. (The preceding chapter by Kolbe et al. has further information and reflection on the applications of PRECEDE-PROCEED in school settings).

Predisposing, Reinforcing, and Enabling Factors. Here the high-priority factors were judged to be the provision of information on symptoms and sources of help for mental disorders and the beliefs of severity and risk for this population.

Using this information, multimedia, a website, and a telephone service were developed as the COMPASS Strategy. Final development with attention to implementation factors took three years and involved audience segmentation strategies, the development of key messages, and the identification of appropriate channels for delivery of those messages. As recommended in the PRECEDE-PROCEED model, a thorough evaluation was planned and conducted. The authors concluded that the measured effectiveness of the campaign "may be attributed to the rigor of the P[RECEDE]-P[ROCEED] Model which facilitated fine tuning of the campaign targets through the population assessment process, the use of evidence-based campaign strategies, and the capacity to refine the campaign elements in response to regular reviews of process evaluation findings" (Wright et al. 2006, 11).

It seems safe to conclude that the PRECEDE-PROCEED model provides a meta-participatory design logic model. Within its assessments, it allows for not only the fine-tuning of application of behavioral theory, but also the hands-on strategies attributed to user-centered design principles. We see these same factors play a role in a related study by Ashton and colleagues (2017).

AN EXAMINATION OF THE FEASIBILITY OF PROMOTING A HEALTHFUL LIFESTYLE IN YOUNG ADULT MEN

Ashton and colleagues (2017) note that unhealthful lifestyles in young adult men can be detrimental to their health trajectories into adulthood, but that there is an absence of clear evidence to guide the development of interactive technologies to alter those behaviors and trajectories. With a focus on three health-related areas—mental health, physical activity, and nutrition—they set out to develop HEYMAN (Harnessing eHealth to Enhance Young Men's Mental Health, Activity and Nutrition). Further, they proposed to test the feasibility and efficacy of HEYMAN in a randomized controlled trial.

The authors indicated that " . . . the development of HEYMAN is based on guidance from a community based participatory research model; PRECEDE-PROCEED . . . [which] includes the target audience in developing the intervention to enhance program effectiveness and ensure that their individual needs and interests are accounted for, a strategy which should also improve reach, retention and engagement of young men" (Ashton et al. 2017, 3).

The results of this study indicated that the participatory nature of their approach, guided by PRECEDE-PROCEED, was essential to overcoming some of the limitations of previous efforts to reach out to this population, as seen in box 14.1.

BOX 14.1
Use of PRECEDE-PROCEED by Ashton and colleagues (2017)

PRECEDE-PROCEED Assessments	Conclusions
• To identify the perceived motivators and barriers for a healthy lifestyle. • To identify end-users' preferences for intervention content and delivery mechanisms.	• Increased the appeal of the program. • Enabled successful recruitment and retention of participants. • Impacted perceived satisfaction of end-users because of responsive design.

TWO CASE REPORTS ON THE USE OF PRECEDE-PROCEED TO CREATE A TAXONOMY USED TO CLASSIFY MHEALTH APPLICATIONS

In addition to being a guide for health promotion planning and evaluation, PRECEDE-PROCEED also can be used as a guide to creating taxonomies in qualitative assessments of mHealth and other technology applications (Payne et al. 2016; Wang et al. 2014; West et al. 2012). Such classification efforts serve two main purposes:

1. By classifying health-related apps according to whether they address predisposing factors, enabling factors, reinforcing factors, or all three, we have more information in our efforts to choose an app appropriately specific to our needs.

2. This process also provides a gap analysis to app developers to assess where opportunities may exist for future app development. In the earlier case reports, we've provided illustration of these.

In this section, we cover two such efforts. First, we look at a study that appraised a selection of apps from the iTunes app store according to their potential for influencing behavioral changes specific to topics as outlined in the Health Education Curriculum Analysis Tool (USDHHS 2008) and an earlier version of Green and Kreuter (1991). There have been other, more directed efforts using these schemas such as Wang et al. (2014). We will examine both here.

There's an App for That: Content Analysis of Paid
Health and Fitness Apps

West and colleagues (2012) posited that with the dramatic increase in mobile applications related to health, there should be a mechanism for classifying these apps to improve both end-user selection as well as a driver for ongoing research to assess the efficacy and effectiveness of these apps specific to their intended outcomes. At the time, there were more than 5,000 apps in the US Apple App Store. Based on their inclusion and exclusion criteria, the researchers settled on a sample of 3,336 apps as their final study sample. The study coders applied the Health Education Curriculum Analysis Tool (HECAT) (USDHHS 2008) to divide these apps into categories of health-related behavior they purported to influence and then further coded each app according to the level of anticipated influence to potentially change behavior. To accomplish the latter, they used PRECEDE-PROCEED's predisposing, enabling, and reinforcing factors as follows:

- **Predisposing factors**: those utilities likely to precede behavior and that were cognitive- or affective-based. Predisposing apps were related to knowledge or awareness of conditions or outcomes providing information; beliefs, values, or attitudes; and confidence or motivation.

- **Enabling factors**: those utilities intended to be used, or which occurred, at or around the same time as the desired behavior and whether they facilitated the behavior through teaching a skill, providing a service, or tracking progress/recording behavior.

- **Reinforcing factors**: those utilities providing the rewards received and the feedback the learner received from others following the adoption of a behavior, which may encourage or discourage continuation of the behavior. These included apps that interfaced with a social networking site, provided encouragement from trainers/coaches (avatar-based or actual), or included an evaluation based upon the user's self-monitoring.

Their sample included a wide array of content areas based on HECAT coding: alcohol, tobacco, and other drugs; healthy eating; mental and emotional health; physical activity; violence prevention and safety; personal health and wellness; and sexual and reproductive health. For our purposes, their theoretical classification based on PRECEDE-PROCEED factors is reproduced in table 14.2.

As can be seen in table 14.2, most apps were classified as predisposing or enabling, with fewer than 7% of the coded apps qualifying as reinforcing. Those coded as predisposing were mostly focused on knowledge provision—though the quality of the knowledge was not assessed. Those coded as reinforcing generally had connections to social media that could encourage reinforcing feedback from

TABLE 14.2. Theoretical classification of apps (*n* = 3,336)

PRECEDE-PROCEED factors	*n* (%) of apps
Predisposing	1,776 (53.24)
Knowledge or awareness	713 (40.15)
Informative	1,372 (77.25)
Beliefs, values, attitudes	378 (21.28)
Confidence or motivation	369 (20.78)
Enabling	2,181 (65.38)
Teach a skill	810 (37.16)
Provide a service or sell something	1,065 (48.85)
Track/record behavior	859 (39.40)
Reinforcing	222 (6.65)
Interfacing with social networking sites for encouragement	101 (45.50)
Encouragement, trainer support, coaching	50 (22.52)
Evaluation based upon self-monitoring	92 (41.44)
All Factors	62 (1.86)

Source: West et al. (2012)

peers on the same social media platforms. Fewer than 2% had elements of all three factors as part of the app design.

The authors suggested that despite any convenience afforded by mobile applications, the apps coded here as predisposing "do not extend beyond what may be accomplished through traditional approaches that employ predisposing factors." Those apps coded as enabling were most often coded as such because of their ability to track progress or record actual behavior. In these cases, the authors felt that this may indeed be preferable to traditional pen-and-paper methods. In the dearth of apps coded as reinforcing, the authors suggest this might be a "missed opportunity given the capacity of emerging technologies" (West et al. 2012, 8).

In summary, the existing apps at the time were often knowledge-based but seemingly not advancing what could already be done in other ways; monitoring and tracking seemed to be an asset of health-related apps; and fewer than 2% of the available apps provided reinforcement essential to maintaining positive behaviors or making positive change. Looking back to the two primary reasons for such a classification, West and colleagues (2012) gave us a roadmap to where opportunities may exist for future app development and tell us where weaknesses exist in the then-current pool of available apps. Two years later, Wang and colleagues (2014) extended this line of research.

A Classification Scheme for Analyzing Mobile Apps
Used to Prevent and Manage Disease in Late Life

Following the next step along this line of using PRECEDE-PROCEED as a classifier of health-related technologies, Wang and colleagues (2014) chose not to apply the HECAT as used earlier (2008), but added two new dichotomous dimensions to their taxonomic schema: (1) health care processes classified as either prevention or disease management-oriented; and (2) health conditions classified as focused on either physical or mental health. They chose to extend the predisposing, reinforcing, and enabling framework as used by West (2012), illustrated in table 14.3.

At the time of this study, there were more than 23,000 apps available in the health and fitness category in the now Apple iTunes Store. Two other elements defined the methodology of this follow-up study: (1) the researchers recognized that the US Food and Drug Administration (FDA) released draft guidance for the development of mobile health apps in July 2011,[1] and as a result, they coded the apps reviewed as either prior to this release or after this release to assess the implications of the new guidance on app development; and (2) the researchers focused on older adults with the intent of addressing the needs of growing demands for aging in place.

The real value of this kind of taxonomy or classification system using the PRECEDE-PROCEED model is illustrated best in figure 14.2. This figure is a

TABLE 14.3. PRECEDE-PROCEED classifiers

PRECEDE-PROCEED factors	Features	Core values
Predisposing apps	Provide health information to impact health perceptions, health beliefs, values, or attitudes toward behavior change (e.g., providing information on risks of diabetes, including obesity).	Promoting correct perceptions about the relation between lifestyle behaviors and the development of chronic disease, as well as about the value of self-management in delaying the onset of disease progression and functional loss.
Enabling apps	Teach a skill (e.g., how to monitor blood pressure); provide a service; record/track behaviors (e.g., an app that records blood pressure values).	Providing useful and direct help to enable people to do something.
Reinforcing apps	Interface with online community using a social network site; provide encouragement from trainers/coaches; evaluate users' self-monitoring (e.g., give an evaluation based on blood pressure values).	Strengthening behaviors through interactions, typically positive feedback; emphasis on support through interaction with users.

Source: Wang et al. (2014)

three-dimensional adaptation of Wang and colleagues' proposed schema (Wang et al. 2014). The x-axis represents the health conditions dimension as physical and mental health applications. The y-axis represents the health care processes of prevention and management. The z-axis represents the PRECEDE-PROCEED factors of predisposing, enabling, and reinforcing factors.

Visualizations of data offer an important way to see relationships that may otherwise be less apparent in tabular format. If we can see through visualizations such as this one that certain multidimensional strategies seem to be more or less effective than others, it helps provide clarity and direction. For example, with the three-dimensional nature of this taxonomy, we are able to see visually that app "A" is focused on the prevention of physical ailments using reinforcing factors. The practitioner could use this information in adapting evidence-based practice to their own setting—and could note that adaptation might be most applicable in these dimensions.

Somewhat surprisingly, the researchers found a significant increase in the development of the apps following the FDA attempt to regulate such development. Unlike the West et al. (2012) study, the most common app classification in terms of the PRECEDE-PROCEED factors was enabling strategies. Again, the least likely characteristic among the apps was those providing reinforcement. The authors conclude that this three-dimensional taxonomy allows for the accurate classification of apps along the most relevant dimensions that might be used for app selection, either for individual use or for researchers looking for technologies as adjuncts to a planned intervention.

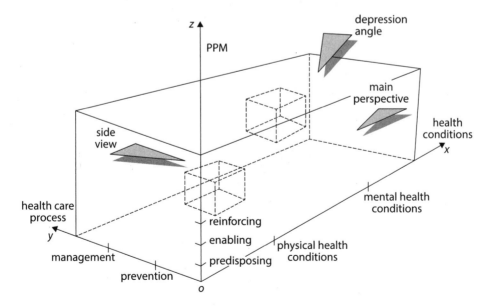

FIGURE 14.2. Schema for App Classification (2014). *Source:* Wang et al. (2014).

A Case Study Regarding COVID-19 and The Use of Technology

A case study illustrating how a PRECEDE-PROCEED study was facilitated by the use of technology during COVID-19 social distancing research restrictions.

Bateman et al. (2021) conducted a study entitled "Confronting COVID-19 in under-resourced, African American neighborhoods: a qualitative study examining community member and stakeholders' perceptions" during a time of COVID-19 research restrictions. The study was intended to examine COVID-19-related barriers to prevention, coping, and testing of African American residents in under-resourced communities in Alabama. As is known, there are serious trust issues in research with African-Americans participating in research dating back to the Tuskegee trials (Brandon et al. 2005). Because of challenges to research posed by COVID-19 restrictions, the authors conducted the study, guided by the PRECEDE-PROCEED model, using Zoom technology to conduct virtual focus groups in five urban and rural Alabama communities. With the permission of participants, the Zoom meetings were audio- and video-recorded, and subsequently transcribed. The authors used the transcripts to conduct thematic analysis based on the model's predisposing, reinforcing, and enabling barriers and facilitators. They further focused on the thematic areas of prevention, coping, and testing. Consistent with COVID-19 guidelines in place at the time for social distancing, it was clear that delivery of health services, schooling, and other needed services was difficult. Moreover, those in low resource communities who had no access or poor access to Internet are often at greater risk.

Among the critical findings (mental health concerns, isolation resulting in decreased access to community ties, church gatherings, education, and health care access), the authors found that technology barriers (e.g., access to the Internet, availability of Internet-capable devices, and the skills and knowledge necessary to effectively utilize these technology opportunities) were significant contributing factors adding to the existing risks. As Benda et al. (2020) stated, living in today's world during times of social distancing, critical access to important social connections, including work, school, church gatherings, and health care providers, relies heavily on technology. Further, access to broadband, closely associated with income, should be considered a social determinant of health (SDOH) because of its mediating influence on access to health care, teleworking capability, and educational opportunities for all ages (Benda et al. 2020). Bateman et al. (2021) conclude that improving access to broadband, ensuring that individuals have Internet-capable devices, and training in using the technology effectively are critical factors that may reduce disparities during the pandemic. Further, limited knowledge on how to access and use the Internet was identified as a predisposing barrier to coping, and access itself emerged as an enabling factor for coping.

In this study, we see another illustration of how the conduct of research using the PRECEDE-PROCEED model was facilitated by today's technologies (e.g., virtual meetings conducted via Zoom). Perhaps more important were the findings that in times of challenge requiring social distancing or other related barriers, knowledge of how to access and use technology, access itself, and training on the effective utilization of available Internet-based technologies are among the critical predisposing, enabling, and reinforcing factors for reducing significant risk to physical, social, and mental health.

SUMMARY

This chapter examines the roles of technology in the application and use of the PRECEDE-PROCEED model. It is very clear that the growth of new technologies and their application to health has been exponential. We illustrated select new technologies that have become available to planners, researchers, and practitioners to enable expanded use of the model. It is also becoming increasingly clear that PRECEDE-PROCEED is being used to develop new applications in a variety of domains, just as it is used for planning, implementing, and evaluating any intervention. Importantly, we also see that the model is being applied in ways that were probably never anticipated at its inception. One example is using its components to evaluate how—and how well—emerging health-related technologies are able to use the foundational principles of health education and health promotion in the PRECEDE-PROCEED framework for public health planning, implementation, and evaluation.

Notes

1. This guidance was updated by the 21st Century Cures Act (H.R.34 12/13/2016) and more clearly defined for current use in FDA Guidances with Digital Health Content (US FDA n.d.).

References

Abujara, F., Alfano, S., Bright, T.J., Kannoth, S., Grant, N., Gueble, M., Peduzzi, P., & Chupp, G. (2018). Building an informed consent tool starting with the patient: The Patient-Centered Virtual Multimedia Interactive Informed Consent (VIC). *AMIA Annual Symposium Proceedings, 2017*, 374–83.

Ashton, L.M., Morgan, P.J., Hutchesson, M.J., Rollo, M.E., & Collins, C.E. (2017). Feasibility and preliminary efficacy of the 'HEYMAN' healthy lifestyle program for young men: a pilot randomised controlled trial. *Nutrition Journal, 16*(1), 2. https://doi.org/10.1186/s12937-017-0227-8

Bateman, L.B., Schoenberger, Y.M., Hansen, B., Osborne, T.N., Okoro, G.C., Speights, K.M., & Fouad, M.N. (2021). Confronting COVID-19 in under-resourced, African American neighborhoods: a qualitative study examining community member and stakeholders' perceptions. *Ethnicity and Health, 26*(1), 49–67. https://doi.org/10.1080/13557858.2021.1873250

Benda, N.C., Veinot, T.C., Sieck, C.J., & Ancker, J.S. (2020). Broadband Internet Access Is a Social Determinant of Health! *Home American Journal of Public Health, 110*(8), 1123–5. https://doi.org/10.2105/AJPH.2020.305784

Brandon, D.T., Isaac, L.A., & LaVeist, T.A. (2005). The legacy of Tuskegee and trust in medical care: is Tuskegee responsible for race differences in mistrust of medical care? *Journal of the National Medical Association, 97*(7), 951–6.

Collins, S., Dykes, P., Bates, D.W., Couture, B., Rozenblum, R., Prey, J., O'Reilly, K., Bourie, P.Q., Dwyer, C., Greysen, R.S., Smith, J., Gropper, M., & Dalal, A.K. (2018). An informatics research agenda to support patient and family empowerment and engagement in care and recovery during and after hospitalization. *Journal of the American Medical Informatics Association (JAMIA), 25*(2), 206–9. https://doi.org/10.1093/jamia/ocx054

De Vito Dabbs, A., Myers, B.A., Mc Curry, K.R., Dunbar-Jacob, J., Hawkins, R.P., Begey, A., & Dew, M.A. (2009). User-centered design and interactive health technologies for patients. *Computers, Informatics, Nursing, 27*(3), 175–83. https://doi.org/10.1097/NCN.0b013e31 819f7c7c

Desmond, D., Layton, N., Bentley, J., Boot, F.H., Borg, J., Dhungana, B.M., Gallagher, P., Gitlow, L., Gowran, R.J., Groce, N., Mavrou, K., Mackeogh, T., McDonald, R., Pettersson, C., & Scherer, M.J. (2018). Assistive technology and people: A position paper from the first global research, innovation and education on assistive technology (GREAT) summit. *Disability and Rehabilitation: Assistive Technology, 13*(5), 437–44. https://doi.org/10.1080 /17483107.2018.1471169

Gartner. (2009). *Gartner EXP worldwide survey of more than 1,500 CIOs shows IT spending to be flat in 2009.* Retrieved June 10, 2018, from https://www.pressebox.com/pressrelease /gartner-deutschland-gmbh/Gartner-EXP-Worldwide-Survey-of-More-than-1-500-CIOs -Shows-IT-Spending-to-Be-Flat-in-2009/boxid/230084

Green, L.W., & Kreuter, M.W. (1991). *Health Promotion Planning: An Educational and Ecological Approach* (3rd ed.). Mayfield Publishing Co.

Green, L.W., & Kreuter, M.W. (2005). *Health Program Planning: An Educational and Ecological Approach* (4th ed.). McGraw-Hill.

Hobson, E.V., Baird, W.O., Partridge, R., Cooper, C.L., Mawson, S., Quinn, A., Shaw, P.J., Walsh, T., Wolstenholme, D., & McDermott, C.J. (2018). The TiM system: developing a novel telehealth service to improve access to specialist care in motor neurone disease using user-centered design. *Amyotrophic Lateral Sclerosis and Frontotemporal Degeneration, 19*(5–6), 351–61. https://doi.org/10.1080/21678421.2018.1440408

H.R.34. (2016). *United States House of Representatives Bill H.R.34—21st Century Cures Act.* Retrieved January 12, 2019, from https://www.congress.gov/bill/114th-congress/house -bill/34/text#toc-H73E766CC72AC4EB8AAF36670EB540164

Ngo, D. (2009, April 29). *First GPS-enabled asthma inhaler prototype.* CNET News. Retrieved June 12, 2018, from https://www.cnet.com/news/first-gps-enabled-asthma-inhaler -prototype/

Payne, H.E., Wilkinson, J., West, J.H., & Bernhardt, J.M. (2016). A content analysis of precede-proceed constructs in stress management mobile apps. *Journal of mHealth, 2*(2), 5. https://doi.org/10.3978/j.issn.2306-9740.2016.02.02

Public Health Informatics Institute. (2018). *Defining Public Health Informatics.* Retrieved February 18, 2020, from https://www.phii.org/defining-public-health-informatics

Rawson, T.M., Moore, L.S.P., Castro-Sanchez, E., Charani, E., Hernandez, B., Alividza, V., Husson, F., Toumazou, C., Ahmad, R., Georgiou, P., & Holmes, A.H. (2018). Development of a patient-centered intervention to improve knowledge and understanding of antibiotic therapy in secondary care. *Antimicrobial Resistance and Infection Control, 7*, 43. https://doi.org/10.1186/s13756-018-0333-1

Sanders, L. (2008). An evolving map of design practice and design research. *ACM Interactions, XV.*6, 1–7. http://www.dubberly.com/wp-content/uploads/2008/11/ddo_article _evolvingmap.pdf

US Department of Health and Human Services (USDHHS). (2008). *Health Education Curriculum Analysis Tool*. Centers for Disease Control and Prevention (CDC).

US Food and Drug Administration (FDA). (n.d.) *Guidance with Digital Health Content*. Retrieved April 20, 2021, from https://www.fda.gov/medical-devices/digital-health-center-excellence/guidances-digital-health-content

Wang, A., An, N., Lu, X., Chen, H., Li, C., & Levkoff, S. (2014). A classification scheme for analyzing mobile apps used to prevent and manage disease in late life. *JMIR mHealth and uHealth, 2*(1), e6. https://doi.org/10.2196/mhealth.2877

West, J.H., Hall, P.C., Hanson, C.L., Barnes, M.D., Giraud-Carrier, C., & Barrett, J. (2012). There's an app for that: content analysis of paid health and fitness apps. *Journal of Medical Internet Research, 14*(3), e72. https://doi.org/10.2196/jmir.1977

Wright, A., McGorry, P.D., Harris, M.G., Jorm, A.F., & Pennell, K. (2006). Development and evaluation of a youth mental health community awareness campaign—The Compass Strategy. *BMC Public Health, 6*, 215. https://doi.org/10.1186/1471-2458-6-215

Yasnoff, W.A., O'Carroll, P.W., Koo, D., Linkins, R.W., & Kilbourne, E.M. (2000). Public health informatics: improving and transforming public health in the information age. *Journal of Public Health Management and Practice, 6*(6), 67–75. https://doi.org/10.1097/00124784-200006060-00010

Frequently Asked Questions about PRECEDE-PROCEED

•

Andrea Carlson Gielen and Vanya C. Jones

We have been teaching PRECEDE-PROCEED as a framework for health behavior change program planning for a combined total of more than thirty years, and we have experience using the model in practice. Common questions and concerns about using the model have emerged for us and for our students. We address those here.

1. Is PRECEDE-PROCEED always used as a linear process?

PRECEDE-PROCEED is an iterative and incremental process. Its structure for systematically developing, implementing, and evaluating public health, social, and behavioral change programs refines and adapts each assessment for a particular set of populations, settings, problems, and resources. For example, during the process of conducting your PRECEDE steps, you may find that supplementary information becomes available (e.g., new data are published, the community receives new resources). Such information may be relevant to a different assessment phase than your current one, but it should be factored into your planning to create a more comprehensive final needs assessment. Similarly, in the PROCEED process, ongoing evaluation may suggest the need for modifications in implementation and measures.

PRECEDE-PROCEED is also both a logical and an intuitive process of reviewing existing data and identifying gaps in information about a health issue. While progressing through the phases, the expert planner is "seeing the whole"—simultaneously working from right to left and thinking from left to right (e.g., "What are the implications of these needs assessment data for the intervention?" and "What have other similar programs done to address this need that my community has identified?")

2. Why are genetics included in the model, as seen in chapter 5?

Increasing evidence shows that relationships between one's environment and one's behavior and genetics influence how a disease manifests and the severity of its outcome. While the relationships and implications for prevention are not fully understood, considering and acknowledging the influence of genetics in program planning can provide practitioners and communities with useful information for targeting their interventions (e.g., identifying and acknowledging populations with genetic predispositions), focusing resources and efforts in a more strategic way (e.g., creating a more tailored approach for behavior change and modification of outcomes), and developing more relevant messages (e.g., communicating what individuals can and cannot control regarding a particular disease).

3. What's the difference between enabling factors and environmental factors, as shown in chapter 5?

Both enabling and environmental factors are those social and physical factors that are external to the individual, plus some internal factors such as new skills and capabilities necessary for a particular behavior change. Both the internal and external enabling factors that influence health or health-related behavior may need to be addressed or modified by your program. Environmental factors describe the *context* in which your assessment and your program take place, and include existing or needed services (e.g., health care), policies (e.g., drunk driving laws), and physical environments (e.g., green space). Enabling factors are those resources and skills that are needed to influence a behavior directly (e.g., offer healthful cooking classes) or indirectly influence a behavior by changing the environment (e.g., adapt licensing policies to reduce the number of alcohol outlets). A comprehensive program will include strategies to address the most important and most changeable environmental and enabling factors for the health problem at hand. It is also important to remember that all behavior occurs within a larger physical and social context, and while your program may not change all facets of the environment, having an understanding of how the environment facilitates or hinders behavior change and promotes or undermines health is important. Assessing the relevant environmental and enabling factors provides opportunities to explore key contextual considerations so you can decide which are most important and most changeable, and thus should be addressed by your program.

4. What's an example of the difference between an enabling factor affecting behavior and an enabling factor affecting an environmental factor, as seen in chapter 6?

Enabling factors are the resources needed in a population or program to address the behavior or environmental factor of interest. For instance, evidence shows that putting children in booster seats before transitioning them to adult seat belts provides lifesaving benefits and that mandatory use laws are effective in increasing their use. If you were building a booster seat promotion program in a jurisdiction that did not require them by law, an important environmental factor you could decide to address would be your state's inadequate child passenger safety law. What will enable you to successfully promote a policy change to make booster seat use mandatory? The resources you would need to promote such a policy change (i.e., resources to conduct an advocacy campaign) would be the enabling factors that address your environmental factor (i.e., the inadequate child passenger safety law). Also, there are enabling skills that relate to a caretaker's ability to put their child in a booster seat—how will your program address the availability and affordability of booster seats for caretakers and their skills in using them? Providing discount coupons or demonstration programs for booster seats would be examples of addressing enabling factors that directly address a behavior.

5. What are some examples of the synergies among predisposing, reinforcing, and enabling factors in their collective impact on behavior, as seen in chapter 6?
The relationships among these factors highlight the importance of the environment (physical and social) on behavior and health. For example, opinions (predisposing factor) are often developed and strengthened through social support (reinforcing factor). The environmental factor or context is the setting in which predisposing and reinforcing factors develop and can facilitate relationships among factors for behavior change. For example, if your program seeks to increase the behavior of eating vegetables at each meal, then you could decide to promote positive beliefs about eating vegetables (predisposing factors) through community meals where friends and peers are eating more vegetables (reinforcing factors), but this would only be effective if there was also a wide array of vegetables available for families to easily purchase in their communities (enabling factors). For another example, consider the uptake of the COVID-19 vaccine when it became widely available a few months after its initial rollout. As it became freely available and accessible in many communities, a major environmental barrier was reduced and enabled anyone over 16 years of age to be vaccinated. Governmental and public health campaigns emphasized the vaccine's effectiveness and safety, which influenced many people's beliefs and opinions about accepting the vaccine (i.e., addressed predisposing factors). High-profile and influential people (e.g., media figures, religious leaders) advertised that they were vaccinated and encouraged others to do so (i.e., addressed reinforcing factors), which in turn further influenced the beliefs and opinions of the public. Additional enabling strategies such as the use of mobile vans came into play to reach communities with special needs (e.g., rural populations, senior centers, and homeless individuals).

6. Why do we start with a social assessment when that rarely happens in practice? What are the benefits of asking those questions, even though you usually know what health problem or what behavior change you will be working on, as suggested in chapter 2?

Conducting a health assessment that builds upon what you already know will often yield additional information that can further refine your program. In conducting your needs assessment, information about health and quality of life will provide valuable knowledge about motivation, including non-health-directed reasons for behavior change, to inform modifications for your program.

Understanding the relationship between health and quality of life is an important consideration for motivating behavior change at the community and individual levels. Individuals are not always motivated by changes in health status (lower blood pressure or reduced cancer risks), but by how successful they are in their life goals (promotions at work or participating in community events). It's easy to understand how being healthy contributes to one's quality of life. Health behavior change programs need to make the link between health and quality of life goals clear, and address it in collaboration with the community.

The social assessment provides an opportunity for experts and program planners to understand how health outcomes are related to life goals in the population being served. Today, the social determinants of health (e.g., education, housing, criminal justice, transportation systems) and equity concerns are being recognized for their importance, and effective health programs must account for and address these quality of life issues now more than ever. The social assessment provides a structured opportunity to do so.

7. Do you always have to measure the health and quality of life impacts of your programs in your evaluations, as seen in chapter 9?

Resources for evaluation are situationally specific and will guide your decisions about what to measure and when. Although you are not required to measure all PROCEED components, the more you are able to include, the more you will understand about how your program changes beliefs, behavior and contributes to improved public health outcomes. All programs can and should document the process evaluation indicators to be able to describe what activities and services were provided and what strategies were used. Process evaluations provide helpful information about the logistics of implementing a health behavior change program and provide program planners with key information about the fidelity of the program implementation. Well-designed programs can have a positive impact on behavior change, but often it requires multiple approaches (e.g., more than one program for several years) to improve public health outcomes, and only rigorous evaluation methods will be able to demonstrate those linkages scientifically. Sometimes the linkages between a health-related behavior and a health outcome (e.g., smoking and lung cancer, seat belt use and motor vehicle crash deaths) have been so well documented that a program evaluation can limit its measures to the behavioral outcomes and infer good estimates of health impact, thereby conserving resources for program services and activities.

8. How much time and money should be spent on needs assessment in each phase of the model? How long does the planning process take? (Chapters 10–14 provide examples of this.)

Needs assessments can be expensive, but they also can be done with few resources. For example, primary data collection is expensive and often a time-consuming process for obtaining needs assessment data. You can reduce costs by starting with a review of secondary data, including examining existing literature and reviewing efforts by previous experts. This approach to your needs assessment will begin to provide direction for program development. The caveat in using only secondary data for your needs assessment is that you need to determine how accurately it reflects the specific population you are working to engage. If you use only national or even state data, you are limiting your knowledge about the differences (or important nuances) that may exist between your population and those larger samples, and as a result potentially reducing the possible impact of your program.

To maximize the potential for your program to succeed, use both primary and secondary data in your needs assessment. Some program planners may feel that if they can't do a representative survey or an in-depth needs assessment with a multitude of their stakeholders, primary data collection is not worth the time and effort. We disagree. It is always better to engage with at least a few key stakeholders during the needs assessment and planning process than to rely exclusively on secondary data. You will undoubtedly gain important insights available only through hands-on engagement with the population you are trying to serve.

In addition, keep in mind that every state in the United States and many nations around the world have both public and private foundations that provide grant support for the development and evaluation of interventions to enhance health, especially among high-risk, underserved populations. Private foundations, in particular, often encourage including both needs assessments and evaluation strategies in community-based programs. Your application of the PRECEDE-PROCEED model gives you an ideal framework with which to propose a well-planned, measurable initiative and increase the likelihood of financial support from such institutions.

There is no timeline for the planning process. It can take as little as a few days to review existing data to years for collecting primary data. The duration is determined by funding, access to information for the planning phase, and your community/agency expectations.

9. How can PRECEDE-PROCEED be used to help identify health disparities and narrow the focus of a health behavior change program, as shown in chapter 4?

PRECEDE-PROCEED provides you with three distinct approaches to identify and address health disparities. First, it provides you with a way to identify the proportion of people affected by the problem within a larger population. For example, one reason for conducting an epidemiological assessment is to understand the scope of the problem, and whether there are disparities for specific populations. Second, the process helps you to determine if and how environmental context explains any differences in the severity of health outcomes or increases in exposure to known health risks. These environmental factors can contribute to exacerbating health disparities, and must be considered in your program planning. These environmental factors also can include historical barriers (including policies or ordinances) that may continue to impact access to programs or services. Lastly, all planning phases, but especially the social assessment (to consider the quality of life and social determinants of health) and the educational and ecological assessments (to understand knowledge, attitudes, beliefs, social and enabling influences), require program planners to consider an approach to health behavior change from the unique perspectives of those who are affected by the problem. By doing so, the planner is better able to tailor the behavior change approach and select effective strategies and interventions that have acknowledged and incorporated to the extent possible all of the most important and changeable determinants of health. Taken together, these three approaches that are at the heart of PRECEDE-PROCEED will result in access to programs that are ethnically and culturally fitting, likely to be maximally effective, and thereby reduce health disparities.

10. What do you do if stakeholders involved in your participatory planning process want to choose something that isn't evidence-based, as seen in chapter 2?

We firmly believe in participatory planning for all the reasons identified in this book. However, this doesn't mean that program planners should ignore their responsibility to provide evidence and facilitate informed decision-making by community partners. This issue can arise in multiple phases in the planning process and is always important to negotiate with respect and with evidence. For example, you may have a group of stakeholders who want to address the problem of pedestrian injury at a preschool by introducing an educational curriculum, whereas the best evidence suggests that children younger than 10 years of age are not developmentally able to learn safe street-crossing skills. By sharing this evidence, the planner should be able to facilitate the development of a more robust, evidence-based strategy to protect the children (e.g., parent education, redesign of the drop-off and pickup process at the preschool).

Compromises that do not result in harm but may not lead to your desired outcome on your timeline should be considered. For instance, what if you recommend a Safe Routes to School (SRTS) walking program as part of a physical activity promotion program for elementary school children in your community, but your stakeholders say it won't work because there is drug paraphernalia on the paths? Addressing this concern first should become a legitimate priority, even though your efforts may be funded by cardiovascular disease prevention dollars, because (1) the SRTS effort would either not be utilized or, if utilized, could result in harms, and (2) partnering with substance abuse prevention and treatment programs to address this concern could bring new partners (and resources) to your issue.

Public Health Competencies by Chapter

•

Darleen V. Peterson

The Council on Education for Public Health (CEPH) sets forth core competencies essential for public health students to meet, endorsed by the Association of Schools and Programs of Public Health (ASPPH). We have gathered these competencies here, in Appendix B. As of 2021, these competencies include 22 foundational competencies for master-level programs; 20 foundational competencies for doctoral programs; and 143 competencies within ten content domain areas covered in the Certified in Public Health (CPH) examination.

To enhance the usefulness of *Health Program Planning, Implementation, and Evaluation* for public health training, we asked our chapter authors to keep these competencies in mind while writing. We also asked them to review their own chapter and to indicate which competencies their chapter addresses. The result of their review is found in the matrix below.

For further information on the CEPH foundational competencies in public health, see https://media.ceph.org/wp_assets/2016.Criteria.pdf.

For further information on the CPH content domain areas and associated competencies, see https://www.nbphe.org/cph-content-outline/.

Specific Competencies	CHAPTER 1	CHAPTER 2	CHAPTER 3	CHAPTER 4	CHAPTER 5	CHAPTER 6	CHAPTER 7	CHAPTER 8	CHAPTER 9	CHAPTER 10	CHAPTER 11	CHAPTER 12	CHAPTER 13	CHAPTER 14
CEPH FOUNDATIONAL COMPETENCIES—MASTER OF PUBLIC HEALTH														
Area 1: Evidence-Based Approaches to Public Health														
A. Apply epidemiological methods to the breadth of settings and situations in public health practice	•			•	•					•		•	•	
B. Select quantitative and qualitative data collection methods appropriate for a given public health context					•	•				•		•		
C. Analyze quantitative and qualitative data using biostatistics, informatics, computer-based programming, and software, as appropriate									•					•
D. Interpret results of data analysis for public health research, policy, or practice	•	•	•	•	•		•			•		•	•	

Specific Competencies	CHAPTER 1	CHAPTER 2	CHAPTER 3	CHAPTER 4	CHAPTER 5	CHAPTER 6	CHAPTER 7	CHAPTER 8	CHAPTER 9	CHAPTER 10	CHAPTER 11	CHAPTER 12	CHAPTER 13	CHAPTER 14
Area 2: Public Health and Health Care Systems														
A. Compare the organization, structure, and function of health care, public health, and regulatory systems across national and international settings													•	
B. Discuss the means by which structural bias, social inequities, and racism undermine health and create challenges to achieving health equity at organizational, community, and societal levels		•											•	
Area 3: Planning and Management to Promote Health														
A. Assess population needs, assets, and capacities that affect communities' health	•	•	•	•	•		•			•	•	•	•	•
B. Apply awareness of cultural values and practices to the design or implementation of public health policies or programs	•	•				•	•			•	•		•	
C. Design a population-based policy, program, project, or intervention	•	•			•	•	•				•	•	•	•
D. Explain basic principles and tools of budget and resource management								•					•	
E. Select methods to evaluate public health programs	•								•		•	•	•	
Area 4: Policy in Public Health														
A. Discuss multiple dimensions of the policy-making process, including the roles of ethics and evidence										•			•	
B. Propose strategies to identify stakeholders and build coalitions and partnerships for influencing public health outcomes	•	•					•			•	•	•	•	
C. Advocate for political, social, or economic policies and programs that will improve health in diverse populations					•		•					•	•	
D. Evaluate policies for their impact on public health and health equity									•		•	•	•	
Area 5: Leadership														
A. Apply principles of leadership, governance, and management, which include creating a vision, empowering others, fostering collaboration, and guiding decision-making		•								•	•	•	•	•
B. Apply negotiation and mediation skills to address organizational or community challenges		•								•				
Area 6: Communication														
A. Select communication strategies for different audiences and sectors		•								•				
B. Communicate audience-appropriate public health content, both in writing and through oral presentation										•				

(continued)

Specific Competencies	CHAPTER 1	CHAPTER 2	CHAPTER 3	CHAPTER 4	CHAPTER 5	CHAPTER 6	CHAPTER 7	CHAPTER 8	CHAPTER 9	CHAPTER 10	CHAPTER 11	CHAPTER 12	CHAPTER 13	CHAPTER 14
C. Describe the importance of cultural competence in communicating public health content		•							•					
Area 7: Interprofessional Practice														
A. Perform effectively on interprofessional teams	•								•			•	•	
Area 8: Systems Thinking														
A. Apply systems thinking tools to a public health issue	•	•	•	•	•	•	•	•		•		•	•	•
CEPH FOUNDATIONAL COMPETENCIES—DOCTOR OF PUBLIC HEALTH														
Area 1: Data and Analysis														
A. Explain qualitative, quantitative, mixed-methods and policy analysis research and evaluation methods to address health issues at multiple (individual, group, organization, community, and population) levels	•					•			•			•		•
B. Design a qualitative, quantitative, mixed-methods policy analysis or evaluation project to address a public health issue									•			•		
C. Explain the use and limitations of surveillance systems and national surveys in assessing, monitoring, and evaluating policies and programs and to address a population's health									•			•		
Area 2: Leadership, Management and Governance														
A. Propose strategies for health improvement and elimination of health inequities by organizing stakeholders, including researchers, practitioners, community leaders, and other partners	•	•	•				•		•	•	•	•	•	•
B. Communicate public health science to diverse stakeholders, including individuals at all levels of health literacy, for purposes of influencing behavior and policies	•	•							•	•		•	•	
C. Integrate knowledge, approaches, methods, values, and potential contributions from multiple professions and systems into addressing public health problems	•	•				•	•		•		•	•	•	
D. Create a strategic plan							•					•	•	
E. Facilitate shared decision-making through negotiation and consensus-building methods		•							•			•	•	
F. Create organizational change strategies							•		•		•	•	•	
G. Propose strategies to promote inclusion and equity within public health programs, policies, and systems		•							•			•	•	
H. Assess one's own strengths and weaknesses in leadership capacities, including cultural proficiency														

Specific Competencies	CHAPTER 1	CHAPTER 2	CHAPTER 3	CHAPTER 4	CHAPTER 5	CHAPTER 6	CHAPTER 7	CHAPTER 8	CHAPTER 9	CHAPTER 10	CHAPTER 11	CHAPTER 12	CHAPTER 13	CHAPTER 14
I. Propose human, fiscal, and other resources to achieve a strategic goal								●				●	●	
J. Cultivate new resources and revenue streams to achieve a strategic goal								●				●	●	
Area 3: Policy and Programs														
A. Design a system-level intervention to address a public health issue	●				●		●				●	●	●	●
B. Integrate knowledge of cultural values and practices into the design of public health policies and programs	●	●	●			●	●			●	●		●	
C. Integrate scientific information, legal and regulatory approaches, ethical frameworks, and varied stakeholder interests into policy development and analysis												●	●	
D. Propose interprofessional team approaches to improving public health	●	●										●		
Area 4: Educational and Workforce Development														
A. Assess an audience's knowledge and learning needs						●	●							
B. Deliver training or educational experiences that promote learning in academic, organizational, or community settings							●							
C. Use best-practice modalities in pedagogical practices						●								
CERTIFIED IN PUBLIC HEALTH SKILL DOMAINS														
Area 1: Evidence-Based Approaches to Public Health														
A. Interpret results of statistical analyses found in public health studies or reports			●	●					●			●		
B. Interpret quantitative or qualitative data following current scientific standards				●	●	●			●			●		
C. Apply common statistical methods for inference				●								●		
D. Apply descriptive techniques commonly used to summarize public data				●	●	●					●	●		
E. Identify the limitations of research results, data sources, or existing practices and programs				●	●	●			●					
F. Use statistical packages or software to analyze data														●
G. Synthesize information from multiple data systems or other sources	●	●	●	●	●	●			●		●	●		●
H. Identify key sources of data for epidemiologic or other public health investigation purposes	●		●	●	●				●			●		●
I. Calculate mortality, morbidity, and health risk factor rates				●	●									

(continued)

Specific Competencies	CHAPTER 1	CHAPTER 2	CHAPTER 3	CHAPTER 4	CHAPTER 5	CHAPTER 6	CHAPTER 7	CHAPTER 8	CHAPTER 9	CHAPTER 10	CHAPTER 11	CHAPTER 12	CHAPTER 13	CHAPTER 14
J. Collect valid and reliable quantitative or qualitative data			•	•	•				•			•		
K. Use information technology for data collection, storage, and retrieval												•		•
L. Illustrate how gender, race, ethnicity, and other evolving demographics affect the health of a population	•	•	•						•			•		
M. Use population health surveillance systems	•		•	•	•							•		•
N. Apply evidence-based theories, concepts, and models from a range of social and behavioral disciplines in the development and evaluation of health programs, policies, and interventions	•	•	•	•	•	•	•		•	•	•	•	•	
Area 2: Communication														
A. Ensure health literacy concepts are applied in communication efforts										•				
B. Identify communication gaps														
C. Propose recommendations for improving communication processes									•					
D. Exercise a variety of communication strategies and methods targeting specific populations and venues to promote policies and programs		•						•		•	•			
E. Communicate effectively and convey information in a manner that is easily understood by diverse audiences (e.g., including persons of limited English proficiency, those who have low literacy skills or are not literate, individuals with disabilities, and those who are deaf or hard of hearing)		•								•	•			
F. Choose communication tools and techniques to facilitate discussions and interactions										•				
G. Assess the health literacy of populations served											•		•	
H. Use risk communication approaches to address public health issues and problems														
I. Set communication goals, objectives, and priorities for a project										•				
J. Inform the public about health policies, programs, and resources										•	•		•	
K. Apply ethical considerations in developing communication plans and promotional initiatives										•				
L. Create and disseminate educational information relating to specific emerging health issues and priorities to promote policy development						•	•	•					•	
M. Communicate the role of public health within the overall health system (e.g., national, state, county, local government) and its impact on the individual	•											•	•	•
N. Communicate with colleagues, patients, families, or communities about health disparities and health care disparities												•	•	•

Specific Competencies	CHAPTER 1	CHAPTER 2	CHAPTER 3	CHAPTER 4	CHAPTER 5	CHAPTER 6	CHAPTER 7	CHAPTER 8	CHAPTER 9	CHAPTER 10	CHAPTER 11	CHAPTER 12	CHAPTER 13	CHAPTER 14
O. Communicate lessons learned to community partners or global constituencies		•							•	•		•	•	
P. Apply facilitation skills in interactions with individuals and groups									•					
Q. Communicate results of population health needs and asset assessments	•	•	•	•	•	•	•				•	•	•	•
R. Communicate with other health professionals in a responsive and responsible manner that supports a team approach to maintaining health of individuals and populations	•	•			•				•		•	•	•	
S. Provide a rationale for program proposals and evaluations to lay, professional, and policy audiences						•	•		•	•	•	•	•	
T. Communicate results of evaluation efforts									•	•		•		
Area 3: Leadership														
A. Utilize critical analysis to prioritize and justify actions and allocation of resources		•				•	•	•			•	•	•	
B. Apply team-building skills								•			•	•		
C. Apply organizational change management concepts and skills								•			•	•	•	
D. Apply conflict management skills								•						
E. Implement strategies to support and improve team performance								•						
F. Apply negotiation skills								•	•					
G. Establish and model standards of performance and accountability								•	•		•	•	•	
H. Guide organizational decision-making and planning based on internal and external assessments	•					•	•	•	•		•	•	•	
I. Prepare professional development plans for self or others		•							•		•	•		
J. Develop strategies to motivate others for collaborative problem-solving, decision-making, and evaluation		•							•		•	•		
K. Develop capacity-building strategies at the individual, organizational, or community level		•			•						•	•		
L. Communicate an organization's mission, goals, values, and shared vision to stakeholders		•									•	•		
M. Create teams for implementing health initiatives		•									•	•		
N. Develop a mission, goals, values, and shared vision for an organization or the community in conjunction with key stakeholders		•							•		•	•		
O. Implement a continuous quality improvement plan								•	•					
P. Develop a continuous quality improvement plan								•	•					
Q. Evaluate organizational performance in relation to strategic and defined goals									•		•	•	•	

(continued)

Specific Competencies	CHAPTER 1	CHAPTER 2	CHAPTER 3	CHAPTER 4	CHAPTER 5	CHAPTER 6	CHAPTER 7	CHAPTER 8	CHAPTER 9	CHAPTER 10	CHAPTER 11	CHAPTER 12	CHAPTER 13	CHAPTER 14
R. Implement organizational strategic planning processes								•				•	•	•
S. Assess organizational policies and procedures regarding working across multiple organizations												•	•	
T. Align organizational policies and procedures with regulatory and statutory requirements												•	•	
U. Maximize efficiency of programs								•		•				
V. Ensure that informatics principles and methods are used in the design and implementation of data systems												•		
Area 4: Law and Ethics														
A. Identify regulations regarding privacy, security, and confidentiality (e.g., personal health information, etc.)												•	•	
B. Design strategies to ensure the implementation of laws and regulations governing the scope of one's legal authority												•	•	
C. Apply basic principles of ethical analysis to issues of public health research, practice, and policy									•	•				
D. Ensure the application of ethical principles in the collection, maintenance, use, and dissemination of data and information				•					•					
E. Manage potential conflicts of interest encountered by practitioners, researchers, and organizations		•							•					
F. Advise on the laws, regulations, policies, and procedures for the ethical conduct of public health research, practice, and policy									•	•				
G. Identify environmental, social justice, and other factors that contribute to health disparities				•			•	•	•					
H. Apply social justice and human rights principles when addressing community needs		•	•					•	•					
Area 5: Public Health Biology and Human Disease														
A. Apply evidence-based biological concepts to inform public health laws, policies, and regulations	•											•	•	
B. Assess how biological agents affect human health	•			•	•									
C. Identify risk factors and modes of transmission for infectious diseases and how these diseases affect both personal and population health	•			•	•	•								
D. Identify risk factors for non-infectious diseases and how these issues affect both personal and population health	•			•	•	•	•					•	•	
Area 6: Collaboration and Partnership														
A. Identify opportunities to partner with health and public health professionals across sectors and related disciplines	•	•				•	•	•		•		•	•	

Specific Competencies	CHAPTER 1	CHAPTER 2	CHAPTER 3	CHAPTER 4	CHAPTER 5	CHAPTER 6	CHAPTER 7	CHAPTER 8	CHAPTER 9	CHAPTER 10	CHAPTER 11	CHAPTER 12	CHAPTER 13	CHAPTER 14
B. Identify key stakeholders	•	•					•	•	•	•	•	•	•	
C. Develop collaborative and partnership agreements with various stakeholders on specific projects	•	•					•	•	•	•		•	•	
D. Establish roles, responsibilities, and action steps of key stakeholders in order to meet project goals and objectives		•					•	•	•	•		•	•	
E. Engage key stakeholders in problem-solving and policy development	•	•					•		•	•	•	•	•	
F. Access the knowledge, skills, and abilities of health professionals to ensure that policies, programs, and resources improve the public's health		•				•	•					•	•	
G. Use knowledge of the role of public health and the roles of other health professions to appropriately address the health needs of individuals and populations	•	•		•	•	•	•					•	•	
H. Manage partnerships with agencies within the national, state, or local levels of government that have authority over public health situations or with specific issues, such as emergency events	•	•		•	•		•	•				•	•	
I. Apply relationship-building values and principles of team dynamics to plan strategies and deliver population health services		•							•		•		•	
J. Develop procedures for managing health partnerships		•												
K. Implement methods of shared accountability and performance measurement with multiple organizations		•							•	•		•	•	
L. Implement strategies for collaboration and partnership among diverse organizations to achieve common public health goals		•						•		•		•	•	
M. Develop strategies for collaboration and partnership among diverse organizations to achieve common public health goals		•						•	•		•	•	•	
N. Identify critical stakeholders for the planning, implementation, and evaluation of health programs, policies, and interventions	•	•	•				•	•	•	•	•	•	•	
O. Engage community partners in actions that promote a healthy environment and healthy behaviors		•	•	•	•	•	•				•		•	•
Area 7: Program Planning and Evaluation														
A. Develop and conduct formative evaluation plans							•	•		•	•	•	•	•
B. Develop and conduct outcome evaluation plans										•	•		•	•
C. Develop process evaluation plans										•	•		•	•
D. Apply qualitative evaluation methods										•			•	•
E. Apply quantitative evaluation methods										•			•	•
F. Evaluate the benefits of qualitative or quantitative methods for use in evaluation							•			•			•	•

(continued)

Specific Competencies	CHAPTER 1	CHAPTER 2	CHAPTER 3	CHAPTER 4	CHAPTER 5	CHAPTER 6	CHAPTER 7	CHAPTER 8	CHAPTER 9	CHAPTER 10	CHAPTER 11	CHAPTER 12	CHAPTER 13	CHAPTER 14
G. Assess evaluation reports in relation to their quality, utility, and impact									•					
H. Assess program performance									•	•		•		•
I. Utilize evaluation results to strengthen and enhance activities and programs									•	•		•	•	
J. Apply evidence-based practices to program planning, implementation, and evaluation	•		•			•	•	•	•	•	•	•	•	
K. Identify challenges to program implementation								•	•	•	•	•	•	
L. Ensure that program implementation occurs as intended								•	•		•	•	•	
M. Plan evidence-based interventions to meet established program goals and objectives	•			•	•	•	•				•	•	•	
N. Implement context-specific health interventions based upon situation analysis and organizational goals	•	•				•	•				•	•		•
O. Design context-specific health interventions based upon situation analysis and organizational goals	•	•			•	•	•			•	•	•	•	
P. Plan and communicate steps and procedures for the planning, implementation, and evaluation of health programs, policies, and interventions	•			•	•	•	•	•	•		•	•		
Q. Design action plans for enhancing community or population-based health					•	•	•	•	•		•	•	•	•
R. Evaluate personnel and material resources		•				•	•							
S. Use available evidence to inform effective teamwork and team-based practices												•	•	
T. Prioritize individual, organizational, or community concerns and resources for health programs	•	•			•	•	•			•		•	•	
U. Design public health interventions that incorporate such factors as gender, race, poverty, history, migration, or culture within public health systems		•	•				•					•	•	
V. Develop a community health plan based on needs and resource assessments		•			•	•	•			•		•	•	
W. Apply evaluation frameworks to measure the performance and impact of health programs, policies, and systems	•								•	•		•	•	
Area 8: Program Management														
A. Develop program or organizational budgets with justification								•	•					
B. Defend a programmatic or organizational budget								•	•					
C. Operate programs within current and forecasted budget constraints								•	•					
D. Respond to changes in financial resources									•					
E. Develop proposals to secure financial support														
F. Participate in the development of contracts or other agreements for the provision of services														

Specific Competencies	CHAPTER 1	CHAPTER 2	CHAPTER 3	CHAPTER 4	CHAPTER 5	CHAPTER 6	CHAPTER 7	CHAPTER 8	CHAPTER 9	CHAPTER 10	CHAPTER 11	CHAPTER 12	CHAPTER 13	CHAPTER 14
G. Ensure implementation of contracts or other agreements for the provision of services								•						
H. Leverage existing resources for program management		•						•						
I. Identify methods for assuring health program sustainability		•						•		•				
J. Give constructive feedback to others about their performance on the team								•						
K. Develop monitoring and evaluation frameworks to assess programs								•	•			•	•	•
L. Implement a community health plan								•				•	•	
M. Implement programs to ensure community health								•		•		•	•	
Area 9: Policy in Public Health														
A. Develop positions on health issues, law, and policy										•		•	•	
B. Establish goals, timelines, funding alternatives, or partnership opportunities for influencing policy initiatives							•	•				•	•	
C. Defend existing health policies, programs, and resources											•	•	•	
D. Educate policy and decision makers to improve health, social justice, and equity								•				•	•	
E. Use scientific evidence, best practices, stakeholder input, or public opinion data to inform policy and program decision-making	•	•	•					•	•		•	•	•	
F. Assess positions of key stakeholders for health policies, programs, and resources	•		•						•			•	•	
G. Promote the adoption of health policies, programs, and resources								•				•	•	
H. Identify the social and economic impact of a health policy, program, or initiative						•			•			•	•	
I. Analyze political, social, and economic policies that affect health systems at the local, national, or global levels						•						•	•	
J. Measure changes in health systems (including input, processes, and output)									•			•	•	
K. Determine the feasibility and expected outcomes of policy options (e.g., health, fiscal, administrative, legal, ethical, social, political)									•			•	•	
L. Analyze policy options when designing programs										•		•		
M. Ensure the consistency of policy integration into organizational plans, procedures, structures, and programs									•			•	•	
N. Implement federal, state, or local regulatory programs and guidelines												•	•	

(continued)

Specific Competencies	CHAPTER 1	CHAPTER 2	CHAPTER 3	CHAPTER 4	CHAPTER 5	CHAPTER 6	CHAPTER 7	CHAPTER 8	CHAPTER 9	CHAPTER 10	CHAPTER 11	CHAPTER 12	CHAPTER 13	CHAPTER 14
Area 10: Health Equity and Social Justice														
A. Apply a social-ecological model to analyze population health issues	●	●	●		●	●	●			●		●	●	
B. Design needs and resource assessments for communities or populations		●	●			●				●		●	●	●
C. Assess how the values and perspectives of diverse individuals, communities, and cultures influence individual and society health behaviors, choices, and practices		●	●		●	●	●		●	●			●	
D. Use culturally appropriate concepts and skills to engage and empower diverse populations		●					●	●	●	●			●	
E. Analyze the availability, acceptability, and accessibility of public health services and activities across diverse populations		●	●					●		●				
F. Address health disparities in the delivery of public health services and activities			●					●	●				●	
G. Conduct culturally appropriate risk and resource assessment, management, and communication with individuals and populations	●	●			●	●		●	●	●			●	
H. Incorporate strategies for interacting and collaborating with persons from diverse backgrounds		●						●	●	●			●	
I. Include representatives of diverse constituencies in partnerships		●						●	●	●			●	
J. Describe the characteristics of a population-based health problem (e.g., magnitude, person, time, and place)	●				●	●	●			●			●	

The Evaluation Standards

A Checklist

Directions: Use the checklist below to help ensure that your evaluation plan will meet the five standards of evaluation.

1. *Utility* — Ensure an evaluation will serve the information needs of intended users.

2. *Feasibility* — Ensure an evaluation will be realistic, prudent, diplomatic, and frugal.

3. *Propriety* — Ensure an evaluation will be conducted legally, ethically, and with due regard for the welfare of those involved in the evaluation, as well as those affected by its results.

4. *Accuracy* — Ensure an evaluation will reveal and convey technically adequate information about the features that determine worth or merit of the program being evaluated.

5. *Accountability* — Ensure the responsible use of resources to produce value.

✓ **Step 1: Engage Stakeholders**

☐ Is it clear *who* will use results of the evaluation? (*Utility*)

☐ Is it clear *how* the results will be used? (*Utility*)

☐ How much time and effort will be devoted to stakeholder engagement? (*Feasibility*) Is it doable? (*Feasibility*)

☐ Have you identified the stakeholders who need to be consulted to conduct an ethical evaluation (e.g., to ensure both the negative and positive aspects of the program are identified)? (*Propriety*)

☐ Do you know broadly you will need to engage stakeholders to paint an accurate picture of the program? (*Accuracy*)

✓ **Step 2: Describe the Program**

☐ Is the logic model either too detailed or not detailed enough for communication with stakeholders? (*Utility*)

☐ Are the program decisions/descriptions clear to those who will plan and implement the evaluation? (*Utility*)

☐ Does the program description include at least some activities and outcomes that are within control of the program? (*Feasibility*)

☐ Is the evaluation complete and fair in assessing all aspects of the program, including its strengths and weaknesses? (*Propriety*)

(continued)

☐ Is the program description comprehensive? (*Propriety*)

☐ Have you documented the context of the program so that likely external influences on the program can be identified? (*Accuracy*)

✓ **Step 3: Focus Evaluation Design**

☐ What is the purpose of the evaluation? (*Utility*)

☐ Who will use the evaluation results, and how will they use them? (*Utility*)

☐ What special needs of any other stakeholders must be addressed? (*Utility*)

☐ What is the program's stage of *development*? (*Feasibility*)

☐ What is the strength of the program "dosage"? (*Feasibility*)

☐ How measurable are the components in the proposed focus? (*Feasibility*)

☐ Will the focus and design adequately detect any unintended consequences? (*Propriety*)

☐ Will the focus and design include examination of the experience of those affected by the program? (*Propriety*)

☐ Is the focus broad enough to detect success or failure of the program? (*Accuracy*)

☐ Is the design the right one to respond to the questions being asked by stakeholders (e.g., attribution)? (*Accuracy*)

✓ **Step 4: Gather Credible Evidence**

☐ Have key stakeholders with access to respondents been consulted? (*Utility*)

☐ Are the methods and sources appropriate to the intended purpose and use of the data? (*Utility*)

☐ Have key stakeholders been consulted on selected methods or sources? (*Utility*)

☐ Are the logistics and protocols realistic given the time and available resources? (*Feasibility*)

☐ Does the evaluation team have the expertise to implement the chosen methods? (*Feasibility*)

☐ Are the methods and sources consistent with respondent characteristics? (*Feasibility*)

☐ Will data collection be unduly disruptive or burdensome? (*Propriety*)

☐ Are there issues of safety or confidentiality that must be addressed? (*Propriety*)

☐ Will respondents answer what they are being asked? (*Accuracy*)

☐ Are enough data being collected to be representative of the population (quantitative) or to answer the evaluation questions (qualitative)? (*Accuracy*)

☐ Are the methods and sources consistent with the nature of the problem, the sensitivity of the issue, and the knowledge level of the respondents? (*Accuracy*)

✓ **Step 5: Justify Conclusions**

☐ Have you carefully described the perspectives, procedures, and rationale used to interpret the findings? (*Utility*)

☐ Have stakeholders considered different approaches for interpreting the findings? (*Utility*)

☐ Is the approach to analysis and interpretation appropriate to the level of expertise and resources available? (*Feasibility*)

☐ Have the standards and values of those less powerful or those most affected by the program been taken into account in determining standards for success? (*Propriety*)

☐ Can you explicitly justify your conclusions? (*Accuracy*)

☐ Are the conclusions fully understandable to stakeholders? (*Accuracy*)

✓ Step 6: Ensure Use and Share Lessons

☐ Do reports clearly describe the program, including its context and the evaluation's purposes, procedures, and findings? (*Utility*)

☐ Have interim findings facilitated their timely use? (*Utility*)

☐ Are findings reported in ways that encourage follow-up by stakeholders? (*Utility*)

☐ Is the format appropriate to your resources and to the time and resources of the audience? (*Feasibility*)

☐ Have you ensured that all evaluation findings are accessible to those affected by the evaluation and others who have the right to receive the results? (*Propriety*)

☐ Have you tried to avoid the distortions that can be caused by personal feelings and other biases? (*Accuracy*)

☐ Do evaluation reports impartially and fairly reflect evaluation findings? (*Accuracy*)

Source: Adapted from US Department of Health and Human Services Centers for Disease Control and Prevention—Office of the Director, Office of Strategy and Innovation. (2011). *Introduction to Program Evaluation for Public Health Programs: A Self-Study Guide.* Centers for Disease Control and Prevention. https://www.cdc.gov/eval/guide/

CDC Evaluation Framework Steps and PRECEDE-PROCEED Phases

Detailed Comparison of Planning and Evaluation Activities

Steps in CDC framework for program evaluation	PRECEDE-PROCEED phases in relation to CDC steps
Step 1: Engage stakeholders. Identify and work with those involved in delivering the program, those served or affected by the program, and the primary users of the evaluation.	**Phase 1: Social Assessment**. Stakeholder engagement initiated to understand needs, priorities, and context. Engagement is sustained through all phases.
Step 2: Describe the program. Describe the program being evaluated, including need, expected effects, activities, resources, stages, context, logic model, and anticipated barriers.	**Phase 2: Epidemiological Assessment**. Health, behavior and environmental needs/priorities identified, outcomes of interest and objectives developed and reflected in model.
	Phase 3: Educational and Ecological Assessment. Priority predisposing, enabling, and reinforcing factors identified, outcomes and measurable objectives developed and reflected in model.
	Phase 4: Health Program and Policy Development. Evidence used to map, match, pool, and patch program activities and resources identified and logic model created.
Step 3: Focus the evaluation design. Assess the issues of greatest concern to stakeholders, using time and resources as efficiently as possible. Consider purpose, users, uses, questions, sample, methods, and agreements.	**Phase 4: Health Program and Policy Development**. Develop evaluation plan and strategies reflecting purpose, intended/uses/users, questions, design, methods, and administrative agreements.
Step 4: Gather credible evidence. Stakeholders need to perceive the evidence gathered as trustworthy and relevant. This can depend on how the questions were posed, the sources of information, the conditions of data collection, the reliability of measurement, the validity of interpretations, and the quality control procedures.	**Phases 5–8**. Implement the evaluation and collect process and outcome data for outcomes according to evaluation plan. Approach to collecting evidence specified in Phase 4 evaluation plan (i.e., type of evidence, amount of evidence needed/sample size, measures, and logistics of implementing the evaluation).
Step 5: Justify conclusions. Link conclusions to the evidence gathered and judge them against agreed-upon values or standards set by the stakeholders.	Apply evaluation plan from Phase 4, linking evidence gathered in Phases 5–7 to evaluation questions and objectives; analyze and synthesize data, interpret results, make judgements, and provide recommendations.
Step 6: Ensure use and share lessons learned. Ensure that stakeholders are aware of the evaluation's procedures and findings, that findings are considered in decisions/actions that affect the program, and that evaluation participants have had a beneficial experience.	Ensure use of the evaluation findings from Phases 5–7 by applying communication strategies in evaluation plan from Phase 4.

Commonly Used Evaluation Designs

This table illustrates the most commonly used designs in program evaluation. The experimental designs include two groups, one of them experimental (where the experimental program is shown by X in the first of the two rows). In both the first and second rows of each design, the R refers to the random assignment of participants and the X indicates the experimental program or intervention. The second row of these designs shows no X because it is a control group. In some situations, a multiple-group interrupted time-series design may be possible by using "naturally occurring" comparison groups or populations for which data are available on the outcome variable. If the program being evaluated includes two or more groups or classes, each working toward the same goals and objectives, you have the opportunity to stagger the introduction of the intervention across the groups.

Experimental designs with control groups

| Pretest-post-test | R | O | X | O | | | | |
| | | | | O | | O | | | |

Pretest-post-test

R O X O
O   O

Post-test only

R   X O
R   O

Time series

R O   O X O O O
R O   O   O O O

Quasi-experimental designs with comparison groups

Pretest and post-test (also used for natural designs)

NR O X O
NR O   O

Time series (also used for natural designs)

NR O O O X O O O
NR O O O   O O O

Nonexperimental design (experimental group only)

Pretest-post-test

O X O

Time series

O O O X O O O

Source: Adapted from Shadish, W.R., Cook, T.D., and Campbell, D.T. (2002). *Experimental and Quasi-Experimental Designs for Generalized Causal Inference* (2nd ed.). Wadsworth Cengage Learning.

R = Randomized; NR = Not randomized; X = Intervention/program; O = Observation

Glossary

This glossary compiles definitions of terms as used throughout the volume. Most terms are highlighted in their first appearance in the text, but not at their appearance in all chapters.

accuracy. That an evaluation or other measure will reveal and convey technically adequate information about the features that determine the worth or merit of the program being evaluated or studied.

action. The conduct of individuals, families, groups, community decision makers and administrators, government or industrial policy makers, health professionals, and others who might influence the health of themselves or others.

adaptations. The alteration of an intervention to make it more suitable for a specific population, culture, or circumstances than for the original research population in which the intervention was experimentally tested.

administrative assessment. An analysis of the policies, resources, and circumstances prevailing in an organizational situation to facilitate or hinder the development of the health promotion program.

advocacy. Working for political, regulatory, or organizational change with or on behalf of a particular interest group or population.

age-adjusted rate. The total rate for a population, adjusted to ignore the age distribution of the specific population by multiplying each of its age-specific rates by the proportion of a standard population (usually national) in that age group, and then adding up the products.

agent. An epidemiological term referring to the organism or object that transmits a disease from the environment to the host.

age-specific rate. The incidence (number of events during a specified period) for an age group, divided by the total number of people in that age group.

allocation. A distribution of resources to specific categories of expenditure or to specific organizations or subpopulations.

analysis of variance. A method for analyzing the differences in the means of two or more groups of cases.

arbitrary standards. Standards set without any rationale.

assessment. An estimation of the relative magnitude, importance, or value of the objects observed. Sometimes used in place of "diagnosis."

attitude. A relatively constant feeling, predisposition, or set of beliefs toward an object, person, or situation.

authorization. A step in the legislative process in which the maximum amount of money to be allocated and the assignment of authority to spend it are decided.

behavior. An action that has a specific frequency, duration, and purpose, whether conscious or unconscious.

behavioral assessment. The delineation of the specific health-related actions that most likely affect, or could affect, a health outcome.

behavioral diagnosis. The identification of factors affecting health that can be attributed to the actions of individuals or groups, rated according to their causal importance and their changeability to set priorities among them and objectives for change in those deemed most important and amenable to change.

behavioral factors. The actions of people associated with and believed to be causal in their relationship to some outcome of interest—in this book, usually health outcomes, but also actions that indirectly affect health through changes in the environment.

behavioral intention. A mental state in which the individual expects to take a specified action at some time in the future.

behavioral objective. A statement of desired outcome that indicates who is to demonstrate how much of what action by when.

belief. A statement or proposition, declared or implied, that is emotionally or intellectually accepted as true by a person or group.

belief in susceptibility. A constellation of perceptions that an individual's health is in jeopardy. One of the three main components of the Health Belief Model.

benefits. Valued health outcomes or improvements in quality of life or social conditions having some known relationship to health promotion or health care interventions.

best practice. Recommendations for an intervention, based on critical reviews of multiple research and evaluation studies that substantiate the efficacy of the intervention in the populations and circumstances in which the studies were done, if not its possible effectiveness in other populations and situations where it might be implemented.

best processes. Proposed as an alternative, or complement, to best practices; emphasizing the diagnosis of needs for change in a specific population, by methods such as PRECEDE or PROCEED, before prescribing and adapting a particular intervention or program tested in other populations.

case study. A focus on a single case or multiple cases of a "bounded system," using detailed inquiry to examine the case(s) over time and with in-depth data collection and analysis.

cash flow. The timing of interventions and budget so as to ensure coverage to the end of the program and for the critical elements within it.

causal theory. The set of testable explanations for the relationship between an independent variable or input and the dependent variable or outcome. See *program theory.*

central location intercept. A survey procedure that seeks interviews with an unsystematic sample of people on the street or in a shopping center to represent the opinions of those likely to be the target of a program.

changeability. Evidence that a factor has evolved based on the results of a previous program, or is assumed that it will evolve on the basis of trends in that factor's prevalence in a population over time.

coalition. A group of organizations or representatives of groups within a community joined to pursue a common objective.

coercive strategies. Preventive methods that bypass the motivation and decisions of people by dictating or precluding choices.

community. A collective of people identified by common values and mutual concern for the development and well-being of their group or geographical area.

community capacity. Pooled assets that include a community's commitment, resources, and skills used to solve problems and strengthen the quality of life for its citizens.

community coalition. An organized group of agencies and individuals working together to share resources and efforts to bring about coordinated actions in the service of a common goal for a population..

community development. A variation on community organization work, usually in developing countries, where the indigenous resources of the community are minimally developed.

community health. The status of, or pursuit of, well-being of a population that shares something (usually local geography) in common.

community organization. The set of procedures and processes by which a population and its institutions mobilize and coordinate resources to solve a mutual problem or to pursue mutual goals.

compliance. Adherence to a prescribed therapeutic or preventive regimen.

compromise standards. What results from negotiation and consensus by multiple stakeholders.

concept mapping. A graphic representation of a concept that depicts the main idea broken down into related subtopics (typically represented as boxes/circles and arrows).

conditions of living. The combination of behavioral and environmental circumstances that make up the lifestyle and health-related social situation of individuals and populations.

confirmable. The extent to which study results can be replicated and attributed to the conditions of the study itself and not the biases of the researchers or their methodology.

construct. Constructs are concepts that represent the building blocks of theories and models. For example, predisposing, enabling, and reinforcing factors are constructs that are operationalized as variables such as health beliefs, attitudes, resources, skills, and rewards.

context analysis. Refers to the systematic assessment and rating of the broad range of environmental factors that may influence the program that is being planned, implemented or evaluated.

convenience sample. A sample in which participants are those most easily reached, typically volunteers.

cost-benefit. A measure of the cost of an intervention relative to the benefits it yields, usually expressed as a ratio of dollars saved or gained for every dollar spent on the program.

cost-effectiveness ratio. A measure of the cost of an intervention relative to its impact, usually expressed in dollars or other currency per unit of effect.

coverage. A ratio (C) of the number of people reached (B) relative to the number in need or eligible (A) for the service or program; also C = B/A can be participants or attendees (B) as a ratio of the target population (A).

credibility. Believability, usually assessed by conducting a study in such a way that results are "believable" by using strong evaluation techniques like random assignment, triangulation, and member checks of trust or the credentials of the producers. The credibility of a qualitative study is judged by the reader/user of study results.

critical element. An element without which the objective(s) cannot be achieved.

critical expectations. How target levels of the objectives can be lowered without jeopardizing the integrity of the program or the expectations of the constituents or sponsors of the program.

critical population groups. Reordering of the people selected as priority target groups to give lower or higher priority to those who are hard to reach or in greater need than those more receptive to the program.

critical timing (cash flow). Target dates are set back to spread the program effort over a longer period—shifting some costs to later periods, or to critical periods when programmatic elements need to be implemented to be most effective. "Cash flow" has two elements: (1) determining what funds are available, and (2) making sure that some are available throughout or at critical periods of the project.

Delphi method. A method of sampling the opinions or preferences of a small number of experts, opinion leaders, or informants, whereby successive questionnaires are sent by mail and the results (rankings or value estimates) are summarized for further refinement on subsequent mailings.

dependable. In qualitative research, dependability refers to the extent to which findings are consistent and could be repeated. In a dependable qualitative study, each step in the study is described in detail such that a different researcher could achieve similar results.

descriptive statistics. Statistics used to describe a population or sample upon which observations were made.

determinants of health. The forces predisposing, enabling, and reinforcing lifestyles and behaviors, or shaping environmental conditions of living, in ways that affect the health of individuals and populations.

diagnosis. Health or behavioral information that designates the "problem" or need; its status, distribution, or frequency in the person or population; and the probable causes or risk factors associated with the problem or need. Sometimes used for "assessment."

Diffusion theory. A theory that offers explanations for why the earlier and later adopters are easier or harder for a program to reach or to effect change in their behavior (modernized by Rogers 1995).

disability. The inability of the human body or mind to perform specific functions, resulting from disease, injury, or birth defects.

dose-response relationship. A term borrowed from clinical trials of drugs; when applied in epidemiology, it refers to a gradient of risk ratios corresponding to degrees of exposure; in health promotion, it refers to the increases in outcome measures associated with proportionate increases in the program resources expended or intervention exposure.

early adopters. People in the population, identified in diffusion theory as those who accept a new idea or practice soon after the innovators (but before the middle majority) and who tend to be opinion leaders for the middle majority.

ecology. Study of the web of relationships among behaviors of individuals and populations and their environments, both social and physical.

ecological assessment. A systematic assessment of the reciprocal determinism of behavior and environment at several levels, where individuals' behaviors influence health or quality of life outcomes and both are influenced by the other.

ecological perspective. A consideration of factors in the physical and social environment and policies that interact with behavior to produce health effects or quality of life outcomes.

economic evaluation . Assesses the costs relative to the consequences of one or more alternative programs or interventions.

economy of scale. The point in the growth of a program or service at which each additional element of service costs less to produce.

educational assessment. (*also* **educational diagnosis**) The delineation of factors that predispose, enable, and reinforce a specific behavior, or through behavior and environmental changes.

educational targets. The cognitions and skills that reside within the individual and groups, and which influence behaviors.

education of the electorate. A process of political change in which those affected by policies are educated so that they will be more likely to vote for candidates or referenda that are in their best interests.

effectiveness. The extent to which the intended effect or benefits that could be achieved under optimal conditions are achieved in practice.

efficacy. The extent to which an intervention can be shown to be beneficial under optimal or experimental conditions.

efficiency. The proportion of people served, reached, or sometimes benefit, which are achieved in practice relative to total costs (e.g., money, resources, time).

Employee Assistance Programs. A confidential, voluntary set of procedures and arrangements to provide information, referral, counseling, and support to workers, and sometimes their family members, to help them deal with personal problems that might interfere with their work.

empowerment education. A process of encouraging a community to take control of its own education, assess its own needs, set its own priorities, develop its own self-help programs, and, if necessary, challenge the power structure to provide resources.

enabling factor. Any characteristic of the environment that facilitates action and any skill or resource required to attain a specific behavior. (Skills are sometimes listed separately as predisposing factors or intermediate outcomes of education if they motivate a person or population to use them.)

environment. The totality of social, biological, and physical circumstances surrounding a defined quality of life, health, or behavioral goal or problem.

environmental diagnosis. A systematic assessment of factors in the social and physical environment that interact with behavior to produce health effects or quality of life outcomes. Also referred to as an **ecological assessment**.

environmental factor. One of the specific elements or components of the social, biological, or physical environment determined during the ecological diagnosis to be causally linked to health or quality of life goals or problems identified in the social or epidemiological diagnosis.

epidemiology. The study of the distribution, incidence, prevalence, and causes of health problems in defined populations, and the application of this study to the control of health problems.

epidemiological assessment. The delineation of the extent, distribution, and interaction among causes of a health problem in defined populations, and the application of this study to the control of health problems.

epidemiological transition. A period in history when the prevailing and prominent diseases and causes of death shifted; most frequently associated with the period in the late first half of the 20th century when chronic diseases began to overtake communicable diseases as the leading causes of death and morbidity.

EPIS (Exploration, Preparation, Implementation, and Sustainment) model. A model from implementation science emphasizing steps in program implementation as a process influenced by multilevel factors over time (Aarons, Hurlburt, and Horwitz 2011).

ethnographic study. Research on the description and interpretation of a cultural group, social group, or system.

etiology. The origins or causes of a disease or condition under study; the first steps in the natural history of a disease.

evaluand. The focus of an evaluation—a program, policy, intervention, product, process, component, or whole system (but not a person).

evaluation. The systematic comparison of an object of interest with a standard of acceptability to provide evidence that is useful to inform decision-making and to demonstrate accountability to social values or policies. In public health, it is also a method for ascertaining whether a program can help confirm that "evidence-based practices" from the literature are consistent with the "practice-based evidence" from the setting in which you are working.

evaluation accountability. Ensuring the most responsible use of resources to produce value.

evidence-based interventions ("best practices"). Program decisions or intervention selections made on the strength of data from research and from the community, concerning needs and data from previously tested interventions or programs concerning their effectiveness, sometimes using theory in the absence of data on the specific alignment of interventions and population needs.

evidence-based practice. Program decisions or intervention selections made on the strength of data from previously tested interventions or programs concerning their effectiveness, ideally from randomized trials, but not necessarily in populations and circumstances similar to those in the proposed setting. See also **practice-based evidence**.

evidence-informed practice. Program decisions or intervention selections made on the strength of data from the community concerning needs and data from previously tested interventions or programs concerning their effectiveness, sometimes using theory and local observations in the absence of data on the specific alignment of interventions and population needs. See also **evidence-based practice**.

excise tax. A tax on the manufacture, sale, or use of certain products such as alcohol or tobacco to generate revenue for a government or to control consumption, or both.

expansionist. An approach to diagnosis or assessment that seeks explanation or causes beyond the immediate determinants at hand; the opposite of *reductionist*, which seeks the minimum number of causes by limiting the explanation of cause to the most proximal or strongest determinant(s). See also **reductionist**.

experimental designs. The random assignment of participants to treatment or control groups so that subsequent differences found between the groups can be attributed to the intervention and not to something else.

external validity. The assurances that the findings or conclusions of a study or series of studies on the effectiveness of an intervention apply to other populations in which they are to be applied.

fear. A mental state that motivates problem-solving behavior if an action (fight or flight) is immediately available; if not, it motivates other defense mechanisms, such as denial or suppression.

feasibility. An estimate of the receptivity, practicality, and manageability of implementing an intervention or program based on pilot tests, conferring with representatives of the population, or simulations in the populations and settings in which it would be conducted.

fidelity. The degree to which an intervention or program adheres to the essential elements that were present in the previously tested or evaluated interventions or programs.

focus group method. Testing the perception and receptivity of a target population to an idea or method by recording the reactions of a sample of eight to ten people discussing it with each other.

formative evaluation. Any combination of measurements obtained and judgments made before or during the implementation of materials, methods, activities, or programs to discover, predict, control, assure, or improve the quality of performance or delivery. (Measurements during implementation are sometimes called process evaluation.)

full operation. A program operation with full implementation and participation from the intended audience and staffing.

Gantt chart. A timetable showing each activity in a program plan as a horizontal line that extends from the start to the finish date of the intervention, so that at any given time a program manager can see which activities should begin, be underway, are about to be, or due to be completed.

genetic factors. Those determinants of physical and physiological features of biological organisms that account for some portion of inheritable diseases and susceptibility to them that are attributable to genes inherited from parents.

grounded theory. A methodology in qualitative research that involves analyzing data to develop a theory describing the phenomenon of interest. In this approach, the researcher avoids any preconceived notions or theories about the phenomenon and examines data with the intent of identifying or developing an explanatory theory.

habituation. The incorporation of a pattern of behavior into one's lifestyle to the degree that it is performed virtually without thought, but does not necessarily entail physical or psychological dependence.

health. The state of an organism's viability and vitality, or the ability to cope with the demands of a manageable quality of life.

Health Belief Model. A paradigm widely used to predict and explain health behavior, based on value-expectancy theory, measures of belief in one's susceptibility to, severity of, or belief that one can have a specific health problem and not know it (the "asymptomatic belief"), and belief in the efficacy of the recommended action to prevent or minimize the disease, injury, or condition (generally attributed to Godfrey Hochbaum as of 1956; Irwin Rosenstock and their colleagues in the US Public Health Service in the 1950s).

health care system. That subsystem of the broader health system that is financed and organized to respond mainly to needs for treatment or continuing care of the illnesses and chronic conditions that compromise health.

health-directed behavior. The conscious pursuit of actions for the purpose of protecting or improving health.

health education. Any planned combination of learning experiences designed to predispose, enable, and reinforce voluntary behavior conducive to health in individuals, groups, or communities.

health enhancement. A dimension of health promotion pertaining to its goal of reaching higher levels of wellness and fitness beyond the mere absence of disease or infirmity.

health equity. The allocation of community resources, services, and opportunities to populations proportionate to their needs.

health field concept. The notion that the factors influencing health can be subsumed under four categories: environment, human biology, behavior, and health care organization. Concept attributed to Marc Lalonde (1974), minister of health for Canada, in presentation to the first International Conference on Health Promotion, and the Ottawa Charter of the WHO.

health outcome. Any medically or epidemiologically defined characteristic of a patient or health problem in a population that results from health promotion, preventive intervention, or care provided or required as measured at one point in time.

health program. A planned set of activities designed to be implemented and maintained for the purpose of applying knowledge and resources effectively to the development of health or the prevention, detection or treatment of disease, illness, or death.

health promotion. Any planned combination of educational, political, regulatory, and organizational supports for actions and conditions of living conducive to the health of individuals, groups, or communities.

health protection. A strategy parallel to health promotion in some national policies; the focus is on environmental rather than behavioral determinants of health, and the methods are more like those of engineers and regulatory agencies than those of educational and social or health service agencies.

health-related behavior. Those actions undertaken for reasons other than the protection or improvement of health, but which may have health effects.

health system. The totality and relationships of individuals, groups, organizations, and sectors of public and private activity that respond to threats to health and opportunities to promote, protect, and repair or palliate health.

hermeneutics. A methodology in qualitative research that focuses on subjective interpretations in the meanings that underlie tests of artistic, cultural, and social phenomena. A hermeneutic approach seeks to understand rather than just explain.

heuristic inquiry. A broad term referring to qualitative methods that focus on the subjective experience of an individual (e.g. social construction, phenomenology, autobiographical).

historical standards. Used by administrators based on past performance of the program.

host. A concept from epidemiology, referring to an individual who harbors or is at risk of harboring a disease or condition in the triad of host, agent, and environment.

immediacy. A criterion for judging the importance of a factor, based on how urgent or imminent the factor is in its influence on the outcome desired.

impact (evaluation). The assessment of program effects on intermediate objectives, including changes in predisposing, enabling, and reinforcing factors and behavioral and environmental changes, and possibly their effect as well on health and social outcomes.

implementation. The act of converting program objectives into actions through leadership, funding, policy changes, regulation, and organization.

implementation outcomes. Results related to implementation, measured via process evaluation or implementation research.

implementation readiness. The stage after administrative assessments of resources needed, available resources, and factors related to implementation, in which the program can be launched.

implementation science. The study of methods to promote the systematic uptake of evidence-based interventions and practice-based evidence into programs and policy, and hence improve health.

importance. The value or relative weight among values placed on identified problems in the health, determinants of health, or other factors in the causal chain to health or quality-of-life outcomes.

incidence. A measure of the frequency of occurrence of a disease or health problem in a population based on the number of new cases over a given period of time (usually one year). An incidence **rate** is obtained by dividing this number by the midyear population and multiplying the quotient by 1,000 or 100,000. See also **prevalence**.

informed consent. A medical-legal doctrine that holds providers responsible for ensuring that consumers or patients understand the relative risks and benefits of a procedure or medicine before it is administered, or an informed electorate in voting before a policy is adopted.

innovators. Those in a population who are the first to adopt a new idea or practice, usually based on information from sources outside the community.

instrumental values. That set of values held by individuals, families, organizations, and cultures that serve to orient their decisions toward behavior that will serve to reflect, protect, or promote their ultimate values. See also **ultimate values**.

internal validity. The degree of certainty that the evidence from research or evaluation adequately controls for biases in the experimental controls. Assurance that the results of an evaluation can be attributed to the object (method or program) evaluated, and not to biased or unrepresentative sampling or measurement bias. Assured particularly with the random assignment of subjects or of multiple groups to experimental and control groups.

intervention. The part of a strategy incorporating method, amount, provider, and technique that actually reaches a person or population.

late adopters. The segment of the population that adopts an innovation or new behavioral norm after the innovators, early adopters, early majority, and late majority, sometimes referred to as the "hard-to-reach" or "vaccine-hesitant" segment of the population in relation to any health practice or innovation.

late majority. The segment of the population more difficult to reach through mass communication channels or to convince of the need to adopt a new idea or practice than the early adopters and middle majority, either because they cannot afford it or cannot get to the source or because of cultural and language differences or other difficulties.

leveraging. The use of initial investments in a program to draw larger investments.

lifestyle. The culturally, socially, economically, and environmentally conditioned complex of actions characteristic of an individual, group, or community as a pattern of habituated behavior over time that is health-related but not necessarily health-directed.

logic model. A diagram and text that describes and illustrates the logical (causal) relationships among program elements and the problem to be solved, thus defining intermediate and ultimate criteria of success.

market testing. The placement of a message or product in a commercial context to determine how it reaches and influences consumer behavior.

matching. A selection of intervention strategies that corresponds to the predisposing, reinforcing, and enabling factors identified in the ecological and educational diagnosis phases of PRECEDE, "as part of an effort to understand the intervention target population, the program setting, and the character of the community, its members, and its strengths" (Bartholomew Eldredge et al. 2016).

mediators. Causal or intermediate variables between interventions and intended effects that can directly affect outcomes.

middle majority. The segment of the population that adopts a new idea or practice after the innovators and early adopters but before the late adopters, usually influenced by a combination of mass media, interpersonal communication, and endorsements by leaders, personalities, or organizations of which they are members.

mixed-method designs. The combination of qualitative and quantitative methods of study or evaluation.

moderators. Characteristics of individuals, settings, channels, and circumstances that can ameliorate or enhance the effect of program variables on mediator variables, or the latter on outcome variables.

morbidity. The existence or rate of disease or infirmity.

mortality. The event of death of an individual or rate of death in a population. Death rates for a specific cause recorded in death certificates or surveys is measured as the numerator relative to the population size in the denominator for a specific time period, usually a year.

motivational factors. People's desires and self-efficacy beliefs that determine their level of motivation, as reflected in how much effort they will exert in an endeavor and how long they will persevere in the face of obstacles (Bandura 2004).

narrative inquiry. A qualitative method that focuses on texts (e.g. stories, documents, journals, field notes) to understand the subjective experience of an individual or population.

natural experiments. Studies that compare a "naturally occurring event" (not under the control of the evaluators or program planners) with a comparison condition.

necessity. A criterion for judging the importance of a factor, based on whether the outcome can occur without this factor. Distinguished from some other factors that are "necessary but not sufficient."

need. (1) Whatever is required for health or comfort, or (2) an estimation of the interventions required based on a diagnosis of the problem and, in populations, the number or proportion of people eligible to benefit from the intervention(s).

nominal group process. An interactive group method for assessing community needs by having opinions listed without critique from the group and then rated by secret ballot, thereby minimizing the influence of interpersonal dynamics and participants' status on the ratings.

non-experimental designs. Assessing outcomes, the evaluator describes a group and assesses a relationship with pre-existing groups or whether there are group differences between those exposed and those not exposed to a presumed determinant of an outcome.

normative effect. The influence of perceived social patterns of and expectations for behavior on the actions taken by individuals and groups.

normative standards. Standards based on performance by comparable organizations, jurisdictions, populations, or programs.

objective. A defined result of specific activity to be achieved in a finite period of time by a specified person or number of people. Objectives state *who* will experience *what* change or benefit by *how much* and by *when*. See also **SMART objective**.

operant conditioning. The view of behavior as a one-way product of the environment that is controlled by consequences.

organization. *verb*: The act of marshalling and coordinating the resources necessary to implement a program; *noun*: A structured entity of multiple positions designed to achieve a specific set of outcomes

organizational development The process of building the capacity of an organization or community to maximize its intended or planned functions.

outcome evaluation. The assessment of the effects of a program on the short-term objectives (key predisposing, enabling, reinforcing factors), intermediate objectives (behavior, environment), but ideally the ultimate outcomes (health, quality of life). Outcome objectives are distinguished from process objectives. See also **process evaluation**.

perceived norms. Beliefs by people about what behaviors are approved or disapproved of by others, or what comparable or desirable other people do.

phenomenological study. Describes the "lived experiences" about a concept or a phenomenon of the research.

photovoice. A qualitative method that involves participants taking pictures or videos that represent their experience or point of view.

planning. The process of defining needs, establishing priorities, diagnosing causes of problems, assessing resources and barriers, and allocating resources to achieve objectives.

point of diminishing returns. A time or amount of invested resources and effort beyond which additional time or resources do not necessarily achieve commensurate gain in impact or outcome.

policy. The set of objectives and rules guiding the activities of an organization or an administration, and providing authority for the allocation of resources.

positional leader. A person whose influence is based, or perceived to be based, on his or her official standing or office, such as an elected or appointed official, executive of a firm, or head of a voluntary organization.

practice-based evidence. The evidence drawn from assessments during the planning, implementation, and evaluation phases of program development, seen as complementary to evidence from controlled research studies that often lack specificity and external validity for the particular program, community, or circumstance of the local situation in which the evidence would be applied.

PRECEDE. Acronym for the diagnostic planning and evaluation model outlined in this book, emphasizing *p*redisposing, *r*einforcing, and *e*nabling *c*onstructs in *e*ducational/*e*pidemiological/*e*cological *d*iagnosis and *e*valuation.

predisposing factor. Any characteristic of a person or population that motivates behavior prior to the occurrence of the behavior, including (for example) knowledge, beliefs, attitudes, and values.

pretesting. An early step in process evaluation in which an intervention or message is assessed for its feasibility, acceptability, comprehension, and other reactions from a sample of people representative of the population in which the intervention or message will be used as part of a program.

prevalence. A measure of the extent of a disease or health problem in a population based on the number of cases (old and new) existing in the population at a given time. See also **incidence**.

principle of intervention specificity. The necessity of aligning interventions with specific characteristics of the individual or population, and with the environment and circumstances in which the program is to be delivered and change is expected to occur.

principle of multiplicity and comprehensiveness. The necessity for successful programs to combine interventions that address at least the three major determinants of change: those that predispose, those that enable, and those that reinforce the necessary changes in behavior or the environment.

principle of participation. The necessity for program relevance, implementation, and sustainability for key representatives of the audience or community to have been engaged in the planning of the program.

priority. Alternatives ranked according to feasibility or value (importance) or both.

problem theory. The presumed determinants of a health or other outcome.

probability sample. A group of cases selected from a population by a random process in which every member of the population has a known, nonzero probability of being selected.

PROCEED. Acronym for *p*olicy, *r*egulatory, and *o*rganizational *c*onstructs in *ed*ucational and *e*nvironmental *d*evelopment; the phases of resource mobilization, implementation, and evaluation following the diagnostic planning phases of PRECEDE.

process evaluation. The assessment of policies, materials, personnel, performance, quality of practice or services, and other inputs and implementation experiences.

process/implementation evaluation. The assessment of policies, materials, personnel, performance, quality of practice or services, and other inputs and implementation experiences.

program monitoring. The determination of whether program inputs and activities have been implemented as intended.

program theory. The combination of causal theory, which explains how one or more mediating variables affect the desired outcome (health effect), and action theory, which links a proposed intervention with the changes needed in the mediating variable. *Also:* The testable assumptions linking the combination of interventions or inputs with the expected outcomes or objectives for their implementation.

propriety. Ensuring that an evaluation will be conducted legally, ethically, and with due regard for the welfare of those involved in the evaluation, as well as those affected by its results.

proximal risk. Those risk factors or conditions in the immediate range of influence, in time or place, over which individuals or communities could exercise control.

program. A set of planned activities over time designed to achieve specified objectives.

purposive sampling. The planner or evaluator recruits participants with particular characteristics according to the planning or evaluation question(s) being asked.

public health system. The authority, organization, resources, and relationships serving a population in support of maintaining and improving the health of a community, state, or nation.

purposive sampling. The planner or evaluator recruits participants with particular characteristics according to the planning or evaluation question(s) being asked.

quantitative evaluation design. Used when the evaluation question includes an object of interest and a standard of acceptability that are measured numerically.

quality assessment. The measurement of a professional or technical practice or service in comparison with accepted standards to determine the degree of excellence.

quality assurance. The formal process of agreeing on and implementing quality assessment and quality improvement in programs to assure stakeholders that professional activities have been performed appropriately.

quality of life. The perception of individuals or groups that their needs are being satisfied and that they are not being denied opportunities to achieve happiness and fulfillment.

quasi-experimental studies. The evaluator identifies a "comparison group," that is, a community or population that is demographically similar to the target population but not receiving the program. Comparisons are made between the two groups, but without random assignment to them, so that the differences might be attributable to the inherent or historical differences between the groups rather than to the program.

random sample. A representation of a larger population by a smaller (and more affordable and manageable) number of people or other subjects in a way that assures that their selection was not biased (i.e., each individual in the larger population had an equal opportunity to be chosen).

rate. A measure of occurrences, such as a disease, injury, behavior, exposure, or death in a population per unit of time.

reach. The number of people attending or exposed to an intervention or program.

reductionist. The approach to diagnosis that seeks to explain and isolate the most important among the causes of a problem or event within the person(s) or population having the problem or within the immediate environment of the event, for the purpose of setting priorities for intervention. See also **expansionist**.

regression (regression analysis). A statistical method for determining the relative association between a dependent variable and one or more independent variables.

regulation. The act of enforcing policies, rules, or laws.

reinforcing factor. Any reward or punishment following or anticipated as a consequence of a behavior, serving to strengthen the motivation for the behavior after (or before, if anticipated) it occurs.

relative risk. The ratio of mortality or incidence of a disease or condition in those exposed to a given risk factor (e.g., smokers) to the mortality or incidence in those not exposed (e.g., nonsmokers). A relative risk (RR) ratio of 1.0 indicates no greater risk in those exposed than in those not exposed.

reliability. The extent to which a measurement instrument or procedure yields consistent, stable, and uniform results over repeated observations or measurements under the same conditions each time.

repeatability of findings. (*also* **test-retest reliability**) Whether the results would be the same if the evaluation were to be done again, exactly as before.

reputational leader. One whose leadership power is based on perceived performance as an influential person, but not necessarily on his or her position.

risk conditions. Those determinants of health that are more distal in time, place, or scope from the control of individuals than the more proximal and malleable "risk factors" such as current behavior.

risk factors. Characteristics of individuals (genetic, behavioral, environmental exposures, and sociocultural living conditions) that increase the probability that they will experience a disease or specific cause of death as measured by population relative risk ratios.

risk ratio. The mortality or incidence of a disease or condition in those exposed to a given risk factor divided by the mortality or incidence in those not exposed. See also **relative risk**.

sampling. The process of selecting representatives from the members of the population, usually to estimate the characteristics of the larger population with statistically known precision or error depending on the size and quality of the sample.

scientific standards. Conclusions based on best practices derived from systematic reviews of research related to the problem and the population.

scale up. The process by which health interventions shown to be efficacious on a small scale under controlled conditions are expanded (or have expandability or replicability) under real-world conditions into a broader population, geography, policy, or practice.

segmentation. The division of a population into segments according to characteristics (demographic, socioeconomic, or localities) that predict their likelihood to respond to one form or another of interventions, such as communication messages. See also **tailoring**.

self-efficacy. A construct from social learning theory, referring to the belief an individual holds that he or she is capable of performing a specific behavior.

sensitivity. The ability of a test to identify all people who have a particular characteristic or condition; that is, the ability to avoid missing cases in a population screening. See also **specificity**.

settings. Organizational or institutional places in which health programs are carried out. More generally, a setting is a milieu in which people gather for schooling, work, cohabitation, or other mutually supportive activities, governed by rules and norms specific to the place.

settings approach. The use of place as a primary consideration in assessing, planning, and organizing health programs, because of the ecological and social exchange and reciprocal relationships that govern the behavior of people in the place, and the potential to restructure those relationships or systems to change behavior and make them more conducive to health (see chapters 10–14).

situation analysis. The combination of social and epidemiological assessments of conditions, trends, and priorities, with a preliminary scan of determinants, relevant policies, resources, organizational support, and regulations that might anticipate or permit action in advance of a more complete assessment of behavioral, environmental, educational, ecological, and administrative factors.

skills. A person's ability to perform tasks that enable a health-related behavior. Absence or insufficiency of the resource blocks the behavior; barriers to the behavior are included in lists of enabling factors to be developed. Skills are sometimes listed separately as predisposing factors if they motivate a person or population to use them (as seen in Bandura's "self-efficacy" concept).

SMART objective. An objective (see above) that includes elements (or meets the criteria of being) *s*pecific, *m*easurable, *a*ttainable/*a*chievable, *r*elevant, and *t*ime-bound.

snowball sampling. The participants refer the evaluator to others in the target population, such as neighbors or friends, who are then recruited into the evaluation.

social assessment. The assessment in both objective and subjective terms of high-priority problems or aspirations for the common good, defined for a population by economic and social indicators and by individuals in terms of their quality of life.

social capital. The processes and conditions among people and organizations that lead to accomplishing a goal of mutual social benefit, usually characterized by four interrelated constructs: trust, cooperation, civic engagement, and reciprocity.

Social Cognitive Theory. A model of emergent interactive agency, in which persons are neither autonomous agents nor simply mechanical conveyers of animating environmental influences; they make causal contribution to their own motivation and action within a system of triadic reciprocal causation (Bandura 1989).

social constructivism. A theory or approach to research that focuses on examining an understanding that is socially co-constructed. The co-construction forms the basis for the way in which the phenomenon is understood by individuals in the population.

social determinants of health. The cumulative effects of a lifetime of exposure to conditions of living that combine to strengthen or compromise optimum health, many of which are beyond the control of the individual. See also **risk conditions**.

social diagnosis. The focus within a *social assessment* or *social reconnaissance* on the social problems and quality of life issues that might be related to health in a population.

social-ecological perspective. This model considers the complex interplay between individual, relationships, community, and societal factors—how factors at one level influence factors at another level.

social indicator. A quality having a numerical value whose change is expected to reflect a change in the quality of life for a population.

socialization. A process of developing behavioral patterns or lifestyle through modeling or imitating socially important persons, including parents, peers, and media personalities.

social problem. A situation that a significant number of people believe to be a source of difficulty or unhappiness. A social problem consists of objective circumstances as well as a social interpretation of their unacceptability.

social reconnaissance. Assessment procedures applied to a large geographic area with the active participation of people having various levels of authority and resources, including government officials and professionals in health and other sectors, and the potential recipients of new programs or services.

specificity. The ability of a test to rule out cases not possessing a particular characteristic or condition—that is, to avoid false-positive results in a population screening. See also **sensitivity**.

specific rates. Morbidity, mortality, fertility, or other rates calculated for specific age, gender, race, or other demographic groupings.

Stages of Implementation Completion (SIC). An eight-stage tool of implementation process and milestones. From Chamberlain, P., Brown, C.H., & Saldana, L. (2011). Observational measure of implementation progress in community-based settings: The Stages of Implementation Completion (SIC). *Implementation Science, 6*(1), 116. https://doi.org/10.1186/1748-5908-6-116

stakeholders. People who have an investment or a stake in the outcome of a program and therefore have reasons to be interested in the evaluation of the program.

standards of acceptability. Statements (preferably quantitative and based on a consensus) of what will be valued or counted as "good" in program objectives or a program evaluation.

stepped approach. A method of intervention following triage, in which minimal

resources or effort are expended on the first group or level, a more intensive effort is applied on the second level, and the most intensive effort is
expended on the third.

strategy. A plan of action that anticipates barriers and resources in relation to
achieving a specific objective, based on a review and pooling of the best experience of prior efforts to achieve the objective in similar populations and
circumstances.

subsystems. The components of a system, each a system unto itself with possible subsystems of its own, overlapping in the network connections with other
systems and subsystems.

summative evaluation. The application of design, measurement, and analysis
methods to the assessment of outcomes of a program or specific interventions within a program.

surveys. Methods of polling a group or population to estimate the norms and
distribution of characteristics from a sample, using direct observations, questionnaires, or interviews.

sustainability. The continued use of program components and activities for the
continued achievement of desirable program and population outcomes. A criterion of importance to funding agencies who want to know that their initial
support for a program will result in maintenance beyond their investment.

system. A set of interlocking relationships where change in one part results in
changes in other parts, with feedback to the part that first changed, resulting
in further change there to establish equilibrium.

tactic. A method or approach employed as a part of a strategy, often in response
to unanticipated circumstances or events.

tailoring. The use of information about individuals to shape the message or
other qualities of a communication or other intervention so that it has the
best possible fit with the factors predisposing, enabling, and reinforcing that
person's behavior. See also **segmentation**.

theoretical sampling. The evaluator purposefully seeks out specific types of
participants, such as a particular age group or geographic location, consistent with a theory of the applicability of the program.

Theory of Planned Behavior. Postulates that behavioral intention is influenced
by three constructs: attitude, perceived norms, and perceived behavioral
control.

Theory of Reasoned Action. Reformulated as the **Theory of Planned Behavior,**
as seen above.

transferable, transferability. The extent to which the results of an evaluation
can apply to or transfer beyond the context in which it is implemented—that
is, whether the results are applicable in similar situations.

Transparent Reporting of Evaluations with Nonrandomized Designs (TREND). A guideline to assist in the reporting standards of nonrandomized evaluations of behavioral and public health interventions; it offers a checklist of 22 areas for reporting about the program or evaluation. The US Centers for Disease Control and Prevention (CDC) maintains a TREND checklist online at *Transparent Reporting of Evaluations with Nonrandomized Designs (TREND)*, https://www.cdc.gov/trendstatement/index.html.

threshold level. A minimum level of investment below which the program, strategy, or method will be too weak to achieve a useful result.

triage. A method of sorting people into (usually three) groups for the purposes of setting priorities in order of intervention and allocation of resources among interventions.

triangulation. Using data from three sources so that if two are inconsistent, a third provides a tiebreak between the other two. More generally, it refers to the use of multiple sources, observers, and methods of data collection to assure that the problem is seen from more than the sometimes-biased single lens.

US CDC Evaluation Framework. A step-by-step guide developed by the CDC to support public health evaluation planning; the framework sets out a series of six actions of steps that are centered around the evaluation standards.

value. A preference shared and transmitted within a family, organization community, or other culture.

ultimate value. As distinct from instrumental values, a preference that justifies more generalizable values and the behaviors associated with them.

vicarious reinforcement. The response to a behavior that strengthens its probability of continuing or being repeated based on the perception of the person that such behavior is similar to that of valued other people who are role models.

wearable technologies. Electronic communication devices designed to be worn as activity monitors, or health-related monitors and collectors or transmitters of data such as heart rate, calories burned, steps or stairs taken, and blood pressure.

wellness. A dimension of health beyond the absence of disease or infirmity, including social, emotional, and spiritual aspects of health.

workplan. A program planning and implementation tool for a specific program, sometimes required for program grant applications.

Index